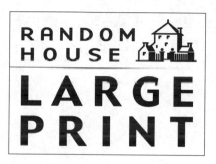

**Also by American Heart Association
available from Random House Large Print**

American Heart Association
Low-Fat, Low-Cholesterol Cookbook

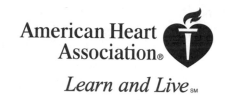

American Heart
Association®

Learn and Live sm

No-Fad
Diet

A **Personal
Plan** for
**Healthy
Weight Loss**

RANDOM HOUSE
LARGE PRINT

The Library of Congress has established a Cataloging-in-Publication record for this title.

ISBN 0-375-43445-3

www.randomlargeprint.com

10   9   8   7   6   5   4   3   2   1

This Large Print edition published in accord with the standards of the N.A.V.H.

contents

acknowledgments

Many people worked together to make the American Heart Association's first-ever comprehensive weight-loss book a reality.

The American Heart Association expresses its sincere gratitude to key volunteers Robert H. Eckel, MD, FAHA; Barry A. Franklin, PhD, FAHA; John M. Jakicic, PhD; and Stephen R. Daniels, MD, PhD, FAHA, for providing expert direction and developing the strategies for our weight-loss plan.

American Heart Association staff members contributing to this book included Rose Marie Robertson, MD, FAHA, FACC, FESC, chief science officer; Robyn Landry, executive vice president, communications; Gayle R. Whitman, PhD, RN, FAHA, FAAN, vice president, science and medicine; and Consumer Publications staff members Jane Anneken Ruehl, director; Deborah Ann Renza, managing editor; Janice Roth Moss, senior editor; Jacqueline Fornerod Haigney, writer/editor; Roberta Westcott Sullivan, assistant editor; and Bharati Gaitonde, senior marketing manager.

The consultants who helped with this book include recipe developers Barbara Seelig Brown,

Christine Caperton, Linda Drachman, Nancy S. Hughes, Nadja Piatka, Carol Ritchie, and Julie Shapero, RD, LD; nutritional analyst Tammi Hancock, RD; and illustrator Katherine Urban.

The American Heart Association gratefully acknowledges the additional expertise provided by Claire M. Bassett; Marc-Andre Cornier, MD; Coni Francis, PhD, RD; Barbara V. Howard, PhD, FAHA; Donna Israel, PhD, RD, LD, LPC, FADA; Penny M. Kris-Etherton, PhD, RD, FAHA; Alice Lichtenstein, DSc, FAHA; F. Xavier Pi-Sunyer, MD, MPH, FAHA; Lawrence Rudel, PhD, FAHA; Frank Sacks, MD, FAHA; Linda Van Horn, PhD, RD, FAHA; Judith Wylie-Rosett, EdD, RD; and Meg Zeller, PhD.

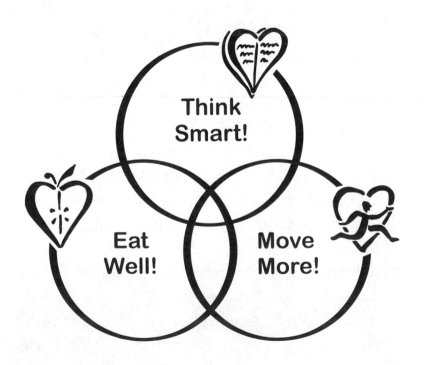

preface

We at the American Heart Association—the nation's most trusted authority on heart-healthy living—are concerned about the growing prevalence of obesity in the United States and around the world and the cardiovascular risks that come as a result. To fight this epidemic, we have written this comprehensive weight-loss book. Its mission is to provide a science-based, **no-fad** approach to losing weight for your better overall health and the accompanying decreased risk of heart disease, stroke, and diabetes.

For many of us, genetics, environment, and emotions act as barriers in our struggle to lose weight. It's important to the American Heart Association to get out the message that it is possible to lose the extra pounds and maintain a healthful weight for life despite these barriers. As you read this book, you'll discover the tools you need to think smart, eat well, and move more to shed unhealthful pounds. You'll read personal stories that will give you the reassurance that you are not alone in this struggle and the confidence that you can overcome your obstacles.

Because you are unique, your approach to losing weight should be tailored to complement you. The American Heart Association, along with leading experts in the medical community, has translated the science behind healthful weight loss into useful strategies that you choose from to best fit into your life. **No-Fad Diet** will provide you with practical ways to assess your current weight and habits, set obtainable goals, and make good health choices for the rest of your life.

We encourage you to make the options in this book your own, integrating them in a way that best suits your personal lifestyle and individual goals. By combining the thinking, eating, and exercise strategies offered throughout this book, along with the sample menus, meal planning guidelines, and recipes, you can build your own customized program to achieve—and maintain—your desired weight. Let this book be your guide and the American Heart Association be your partner on your journey to losing weight—and keeping it off—realistically, healthfully, and successfully for years to come. Do it for you, and encourage those you love to join you. Years of added life may well be the outcome!

Robert H. Eckel, MD
President, American Heart
Association, 2005–2006

INTRODUCTION:
welcome to a no-fad way of life

Our mission at the American Heart Association is to help you **learn and live.** We have designed this book to help you **learn** to make wise decisions about your weight and **live** well. If you're looking for a long-term, livable way to lose weight and keep it off, we're here to help.

You may have tried several times before to lose weight, but without much long-term success. There's no point in feeling bad about yourself, because the truth is, losing weight is not easy. No magic formula will trim away extra pounds and keep them off. Gimmicks and get-thin-quick schemes don't work. That's why, over the long haul, the fads—the grapefruit diet, the very low fat diet, the low-carb diet—are not the answer.

We aren't offering any magic, either—quite the opposite. Instead, we offer you the right tools you need to personalize a weight-loss plan to fit your lifestyle. You can design your own approach using three key concepts:

- **Think smart**
- **Eat well**
- **Move more**

We think of these concepts as interlocking circles: the Circles of Success (see page xii). Each component is an essential part of the plan that will lead to no-fad and lifelong weight control.

No matter what else may change as different fads come into vogue, the bottom line is still the same:

To keep your weight from rising, you must balance the food calories coming into your body with the calories your body uses up. We call this Energy Balance, or Calories In/Calories Out.

Like our colleagues at many other major health organizations, we want to help you achieve a healthful lifestyle based on a positive attitude about food, activity, and body image. Your efforts to lose weight should not endanger your long-term health, no matter how enticing the promises of a quick and easy fix may be. In these times of conflicting and confusing messages about diet, exercise, and health, you can turn to this book with confidence. Our recommendations reflect the opinion of many experts—physicians, nutritionists, and specialists in physical activity and behavior modification—not a celebrity or just one physician. Our panel of scientists has reviewed the research and come to a consensus for you. Our message is backed by the science community of the American Heart Association.

We know it isn't easy to lose weight, but we offer you a simple approach that can bring you success—now and for your future. Fads come and go, just like the weight loss they promise.

Instead, we will help you create your own work-able plan to reach a healthful weight and maintain it. It's time to try our no-fad approach to a lifetime of good health!

the three circles of success

If you're reading this book, most likely your immediate goal is to be thinner. That idea is a good place to start, but the question is how to really achieve lasting success. To make a real difference, direct your attention inward, to the specific things you can control. You need to embrace all of who you are—heart, mind, body, and soul—not

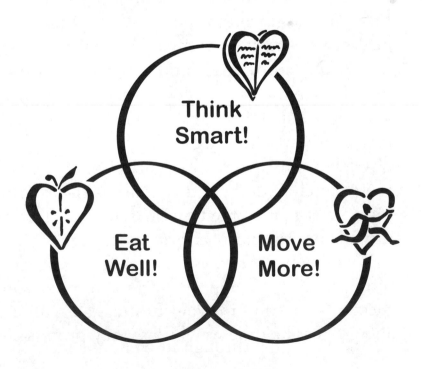

focus just on the extra pounds you see when you look in the mirror.

To lose weight effectively, you need realistic goals and a personal action plan. Instead of a one-size-fits-all approach, we offer you a menu of choices. Your planning should focus on you, your commitment to yourself, and the three essential circles in our plan—thinking, eating, and moving. What kind of attitude do you bring to the process of losing weight? How much weight do you want to lose and at what rate? How do you want to tailor your activity plan? You make these choices to fit your environment, individual needs, and comfort level. Keep in mind that your plan needs to work for you. You need a plan that will inspire the same commitment you make to other important areas in your life. Are you ready to commit to a healthier you and develop that plan?

If your answer is yes, consider the three key Circles of Success. Each circle plays an important part in your personal action plan and they will overlap as you work toward your goals. You will need to include all three circles to achieve successful weight control for life. To address each circle, you have several options to choose from. Because your choices reflect **your** individual needs, the actions you take will become part of **your** new life. It may not happen overnight, but if you follow through, it will happen!

circle 1: think smart!

Making good choices is the cornerstone of success. If negative thinking is affecting your choices, we want to help you learn to change the way you think. The power of thought works both ways. Just as you can talk yourself into having that extra piece of pie, you can also talk yourself into a new attitude and ultimately new behavior that will lead to successful weight loss. Chapter 1, "Think Smart: Find a New Start," will give you different strategies to rework your current mind-set so you can recognize and change the thought patterns that lead you away from your goals.

When you start to think of yourself as a thinner, healthier person, you will help yourself become one. You will think about and make the choices that support that image. For instance, instead of ordering a soft drink, you'll order something else you like—perhaps unsweetened iced tea or sparkling water—not because you are depriving yourself but because you are making smart substitutions and see yourself as a person who chooses wisely.

circle 2: eat well!

You already know that if you take in fewer calories than you expend, you will lose weight. The amount of food you eat each day is the Calories In side of Energy Balance. But as you reduce calories, you also need to pay attention to the essentials of good nutrition. **Remember: Quality first, then quantity.** Chapter 2, "Eat Well: A Personal Approach to a Healthful Weight," gives you tools to assess your current eating habits and how they contribute to your current weight. The first step in your action plan is to understand how all the facets of your eating patterns work together to cause you to eat the way you do. We offer three different strategies for eating well to lose weight. We will help you decide which strategy will work best for you.

circle 3: move more!

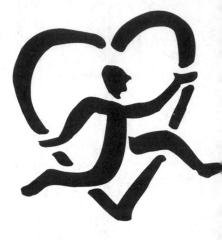

You may think that physical activity is just too much trouble to fit into your hectic life. It's true that calorie reduction is the key to weight loss, but to keep off the pounds for good, you have to get moving and keep moving. Physical activity is the Calories Out side of Energy Balance and is an essential part of maintaining weight loss and good health.

In Chapter 3, "Move More: More Fit and Less Fat," we outline three practical ways to live a more active life and maintain your weight loss for the long term. We will help you choose which strategy will help you live a more active lifestyle, even if you rarely walk farther than your office parking garage. As you work toward your weight-loss goal, we suggest you start by including at least 10 minutes of activity, such as walking, in your daily routine. Chapter 3 explains how to progress from this starting point to a more active lifestyle. Especially if you are not active now, this is a good way to get past the feeling of inertia, get energized, and get used to the benefits of moving more. You are paving the way for your future well-being as a more active person.

how did we get so heavy?

One thing is certain: If you want to lose weight, you are not alone. The spread of overweight and obesity has covered the country. How did so many people get into this predicament of weight gain? The simple answer is that we regularly take in more calories than we burn through physical activity. Our bodies are programmed to defend stored fat as insurance against future famine. What may have been a survival technique for cave dwellers works against us in our modern environment. Once fat is stored, some people's bodies are especially good at keeping it. Most important, environmental factors—such as new technology and labor-saving devices, easy access to fattening fast food, increasing portion sizes, more frequent meals in restaurants, and changing food trends—have contributed to the steady rise in weight gain and the decreasing level of physical activity in the United States.

easy eating: convenience foods and portion distortion

These days, we have lots of easy access to low-cost, high-calorie foods that are heavily marketed to us on a daily basis. For most mod-

"Never eat anything larger than your head."
—MISS PIGGY

changes in serving size

20 YEARS AGO	TODAY

blueberry muffin

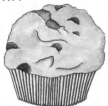

210 calories	500 calories

cheeseburger

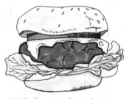

333 calories	590 calories

spaghetti and meatballs

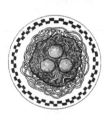

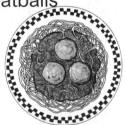

500 calories	1,025 calories

soda

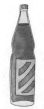

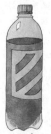

85 calories	250 calories

ern families with little time after work, school, and the infamous soccer games, fast food is a convenience they can't imagine living without. Not only are we eating out more often than before but we are eating much larger servings than we did twenty-five years ago. **Portion distortion** is a major contributor to many expanding waistlines. How do we know? Take a look at the graphic examples opposite.

Many restaurants in the United States serve huge single-serving portions, large enough for two or more people. That's a great value if customers are prepared to take half home, but more often than not, people eat more than they need just because it's in front of them. Gradually we're coming to expect more and more food on our plates. You don't need to avoid restaurants or even fast-food places when you're taking a no-fad approach to weight loss. The key is knowing how to make sensible choices when eating out. For helpful suggestions, check out our tips in Appendix C.

low-fat versus low-calorie

The mixed messages coming from product labeling and food advertising may have contributed to the escalating prevalence of overweight and obesity. With so many claims being made, it's no wonder there's confusion about what to eat. For the past few decades, you've heard a lot about reducing the amount of total fat in the average diet. The idea was that lowering the total percentage of fat in your diet (which is very high in the typical American diet) would help your heart because you would be eating less saturated fat. By cutting back on fat, you would also find it easier to maintain a healthful weight because you would be able to replace the high-calorie fats with foods of larger volume but fewer calories, such as vegetables and complex carbohydrates.

The subtleties of this concept were overshadowed by the mistaken message that fat is "bad" and carbohydrates are "good." This oversimplistic view led to a glut of low-fat but high-calorie products. People thought they were eating "diet foods" and didn't realize that in many cases they were actually getting more calories than the full-fat versions provided. Likewise, under the impression that all carbohydrates are equal, people filled up on white bread, white-flour pasta, and other simple carbs instead of the fiber- and nutrition-rich whole grains.

Yet there is no mystery. Studies show that the primary way to achieve weight loss is through a reduction in calorie intake, regardless of which foods are eaten. Read product labels carefully, and don't assume that low-fat means low-calorie. We'll show you how to develop eating and activity strategies that will trim the calories, keep your fat intake in bounds, and fit comfortably into your lifestyle.

environmental challenges

At the same time that we are eating more, modern technology is conspiring to keep us less active. At work we may sit at a desk for hours. Typically, our leisure time revolves around passive entertainment, such as watching television, going to movies, and playing video games. As for sports, many people are more likely to watch games than play them. The addition of computers to the workplace and at home practically guarantees that we sit for several, if not most, of our waking hours. This not only makes it harder to control weight, it also can predict the risk of cardiovascular disease. According to a recent report, the risk of developing heart disease was nearly twice as great among women who spent the major portion of their day sitting when compared with women who spent less than 4 hours seated.

physical activities replaced by labor-saving devices

1905	2005
Walking	Riding in cars; sidewalks eliminated
Climbing stairs	Taking elevators and escalators
Cleaning by sweeping and dusting	Cleaning using vacuum cleaners
Working fields with plows	Riding a tractor
Picking crops	Harvesting using mechanized equipment
Mowing the lawn	Riding a mower
Carrying messages	Using telephones, faxes, and e-mails
Sawing wood	Using a power saw
Washing and hanging clothes	Using a washer and dryer
Shoveling snow	Using a snowblower
Finding and shelving books in	Searching the Internet the library

Even for school-age children, the situation is hardly better. Physical education has been reduced or even eliminated in many schools. The school programs that remain often do not provide sufficient activity. The issue of concern for children's safety restricts their outdoor activity even more. More often than not, parents drive their children to school or other activities. It is harder than ever for children to learn lifetime habits that incorporate physical activity.

positive momentum to move forward

The good news is that you **can** do something about these trends, but not with grapefruit or cabbage soup (remember those diets?), "fat-blocker" pills, or fraudulent gadgets. Instead, focus your attention on yourself, listen to your body, truly understand how you gained extra weight, and identify the best ways to control your weight for life.

" We want to encourage people to lose weight for all the right reasons and for all aspects of their health. Obesity poses a great risk for cardiovascular disease and stroke, and the time is ripe for us all to

find the lifestyle approaches that will have long-lasting benefits. "

ROBERT H. ECKEL,
MD, FAHA
Professor of Medicine
and of Physiology and
Biophysics
University of Colorado Health
Sciences Center

Think smart, eat well, and move more! Once you believe that weight control is possible, you can be a successful loser. Any step you take in the right direction in mind and in body—no matter how small—moves you closer to your weight-loss goals and a healthier life.

Part I

LOSING WEIGHT AND KEEPING IT OFF

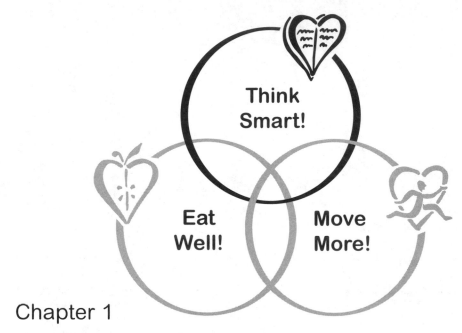

Think
Smart!

Eat
Well!

Move
More!

Chapter 1

THINK SMART:
find a new start

"Change your thoughts
and you change your world."

—NORMAN VINCENT PEALE

Despite what you may believe, good planning, not sheer willpower, is the key to losing weight for good. When you plan your day-to-day activities to support your efforts, you will find it much easier to reach and maintain your target weight. Think about how your current behavior fits with your planning. If you see a disconnect, find ways to change that behavior at the first opportunity. Planning is crucial to success.

When you consider the process of losing weight, what do you think about? If you think of a few weeks of being hungry as the quick fix, or rationalize your typical eating patterns, you're not planning like a successful loser. We want to help you learn to change the way you think as you experience the process of losing weight.

Identify what thoughts you have as you go through the process of following a diet plan. By using simple mental strategies, you can recognize destructive thinking, analyze your situation, find positive solutions to obstacles, and work toward modifying your lifestyle to match your weight-loss goals. Your mind is a powerful tool. To make effective changes, you need to change your mind-set. If you want to be in control, learn to think smart!

If you fail to plan, you plan to fail!

do it now: take the first opportunity

Thinking smart means finding ways to deal with the thoughts that lead you away from your goals. It does NOT mean putting things off until tomorrow. For example, if you know you indulged at a Friday-night dinner, you might react in one of several ways:

Tonight I ate so much at dinner,

1. I have totally blown it. I'll never be able to lose weight anyway. I give up!
2. I might as well eat two desserts! Then I'll get back on track on Monday.
3. I guess it won't matter if I eat dessert. Then I can start again tomorrow.
4. I'll choose not to have dessert.

Or, what if you haven't been as diligent as you'd planned:

I haven't been to aerobics class in weeks.

1. I'm so out of shape that I'll never go back!
2. I guess I can start over again next month.
3. It won't matter if I wait until next week.

4. I'd better pack my gym bag and go to the very next class.

As the first three statements in each situation show, there are lots of ways to delay taking action. Only the last approach is an example of taking the first opportunity to work toward your goal. Consider what your thoughts are in these situations. Ask yourself, "What are the implications of each thought?" Now think about the specific behavior that resulted from your thinking. The better choice here is to **change your behavior at the first opportunity**, not to wait until later.

believe: you will succeed

Increasing scientific evidence supports the idea that you become what you think about. Successful people—athletes, for example—use the technique of visualizing their goals to bolster their confidence, and they revisit those goals often. Don't let fear of failure keep you from starting toward your weight-loss goal. Action is the best way to sidestep misgivings and cure procrastination!

visualize: see through your mind's eye

You've often heard the saying "What you see is what you get." You can use that phrase in a new way. What you visualize by using some simple techniques lets you see your way through to successful weight loss.

- **Picture positive.** Take a minute to think about something that represents inner strength to you. Perhaps it is a person or a memory of the pride you felt when you accomplished something. No matter where you are or what you're doing, you can call up that image for a boost of resolve whenever you need a source of strength.

- **Picture the ultimate outcome.** Close your eyes and picture how you want to look when you've reached your target weight. How does this make you feel? When you hit a hurdle, focus on the image of a new you and the feelings this image evokes. Imagine how it will feel to be able to do the things that are not easy for you now.

talk back: retrain your brain

Do these statements sound familiar? "I just don't have enough time to walk around the block." "I'll exercise later." "It's OK to have french fries now. I'll just have a salad for dinner." Does the voice inside your head make excuses, rationalize, and justify why you did or did not do something? Unfortunately, that inner voice doesn't always steer you in the best direction. But just as you can talk yourself into bad behavior, you can talk yourself into doing things that will help you in the long run. Here are some strategies to retrain your brain and think smart:

- **Be conscious of self-talk.** Acknowledge that your inner voice feeds you information or messages more often than you may realize.

- **Evaluate.** Once you are aware of your self-talk, listen critically to what it is saying. Differentiate what you tell yourself from other sources of information.

- **Rephrase negative messages.** If you are sending yourself a negative message, such as "I had a bad day at work. I'm not in the mood to take a walk," choose not to accept the message. Instead, rephrase it into a positive statement: "I had a bad day at work. A thirty-minute walk will help me clear my head and focus on me."

energize your efforts

For every negative or unproductive thought you notice, find a positive image or saying to counter it. See yourself changing the negative thoughts into positive ones, and practice in your mind before the next negative thought arises.

set your goals

How are you **actually** going to accomplish the things you want? Here are some strategies to help you create effective goals.

- **Be reasonable and realistic.** It is natural to be enthusiastic about a new weight-loss plan. You may think to yourself, "I'm going to try all the recipes in this book and go every day to the new gym across town!" Along with being enthused, also be realistic about your expectations and the changes that will best fit your lifestyle. You need a reasonable goal so you will be pleased with realistic results.

How do you know whether the goals you set are realistic and reachable? Ask these questions:

- Is this something I really want to do for myself? A personal commitment is more motivating than the feeling of "I should."
- Is each of my goals measurable? How will I know when I'm there? Make sure your goals are clearly defined in terms of what, when, and how.

As you choose your target goals, think about the barriers you may meet. Work out specific strategies to remove the obstacles that might keep you from effectively changing your behavior, now and in the future. For example, if you prefer to exercise in the morning but you drive your children to school instead, try to arrange a morning carpool that would allow you more time. Good planning is essential for your success.

- **Set short-term milestones.** A short-term goal is something specific that happens every day, every few days, or even once a week and is tied to a specific action. Short-term milestones help you move toward your larger goal. When you set your short-term milestones, choose a time frame that will allow you to see progress. For example, you might decide your goal is to skip dessert every day, have a low-calorie lunch twice a week, and cook a healthful dinner once a week. Other examples include planning to walk after dinner instead of turning on the television, or going to the park to play with your dog twice a week.

- **Set long-term milestones.** When you set your long-term goals, choose an amount of time that is manageable but flexible enough to accommodate the inevitable ups and downs of life. For most of us, a year seems too far to feel an immediate sense of accomplishment. If you continue to reevaluate your progress and set new short-term goals every six weeks or so, however, you will reach your ultimate goal: maintaining your target weight for a lifetime!

- **Set intermediate checkpoints.** Short-term goals are the small steps that lead you to your desired long-term result. To be able to see the payback from your efforts along the way, plan checkpoints to assess or reassess your progress every six weeks. Have you reached your short-term goals? If so, celebrate your achievements, but don't stop there. Continue to set new goals that keep you moving in the right direction. If not, take another look at the information in this book. Then adjust your goals and your strategies accordingly.

anticipate: expect the unexpected

Food comes into play in many different business and social settings in our lives. These situations can present bumps on the road to successful weight control. Plan how you want to react in these situations. Consider what you might be thinking when you have to make a choice to eat or not. Be prepared to stop a negative thought from derailing you.

- **Say "Thanks but no thanks."** What if your boss brings in doughnuts for the office and personally hands one to you? Knowing that the doughnut does not fit into your eating strategy, how do you respond? Mentally rehearse your answer so that you will feel comfortable declining food. For example, you might say, "Thank you, Ms. Smith, but I'm trying to cut back." Most people will be understanding and glad you were honest. Even if they unthinkingly press you to accept foods you try to refuse, remain firm. Your first responsibility is to your own well-being.

- **See the situation.** What if you are invited to a neighbor's house for dinner? How will you handle the holidays? Visualize potential troublesome scenarios and prepare your actions and reactions. You can use positive thoughts to keep yourself on track. Let's say you've lost several pounds and are feeling pretty proud of being so "good." Remind yourself that sticking to your plan was how you got "good" in the first place!

- **Don't get sidetracked.** What if your colleagues ask you out to a movie on Wednesday evening, but you've been diligent about working out every Monday, Wednesday, and Friday right after work? Think about whether you can go out for a quick drink and then work out. You can also consider whether you can work out at lunchtime on Wednesday or Thursday instead. Think ahead so you'll have options when you'd like to change your plans.

- **Ask for what you need.** Don't hesitate to speak up and politely request something different from what's offered, such as a diet drink or sparkling water instead of sugar-filled lemonade or soda. Most people are more than happy to help you, but they can't know how unless you ask.

write it down: keep a personal weight-loss diary

As you develop your action plan, you should keep a journal of your weight-loss efforts. It is important to put your thoughts and goals onto paper because writing focuses your attention. When you transfer your thoughts from brainwaves to ink and paper, they become real.

Your journal provides a record of the thoughts that lead to your behavior at specific moments. Analyzing the entries in your journal will tell you how your thoughts work for or against your weight-loss goals. The chapters "Eat Well" and "Move More" provide more information on the specifics of goal setting for weight loss and weight control. We also have included sample pages for a food and activity diary (Appendixes E and F) to help you reach the goals you set.

Here are some important things you should include in your diary:

Self-assessment

- What, how much, and when you eat now
- How much and what type of activity you get now
- Your thoughts—both positive and negative

Goals

- Short- and long-term milestones
- Checkpoints at regular intervals
- How to make eating well a part of your lifestyle
- How to make physical activity a part of your lifestyle

Tracking and Progress Reports

- Daily entries of food intake and physical activity as you proceed through the weight-loss process
- Results achieved at your chosen checkpoints

be persistent: practice makes perfect

All these techniques are skills that need practice to become habit, just like playing the piano or shooting baskets. You won't become proficient unless you put the words into action on a daily basis.

66 Modifying your behavior is the cornerstone of any approach to weight control. It is not enough to simply understand that body weight results from the balance between calories eaten and calories burned

through different activities. Rather, it is critical to know how to make the lifestyle changes that will allow you to adopt and maintain new behaviors over time. Finding the right strategies that lead to realistic and sustained behavior change will ultimately result in the most successful weight control. **"**

JOHN M. JAKICIC, PhD
Chair, Department of Health
and Physical Activity
Director, Physical Activity and
Weight Management
Research Center
University of Pittsburgh

As you learn to think smarter, it will be easier to put the other two Circles of Success into motion. In the next chapters, you'll learn to make smart choices about how to eat well, move more, and make weight control a permanent part of your life.

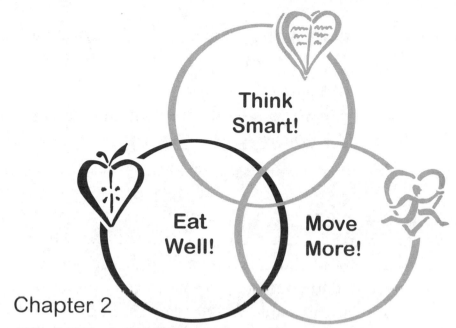

Think
Smart!

Eat
Well!

Move
More!

Chapter 2

EAT WELL: a personal approach to a healthful weight

Good food and good health: They **do** go together! Eating well is a lot more than following a diet plan until you've lost weight—it is the commitment you make to choose foods wisely. We offer you three simple strategies to cut back on extra calories and transition to a healthful way of eating at the same time. We'll help you decide which approach best fits your preferences and your individual weight-loss needs. You can then adopt the one that is right for you.

Nutritionally balanced meals are an important part of maintaining a healthful lifestyle for yourself and those you love. That's why we strongly encourage you to avoid the fads and choose a reasonable eating plan based on sound nutritional guidelines you can follow for a lifetime. No matter which hook the fad diets are using, it isn't reasonable to expect miraculous weight loss that will last. No foods by themselves burn away calories. Eating only foods from certain groups and cutting way back on foods from other groups leads to nutritional imbalance. **You don't need to think in terms of "good" or "bad" foods.** Rather, think about finding the right combination of foods to reach the right number of calories to fuel your body.

The diets you may have tried before worked at first because you were motivated and because you cut back on calories, not because there was anything magical about the specific diet you chose. Many different food combinations or theories can lead you to eat fewer calories each day and therefore lose weight. Over time, however, for various reasons you often regain the weight you lose, and perhaps even a few extra pounds.

❝ I never had to think about my weight when I was young. I could eat anything I wanted, and I never gained a pound. Then I had my first child, and suddenly I noticed that I couldn't lose the weight I'd

---

simple steps to healthful weight loss

1. Self-assess: What are you eating now—and why?

2. Decide on your personal weight loss goal: First lose 10 percent of your body weight, then aim for a healthful target weight.

3. Choose an eating strategy to lose 1 to 2 pounds each week.
   - The Switch and Swap Approach
   - The 75% Solution
   - The American Heart Association Menu Plans

4. Monitor your progress and reassess at six weeks.

---

gained. By the time my second child was born, I knew I had to do something. If a friend told me about some new diet, I'd get all enthusiastic and try it. I bought whatever food was supposed to melt away the fat, or I completely cut out fat or carbs. I tried it all. I always lost a few pounds at the beginning, but gradually the weight came back, sometimes with a vengeance. I'd feel discouraged until I heard about another diet plan. Then I'd start all over again.

This has gone on for about 10 years now. I have three distinct wardrobes in my closet—one for each stage in my weight-loss-and-gain cycle! What I really want is to be able to throw away the 'fat' clothes for good, but nothing I do seems to really work. **99**

32-YEAR-OLD MOTHER, ALBANY, NEW YORK

What's wrong with this picture? This woman is looking so hard for the one "right" diet that she isn't looking at her habits or her personal needs. If you've had the same experience, don't be discouraged. By using the right eating strategies, you can tailor a no-fad weight-loss plan to your lifestyle and avoid the yo-yo effect.

> **You—not a steak or a carrot or a secret formula—are at the center of weight-loss success. It's time to focus less on the diet and more on you!**

energy balance

A major component of lifelong weight control is understanding the concept of Energy Balance. To make a successful transition from your current eating habits to a healthful eating plan, you must learn how those habits contribute to your personal Energy Balance. Imagine a scale with your daily Calories In (the food you eat) on one side and your Calories Out (the average of calories you burn through both basic metabolic function and physical activity) on the other. No matter how much you weigh, that scale looks like this if your weight stays relatively stable:

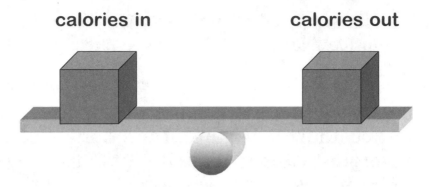

To create weight loss, you must upset the balance in favor of Calories Out:

calories in   **calories out**

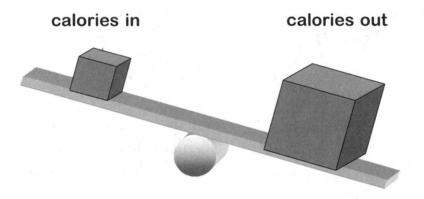

It doesn't take a lot to affect the balance of Calories In and Calories Out. Eating merely 100 extra calories per day can add up to about 10 pounds of weight gain in one year. But just think—it also means that **subtracting** an extra 100 calories a day can bring you a 10-pound weight loss in one year! That's as easy as walking an extra mile or cutting out 8 ounces of regular soda each day. In light of your Energy Balance, it's easy to see that small changes can make a meaningful difference.

the basics: calorie reduction and nutritional balance

Our plan for safe and long-lasting weight loss is based on a simple core principle: to lose weight, you must consume fewer daily calories than the number of calories it takes to maintain your current weight. For most people, these general guidelines apply:

- **If you subtract 500 calories per day, you will lose about 1 pound per week, or 5 to 6 pounds in six weeks.**

- **If you subtract 1,000 calories per day, you will lose about 2 pounds per week, or 10 to 12 pounds in six weeks.**

The idea is that you can "subtract" calories by eating less, moving more, or combining the two.

You might wonder how this can work for so many different people. Interestingly, research shows that when you reduce your average daily calorie intake by 500 to 1,000 calories, you will lose about the same amount of weight at about the same rate as most other people, regardless of how much you might weigh at the time. In fact, as a general rule, we don't recommend that you try to lose more than 2 pounds per week without the guidance of a health-care professional.

Reducing calories, no matter how you do it, will result in weight loss. In most cases, the loss will make you healthier. But as you learn to cut calories, it's important to learn to find a good balance of healthful foods as well. After all, your body can't function properly for long without the essential nutrients it needs. We suggest you first make small changes to find workable ways to cut calories. As soon as you've adjusted to eating less and celebrated your initial weight loss, transition to incorporating nutritional balance into your food choices. See "Food Sense: What Every Body Needs" (page 66) for specific information on the American Heart Association guidelines for good nutrition. As you concentrate more on eating well, you will learn to find options that are both low in calories **and** high in nutrition. As a reminder to get focused on the big picture, you can use the catch phrase **"quality first, then quantity."** By recommending "quality," we mean that you should choose a combination of foods that provides a complete nutritional package over time.

exceptions to the rule

There are always situations that don't fit the usual pattern, and weight loss is no different. These general guidelines may be less applicable to very small or very large people. For example, a 140-pound, 30-year-old woman who is 5 feet tall and not active will not be able to reduce her calorie intake by much more than 500 calories because she is now eating about 1,800 calories a day to maintain her present weight. Because she needs at least 1,200 calories a day for good nutrition, she should not cut more than 600 calories from her daily diet.

In a recent comparison of the most popular weight-loss plans, researchers found that long-term success had much less to do with the type of diet than the perseverance of the participants. People who make changes to their lifestyle, not just their diet, are the ones who will be able to maintain their weight loss for life. Researchers also found that successful losers set reasonable goals, tracked their progress, became accustomed to eating less, and transitioned to healthful eating habits that promote good nutrition. They also focused on developing long-term plans for overall good health that they could stick with for the rest of their lives. You will find all these elements in our plan for healthy weight loss.

self-assess: what are you eating now—and why?

The following pages will help you develop an effective, personalized approach to weight loss and will lead you to a better understanding of yourself. Before you can head in the right direction, you need to know your starting point. The best way to find out what you're really eating is to keep a food diary. Write down everything you eat and drink for one week, even if you think the amount is too small to matter, and make a note of what you are thinking at the time.

As you track your eating habits, don't forget the "hidden" calories. These calories come from the foods you eat either without realizing it or in such small amounts that you think they "don't count." For example, when you are cooking, do you often taste for seasoning or automatically add margarine to vegetables? Do you chew gum after lunch every day? Do you "help" your children clean their plates? Do you eat the last few mouthfuls of mashed potatoes because you think it isn't right to waste food? One bite may not seem to make much difference, but these tidbits do add up. If you eat it or drink it, write it down! It takes only a few minutes each day to keep track, but the payoff can be huge.

We've provided a blank log page that you can copy and use to create your own food diary (page 702). We've also included a sample page of entries to show you how one person's diary entries might look. Later in the chapter, we show how this person's diary would look as he or she applies some of the weight-loss strategies.

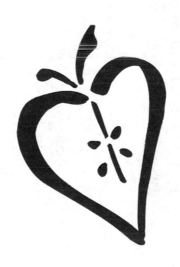

sample food diary page of original eating habits

Date: January 11 ☐ Mon. ☒ Tues. ☐ Wed. ☐ Thurs. ☐ Fri. ☐ Sat. ☐ Sun.

TIME & PLACE	FOOD OR BEVERAGE (type and amount)	CALORIES	WHAT PROMPTED YOU TO EAT?
breakfast 8:00 A.M. Home	1.9-oz. slice pecan coffee cake	230	Hunger—needed fuel for the day
	8 oz. low-fat strawberry yogurt (with fruit)	240	
	6 oz. orange juice	89	
	6 oz. coffee with		
	2 Tb. half-and-half	44	
snack 10:30 A.M. Work	22 animal crackers	252	Needed a break
	8 oz. whole milk	150	

lunch 12:00 P.M. Fast-food restaurant	8 chicken nuggets (3.9 oz)	290	Hunger—wanted to escape from the office
	3 oz. waffle fries	290	
	1/2 cup coleslaw	130	
	1 fudge nut brownie (2.6 oz.)	350	
	16 oz. regular cola	150	
snack 2:30 P.M. Work 5:30 P.M. Work	1 oz. Cheddar cheese	114	Stress
	6 saltine crackers	73	
	1 apple	81	
	1 candy bar (2.1 oz.)	280	Sugar craving—treat for end of workday
dinner 6:30 P.M. Home	3 oz. T-bone steak	253	It was "time" for dinner—wanted to eat with my family
	1 baked potato with skin (6.5 oz.) with 1 Tb. sour cream and 1 Tb. stick margarine	346	
	1/2 cup canned green beans with 1 Tb. stick margarine	120	

27

TIME & PLACE	FOOD OR BEVERAGE (type and amount)	CALORIES	WHAT PROMPTED YOU TO EAT?
	1 cup green salad with 2 Tb. creamy Italian dressing	145	
	1 slice garlic bread	95	
	1/2 cup canned fruit cocktail (in heavy syrup)	93	
snack 10:00 P.M. Home	1/2 cup mint chocolate chip ice cream	250	Habit while watching TV at night

TOTAL Daily Calories: 4,070

why are you eating that bag of chips?

Once you've collected about a week's worth of information, read it over and look for patterns. Analyzing this information is crucial to understanding why you eat the way you do. Are you surprised by how many times you grabbed a candy bar for a quick pick-me-up or downed a high-calorie soda? Did you realize how often you went back for extra helpings or how few whole grains you actually eat?

As part of your self-assessment, identify the different reasons you find yourself eating. Are you responding to physical cues, such as hunger pangs? Do emotional triggers make you think you're hungry when what you really need is reassurance or distraction? Almost everyone experiences cravings. How do you deal with them? Ask yourself, What thoughts and triggers drive me to eat when I'm not hungry?

Many of these behaviors and responses (or reasons for eating the way you do) are learned, and they become habits over time. But you can unlearn them or replace them. Make a list of your eating habits and cravings. Try to make notes in your food diary about why you made certain food choices. What does this information tell you about the type of eater you are? That is, do you eat because you feel hungry?

Are you a grazer who needs small amounts of food all day long? Be honest with yourself, and it will be easier to find a workable strategy to satisfy a craving without caving. Many avenues to successful, healthy weight loss are available to you. If you pay attention to your own needs, you will know which one to follow. After a week of keeping track and some time spent reviewing your eating habits, you'll be able to see ways to change your patterns of thought and behavior. That's the power of keeping a food diary.

did you know . . .

that some people really do feel hungry all the time? They can't help it; it's in their body chemistry. If you think you are one of these people, ask your healthcare professional for advice on controlling your hunger pangs.

As you review your diary entries, you don't need to add up the actual calorie total, or Calories In, unless you want to. The real purpose of the diary is to provide a record of exactly what you are eating so you can analyze that information. Instead of adding up the calories, use the formula below to easily estimate the number of calories you are eating to maintain your current weight. You'll need this information to know how many calories to cut out of your diet for safe and effective weight loss.

calories needed to maintain your current weight

Before you can decide how many calories you should eat each day to lose weight, you'll need to determine how many calories you are eating now to maintain your current weight. To do this, use the following formula. Multiply your current weight in pounds by 10 to find a number of Base Calories. Multiply your current weight by 3 (not active), 5 (moderately active), or 8 (very active), depending on your activity level, to find a number of Activity Calories.

When you add your Base Calories and Activity Calories, the total will tell you **about how many calories** you need on an average day to maintain your weight. At middle age, you may experience a decrease in metabolism. To accommodate for that decrease, subtract 10 percent of your total if you are over 50 years old. The final adjusted total is your baseline, or the number of calories you need to maintain your current weight. To lose weight, you'll need to eat fewer calories.

Multiply current weight in pounds _____
X 10 = Base Calories _____

Multiply current weight in pounds _____
If not active: **X 3**
If moderately active: **X 5**
If very active: **X 8 = Activity Calories** _____
Add Base + Activity Calories =
  Total Calories to Maintain Weight _____
If you are older than 50 years, subtract 10%
of that total.   (−10%) _____
Total Adjusted Calories _____

For example, here's what this calculation would look like for a woman who weighs 180 pounds, is not active, and is 55 years old. To lose weight, this woman must reduce her calorie intake to an average of less than 2,106 calories each day. The more calories she subtracts, the faster she will lose.

Multiply current weight in pounds __180__
  X 10 = Base Calories __1,800__
Multiply current weight in pounds __180__
If not active: **X 3**
If moderately active: **X 5**
If very active: **X 8 = Activity Calories** __540__
Add Base + Activity Calories =
  Total Calories to Maintain Weight __2,340__
If you are older than 50 years, subtract 10%
of that total.   (−10%) __234__
  Total Adjusted Calories __2,160__

The following sections will help you determine a reasonable and healthy target weight for yourself and set a personal weight-loss goal. You will use your baseline calorie intake and your current weight to decide how fast you want to lose and which weight-loss strategy is the best for you.

Remember, a good rule of thumb is to lose no more than 2 pounds each week. That's a sensible amount of weight loss that is much more likely to become habit for the long term. As you make your choices, consider this: Behavior experts tell us that starting your program with a greater calorie reduction per day will help "train" you and make it easier to stick to the program—even if you cut back that much for only the first two weeks. It's okay, too, if you just want to take it slowly, since smaller changes may fit more easily into your lifestyle. You can always switch to a greater calorie reduction if you find that you want to lose weight faster. Be aware, however, that if you eat fewer than 1,200 calories per day, you run the risk of not getting all the nutrients you need.

what if i don't lose weight?

Our recommended calorie intake levels are averages and apply to most people. If these recommendations do not produce the weight loss you expect, you will need to further restrict calories. To help you do that, find a healthcare professional who advises patients on how to lose weight. He or she can work with you to determine an ideal daily calorie intake level based on an your individual needs. That recommendation may differ from the results of these general guidelines, especially for higher weight ranges.

decide on a personal weight-loss goal

It seems everyone wants to have a picture-perfect body. After all, the entertainment industry and advertisements are full of them. When setting your goals, bear in mind that movie stars and models benefit from lots of professional help, both behind the scenes and in front of the camera. The work of personal chefs and trainers, make-up artists, and lighting experts—as well as careful editing, cropping, and airbrushing—all help create the illusions that we have come to see as real. It just isn't fair to expect your mirror to show the same results!

how much weight should you lose?

First, start with reasonable expectations. When most people go on a diet, they usually want to lose a lot of weight and lose it quickly. Probably they gained those pounds in small increments over a long time, and, realistically, it will take time to lose them. To avoid setting yourself up for failure, allow yourself enough time to be a successful loser in the long run. Armed with a good (and honest) understanding of what you are eating now, you can make an educated decision about how much weight you want to lose.

We recommend that you start with an initial goal of losing about 10 percent of your body weight.

The good news is that you don't have to lose every pound before your health will benefit. Studies have shown that losing even 10 pounds may help reduce your risk of heart disease, stroke, and diabetes.

Let's use our 180-pound, 55-year-old woman as an example. She is currently eating an average of 2,100 calories each day. If she cuts back by only 500 calories each day, she will lose 18 pounds, or 10 percent of her body weight, in about 18 weeks. If she increases her activity level, she also will increase the likelihood of maintaining that weight loss for good. As she chooses how to eliminate those 500 calories, she can also gradually start making more healthful choices to reap better nutritional benefits from the foods she does eat. Again, small changes lead to big rewards!

Additionally, ask yourself whether you have enough energy to do the things you need and want to do in your life. These are the important issues to consider. Instead of fretting about whether you will ever fit into the clothes you wore in college, realize that people come in all different shapes and sizes. Ten women who each weigh the same 130 pounds will offer ten completely different looks. Focus on what you like about your body, not what you wish you could change. What look is right for **you?** Think smart: See yourself in your mind's eye as the person you want to be—at the weight that feels right to you—and make it so. Learn to love what you are proud of, and let go of what you can't change. Remember that your long-term goal should be to reach a healthful weight.

how is a healthful weight defined?

Healthcare professionals often use body mass index (BMI) to classify levels of overweight and obesity. A BMI of less than 25 indicates that you are at a weight that is healthful for you (less than 18.5 is considered underweight, however). If your BMI is between 25 and 29.9, you are considered overweight. A BMI of 30 or more indicates obesity.

The chart below shows you how to determine your BMI. Find your height in the left-hand column and see whether your weight falls into either range listed. If you prefer to calculate your exact BMI, multiply your weight in pounds by 705. Divide by your height in inches; divide again by your height in inches.

body mass index

HEIGHT	OVERWEIGHT (BMI 25.0–29.9)	OBESE (BMI 30.0 and above)
4'10"	119–142 lb	143 lb or more
4'11"	124–147	148
5'0"	128–152	153
5'1"	132–157	158
5'2"	136–163	164
5'3"	141–168	169
5'4"	145–173	174
5'5"	150–179	180
5'6"	155–185	186
5'7"	159–190	191
5'8"	164–196	197
5'9"	169–202	203
5'10"	174–208	209

HEIGHT	OVERWEIGHT (BMI 25.0–29.9)	OBESE (BMI 30.0 and above)
5'11"	179–214	215
6'0"	184–220	221
6'1"	189–226	227
6'2"	194–232	233
6'3"	200–239	240
6'4"	205–245	246

You can use the BMI chart to help set your weight-loss goals. If you are 5'7", for example, your ultimate goal may be to reach a BMI of less than 25, so your goal weight would be 155 pounds.

write down your goals and checkpoints

You know from Chapter 1 how important it is to identify your goals and write them down. Plan checkpoints at two-week intervals. Use the following sample "contract" to record your goals, both long- and short-term, and the rewards you will enjoy as you reach each of your targets. Write down your specific objectives for the two-week, four-week, and six-week target

"If you don't know where you're going, you might wind up someplace else."
—YOGI BERRA

dates in the numbered spaces on the "contract" that follows. As the pounds disappear, you'll be able to track and celebrate your progress. Be sure to keep track of your progress in your diary. Persistence is the key: Even if you don't reach your target on occasion, realize that every step you make toward your goal is a sign of success.

my weight-loss goals

Date: _____

My long-term weight-loss goal is to lose _____ by _____.

My short-term weight-loss goals are to lose

1. _____ by _____ and

2. _____ by _____ and

3. _____ by _____.

I plan to achieve my goals through these specific actions:

_____

_____

_____

The rewards for reaching my goals are:

1. _____ and

2. _____ and

3. _____.

Signature: _____

choose the eating strategy that works best for you

We offer three different approaches to keeping your calories in line: the Switch and Swap Approach, the 75% Solution, and the American Heart Association Menu Plans. It's your choice—not someone else's rigid diet plan—that determines the method that best suits your eating habits and your individual lifestyle. Think of these options as three tools in a toolbox at your disposal. As everyone knows, there is a right tool for every job, and there is a right strategy for you!

Start with the following questionnaire. Your honest answers to these questions will help you identify the plan that will work best for you.

Which Strategy Will Work Best for You?

1. How often do you eat out (don't forget to count breakfasts, brunches, and lunches, as well as dinners)?
   A. Three to five times a week
   B. More than five times a week
   C. Once or twice a week _____

2. How aware are you of the number of calories you are consuming?
   A. Haven't a clue
   B. Sort of aware
   C. Very aware _____

3. Do you like to plan ahead or go with the flow?
   A. Go with the flow
   B. Plan when I can
   C. Planning is my strong suit   _____

4. Do you feel like you have already cut out high-calorie foods from your diet?
   A. Haven't really paid attention
   B. Somewhat
   C. Absolutely   _____

5. Do you read food ingredient labels?
   A. Sometimes
   B. Can't be bothered
   C. Always   _____

6. Do you enjoy cooking at home?
   A. When I have time
   B. Not really
   C. Love it   _____

7. Do you like to look up nutrition facts (in brochures, books, or on the Web) about the food you're eating?
   A. Can't be bothered
   B. Sometimes
   C. Love it   _____

8. How often do you eat fast food?
   A. A few times a week
   B. Every day
   C. Seldom or never   _____

9. Do you like to try new foods and new cooking methods?
   A. Somewhat
   B. Not really
   C. Absolutely   _____

10. How balanced are your meals?
    A. Somewhat
    B. Very
    C. Haven't a clue   _____

Total Number of As   _____
Total Number of Bs   _____
Total Number of Cs   _____

What Your Score Means

6–10 As   See page 44 for the Switch and Swap Approach.

6–10 Bs   See page 53 for the 75% Solution.

6–10 Cs   See page 155 for the American Heart Association Menu Plans.

What if your scores are fairly evenly split? Try combining the two methods that have the highest number. For example, if you have mostly As and Bs, try both the Switch and Swap Approach and the 75% Solution.

basic rule to post on the refrigerator:

EAT LESS WHEN YOU'RE HUNGRY, STOP WHEN YOU'RE NOT.

STRATEGY 1: the switch and swap approach

SUBSTITUTE LOWER-CALORIE FOODS FOR HIGH-CALORIE FOODS

The first strategy is based on the idea that you can subtract calories by making small but effective changes in your daily eating patterns. Where are your daily calories coming from? What can you replace with a lower- or no-calorie substitute? We have included a list of some easy alternatives to get you started on page 46. Find about 500 calories of substitutions each day for the high-calorie foods you eat frequently, and you're already on your way to losing about 1 pound each week. You can also refer to the list of common foods by calorie count in Appendix D (page 695).

> **❝ I knew I should drink more milk for the calcium—the doctor had told me often enough—but I just don't like milk. Instead, I ate two containers of low-fat fruit yogurt each day, thinking the lower fat content would keep the calories down too. But when I started keeping a food diary, I realized I was getting a whopping**

190 calories from each of those containers—380 calories a day! So I switched to nonfat, no-sugar-added yogurt. I still get the calcium I need, but for only a fraction of the calories. **"**

46-YEAR-OLD
ADVERTISING EXECUTIVE,
CHICAGO, ILLINOIS

Keeping a food diary is an essential part of the substitution approach. Base your switches on the information and patterns you find there. It's easy to skip the margarine on your daily toast and use a tablespoon of all-fruit spread instead when you realize that you'll save about 75 calories. If you switch from whole milk to fat-free, you'll save another 60 calories per cup. That's a 135-calorie reduction just for breakfast! Keep in mind that you need to try to eat enough servings from all the food groups. Using the entries from your food diary and the information on balanced nutrition on pages 66–70, you will be able to see where you can cut calories without cutting nutritional quality.

sample food substitutions

INSTEAD OF…	HOW ABOUT…	CALORIE SAVINGS
1 cinnamon roll	1 cinnamon-raisin English muffin with 2 teaspoons light tub margarine	312
1 milk chocolate bar (1.55 ounces)	10 chocolate-covered raisins	187
½ cup Alfredo sauce	½ cup marinara sauce	185
Bacon, lettuce, and tomato sandwich, made with 2 slices white bread, 4 slices bacon, 1 tablespoon mayonnaise, 2 lettuce leaves, and ½ medium tomato	Turkey bacon, lettuce, and tomato sandwich, made with 2 slices light white bread, 4 slices turkey bacon, 1 tablespoon light mayonnaise dressing, 2 lettuce leaves, and ½ medium tomato	161
16 ounces regular cola	16 ounces diet cola	149
2 ¼ cups Caesar salad with dressing	3 cups tossed salad with 2 tablespoons light Italian salad dressing	140

	Calories	
½ cup vanilla ice cream	139	½ cup sorbet
1 medium baked potato with skin, topped with 1 tablespoon each sour cream, stick margarine, shredded Cheddar cheese, and chopped chives	104	1 medium baked potato with skin, topped with 2 tablespoons each light sour cream and salsa
½ cup granola	92	½ to ⅔ cup low-fat granola
8 ounces low-fat vanilla yogurt	89	3 ounces fat-free, sugar-free vanilla yogurt
½ cup prepared instant vanilla pudding made with 2% milk	80	½ cup prepared fat-free, sugar-free instant vanilla pudding, made with fat-free milk
8 ounces whole milk	66	8 ounces fat-free milk
½ cup fried rice	53	½ cup steamed rice
1 tablespoon regular stick margarine	52	1 tablespoon light stick margarine
6 ounces orange juice	51	6 ounces tomato juice
1 medium egg	36	¼ cup liquid egg substitute

Here's an example of how you could apply the principles of Switch and Swap to your eating plan. Compare the diary pages 49–51 with the one on pages 26–28. You can see how many calories you can save just by making easy substitutions (shown in bold) for foods or items that are part of a routine or habitual pattern. It's really just a matter of swapping one habit for another.

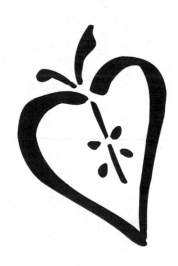

sample food diary page using the switch and swap plan

Date: January 11 ☐ Mon. ☒ Tues. ☐ Wed. ☐ Thurs. ☐ Fri. ☐ Sat. ☐ Sun.

TIME & PLACE	FOOD OR BEVERAGE (type and amount)	CALORIES	WHAT PROMPTED YOU TO EAT?
breakfast 8:00 A.M. Home	1.9-oz. slice pecan coffee cake	230	Hunger—needed fuel for the day
	8 oz. low-fat strawberry yogurt (with fruit)	240	
	6 oz. tomato juice	**38**	
	6 oz. coffee with		
	2 Tb. fat-free half-and-half	24	
snack 10:30 A.M. Work	22 animal crackers	252	Needed a break
	8 oz. fat-free milk	**84**	

49

TIME & PLACE	FOOD OR BEVERAGE (type and amount)	CALORIES	WHAT PROMPTED YOU TO EAT?
lunch 12:00 P.M. Fast-food restaurant	8 chicken nuggets (3.9 oz.) 3 oz. waffle fries ½ cup coleslaw 1 fudge nut brownie (2.6 oz.) **16 oz. diet cola**	290 290 130 350 **1**	Hunger—wanted to escape from the office
snack 2:30 P.M. Work 5:30 P.M. Work	1 oz. Cheddar cheese 6 saltine crackers 1 apple 1 candy bar (2.1 oz.)	114 78 81 280	Stress Sugar craving—treat for end of workday

dinner 6:30 P.M. Home	3 oz. T-bone steak 1 baked potato with skin (6.5 oz.) with 1 Tb. light sour cream (no margarine) 1/2 cup canned green beans with 1 Tb. stick margarine 1 cup green salad with 2 Tb. creamy Italian dressing 1 slice garlic bread 1/2 cup canned fruit cocktail (in heavy syrup)	253 346 120 145 95 95	It was "time" for dinner—wanted to eat with my family
snack 10:00 P.M. Home	1/2 cup mint chocolate chip ice cream	250	Habit while watch-ing TV at night
	TOTAL Daily Calories:	3,573	**Calories Saved: 497**

The Switch and Swap Approach is especially good for people who usually follow a routine and can see how their eating habits may be contributing to weight gain. You can change the way you think about eating and food when you move toward making better choices. If you look at the entries in your daily food diary and can find several foods to replace with lower-calorie, higher-nutrition options, the substitution plan may be just the way to find a leaner, trimmer you!

STRATEGY 2:
the 75% solution

EAT THREE-QUARTERS OF THE AMOUNT OF FOOD THAT YOU EAT NOW

Portion control is a major issue for most people. If you are one of the many who have gotten into the habit of eating too much too often, the 75% Solution may be the simplest way for you to start working toward a healthful weight. Although we don't recommend that you continue indefinitely to eat many foods that have little nutritional value, the simplicity of just cutting back across the board can be a great help in starting to change lifetime habits.

You might be pleasantly surprised at how easy it can be to cut out 500 to 1,000 calories each day if you cut back on the amount of food you eat overall. You don't need to think too hard about this approach: Just concentrate at first on reducing your daily calorie intake. You can continue to eat most of the things you like—just eat less of each one.

As you serve yourself each meal, mentally draw a line on your plate to portion out 75 percent of what you normally eat. Compare that amount to what we consider a reasonable serving, using the size estimates below. You will probably find that the smaller portion (the 75 percent portion) is close to a reasonable serving size.

3 ounces meat = a computer mouse

3 ounces grilled fish = a checkbook

1 ounce cheese = four stacked dice

1 teaspoon mayonnaise = the tip of a thumb

1 medium fruit = a baseball

$\frac{1}{2}$ cup cooked pasta = a baseball

1 cup = the tight fist of a small hand

Need to grab a meal on the run? You can still enjoy your favorites if you commit to eating less. Order what you would usually choose and remove one-quarter of it. Eat the three-quarters that remains—free of guilt. We think you'll find that you are quite satisfied, but you will have eliminated those crucial extra calories. Hate the waste? Take the leftovers home for a snack or to add to another meal. If that's not feasible, recognize that a few cents' worth of waste is a small price to pay if you also hate your waist! You can make a few changes to your order as well. Choose a single burger instead of a double. Select a small order of fries instead of a medium, or share your usual order with someone else. Check out the helpful tips for eating in restaurants in Appendix C (page 688).

Take another look at the sample diary page on pages 46–51. Compare it with the one following to see one example of how the 75% Solution can work for you.

sample food diary page using the 75% solution plan

Date: January 11 ☐ Mon. ☒ Tues. ☐ Wed. ☐ Thurs. ☐ Fri. ☐ Sat. ☐ Sun.

TIME & PLACE	FOOD OR BEVERAGE (type and amount)	CALORIES	WHAT PROMPTED YOU TO EAT?
breakfast 8:00 A.M. Home	¾ slice pecan coffee cake (1.4 oz)	173	Hunger—needed fuel for the day
	6 oz. low-fat strawberry yogurt (with fruit)	180	
	4.5 oz. orange juice	67	
	4.5 oz. coffee with 1½ Tb. half-and-half	34	
snack 10:30 A.M. Work	17 animal crackers	195	Needed a break
	6 oz. whole milk	113	

lunch 12:00 P.M. Fast-food restaurant	6 chicken nuggets (2.9 oz)	213	Hunger—wanted to escape from the office
	2¼ oz. waffle fries (³⁄₄ of an order)	213	
	³⁄₈ cup coleslaw	93	
	³⁄₄ fudge nut brownie (2 oz.)	263	
	12 oz. regular cola	113	
snack 2:30 P.M. Work	³⁄₄ oz. Cheddar cheese	86	Stress
	4½ saltine crackers	59	
	³⁄₄ apple	61	
5:30 P.M. Work	³⁄₄ candy bar (1.6 oz.)	210	Sugar craving—treat for end of workday
dinner 6:30 P.M. Home	2¼ oz. T-bone steak	190	It was "time" for dinner—wanted to eat with my family
	³⁄₄ baked potato with skin (4.9 oz.) with 2¼ tsp. sourcream and 2¼ tsp. stick margarine	260	

TIME & PLACE	FOOD OR BEVERAGE (type and amount)	CALORIES	WHAT PROMPTED YOU TO EAT?
	3/8 cup canned green beans with 2¼ tsp. stick margarine	90	
	3/4 cup green salad with 1½ Tb. creamy Italian dressing	109	
	3/4 slice garlic bread	71	
	3/8 cup canned fruit cocktail (in heavy syrup)	70	
snack 10:00 P.M. Home	3/8 cup mint chocolate chip ice cream	188	Habit while watching TV at night
TOTAL Daily Calories:		3,066	**Calories Saved: 1,004**

This approach to cutting back seems to work especially well for people on the go. Do you find yourself eating three slices of deep-dish pizza at your kid's football game every Friday night? Try cutting back to two pieces of pizza, and have a large salad if it's available. You can't always control where or what you are going to eat, but in most circumstances, you are the only one who decides how much you will eat of the food you are served. Knowing that you are in control may be just the ticket to putting the 75% Solution to work for you!

As you make your meal choices, gradually transition to include enough servings from each important food group. Remember our recommendation to consider quality before quantity. If you focus on nutrient-rich foods and reduce the amount of high-calorie, nutrient-poor foods, you'll have more leeway to eat other things you enjoy. It takes about six weeks to form new habits, so make it part of your six-week strategy to replace those foods that aren't contributing nutrients to your diet. Your food diary will help you see which foods to replace. If you usually have a dough-nut for breakfast, start cutting calories by eating only three-quarters. These small changes do add up. But once you've adjusted to eating less, find an alternative food for breakfast, such as a small whole-grain muffin. Try a grilled chicken sandwich and a side salad for lunch instead of a burger with fries. (For more ideas, see pages 46–47.) Those changes will give you the ultimate benefit of better nutrition for better health.

STRATEGY 3:
the american heart association menu plans

follow our easy-to-use two-week menu plans

For the many people who prefer a defined and well-planned program, we offer two weeks' worth of delicious menu plans to take the guesswork out of shopping and calorie counting. These menus, developed using some of the more than 190 recipes found on pages 244 to 669, are based on the American Heart Association dietary guidelines. To promote heart health, the menus and recipes are all low in saturated fat and moderate in sodium as well.

Using the formula on page 18 to establish your current calorie intake, you can decide which menu plan to follow. Depending on your calorie needs, choose from the 1,200-, 1,600-, or 2,000-calorie menus to safely lose between 1 and 2 pounds each week. Let's return to our 180-pound woman as an example. Since she is now eating about 2,100 calories, she could choose the 1,600-calorie menus to subtract 500 calories each day to lose 1 pound a week. If she wants to lose faster, she could follow the 1,200-calorie plan, reducing her intake by about 900 calories for a loss of just under 2 pounds per week. For more information, turn to "Part II: Menu Planning and Recipes," starting on page 149, for the details on how to make this weight-loss strategy work for you.

developing your own menu plans

Planning your own menus allows you not only to be creative but also to control your calorie intake. Take some time to organize your meals in advance to avoid the stress of wondering what to have for dinner and making last-minute shopping trips. Once you are familiar with the basics of our nutrition guidelines, you will be able to construct your own healthful, low-calorie menu plans. Have fun . . . and get started making smart, healthful choices every day.

We encourage you to use the recipes in this book to create your own menus. To make it easier to find the recipes that fit into your daily calorie balance, you will find a quick-reference visual, a "calorie bar," with each recipe. Each calorie bar represents a total of 400 calories, divided into eight parts of 50 calories each. The shaded area shows you at a glance about how many calories one serving will yield. For example, Asian Citrus Salad (page 317) has 90 calories per serving, so the calorie bar looks like this:

100   200   300   400

You may want to start with our two-week plans and then create your own menus for at least two more weeks. You'll have plenty of variety without having to take the time to make a new plan for each week. Use the calorie bars to find recipes that have about the same number of calories as those in our menus. By keeping a grocery list of the core items used in these plans, you'll be sure you have what you need in your pantry.

planning for emergencies

It's a good idea to keep some basic supplies on hand for quick and easy meals. We've included a pantry list for your reference on page 679. These foods fit right into a low-calorie eating plan and are quite versatile. With a wide selection of items in your kitchen, you can put together many simple combinations with a variety of seasonings on the spur of the moment. Appendixes A (page 672) and B (page 684) will give you lots of ideas and helpful information on shopping and cooking. The list of common foods by calorie count in Appendix D (page 695) will also help you plan your meals and track your calories.

eating well for good health

Because the concept of Energy Balance—Calories In/Calories Out—is the key to maintaining a healthful weight, it is also at the heart of any weight-loss program. But once you've chosen a strategy to trim calories, we'll also help you learn to eat in a healthful way at the same time. We want you to transition from the first phase—getting used to eating less—to ultimately making good food choices for a healthy life. How much do you really know about the calorie counts of different foods? Are you familiar with the basic nutritional guidelines? Many people make assumptions that turn out to be quite wrong.

A basic knowledge of calorie levels and good nutrition will be a big help no matter which eating strategy you choose. Take the following quiz and see if you can find the lowest-calorie foods—you may be surprised by the results.

test your calorie sense

For each pair below, choose the one you think has fewer calories. You will find the correct answers in bold type, as well as the calorie counts for both choices, at the end of the quiz.*

1. (a) $\frac{1}{2}$ cup cooked cauliflower with cheese sauce
   (b) $\frac{1}{2}$ cup canned pickled beets

2. (a) 10 chocolate-covered peanuts, 1.4 ounces total

(b) 2 mini peanut butter cups, 0.28 ounce each

3. (a) 10 small jelly beans, 0.4 ounce total
   (b) 10 small gumdrops, 0.4 ounce total

4. (a) 1 ounce feta cheese
   (b) 1 ounce Cheddar cheese

5. (a) 1 cup grapefruit juice
   (b) 1 cup tomato juice

6. (a) 13 ounces take-out latte with whole milk
   (b) $\frac{1}{2}$ cup trail mix

7. (a) 12 ounces club soda
   (b) 12 ounces tonic water

8. (a) 1 take-out hamburger, regular size, double patty with cheese and bun
   (b) 3.25 ounces fried chicken tenders

9. (a) $3\frac{1}{2}$-inch cinnamon-raisin bagel with $\frac{1}{2}$ ounce cream cheese
   (b) $\frac{1}{2}$ cup granola with $\frac{1}{4}$ cup fat-free milk

10. (a) 2 ounces deli turkey breast on small whole-wheat pita with 2 teaspoons mayonnaise, lettuce, and tomato
    (b) 2 ounces American cheese on 2 slices seven-grain bread with 2 teaspoons mustard, lettuce, and tomato

*We are not recommending that you choose the entries in this quiz. We've listed them to give you an idea of some surprising comparisons of calorie content.

ANSWERS

The bold type indicates the correct answer.
1. (a) **60,** (b) 75; 2. (a) 208, **(b) 80;** 3. (a) **40,**
(b) 135; 4. **(a) 75,** (b) 114; 5. (a) 100, **(b) 42;**
6. **(a) 152,** (b) 353; 7. **(a) 0,** (b) 125; 8. (a)
457, **(b) 264;** 9. **(a) 244,** (b) 325; 10. **(a) 198,**
(b) 336.

food sense: what every body needs

As you work toward your goal weight, be sure
to consider the nutritional quality of the sources
of your daily calories: Quality first, then quantity. Choosing a wide variety of foods on a regular basis gives you the best chance of consuming
the many nutrients your body needs. Eating
plans that eliminate one or more food groups
deprive your body of essential nutrients.

The American Heart Association recommends a balanced diet that is rich in vegetables,
fruits, and whole grains. It's also important to
control the amount of saturated and trans fats
in your diet. As you make your meal choices,
include lean meats, skinless poultry, and
seafood, especially fatty fish that are rich in
omega-3 fatty acids. In fact, we recommend
that you include at least two 3-ounce servings
of fish (preferably fatty fish) each week.

For more information on these recommendations for heart-healthy nutrition, refer to
the American Heart Association website

healthy-heart basics

- Replace saturated fats (such as those found in foods from animal sources) with healthful polyunsaturated and monounsaturated fats (such as corn, safflower, soybean, sunflower, olive, and canola oils).

- Avoid trans fats.

- Limit your daily intake of dietary cholesterol to less than 300 milligrams.

- Limit your daily intake of sodium to less than 2,300 miligrams. (Watch both table salt and sodium levels in prepared foods.)

- If you drink alcohol, limit your daily intake to one drink for a woman, two for a man.

- Aim for a daily intake of 25 to 30 grams of fiber (from whole grains, fruits, and vegetables).

(americanheart.org) or call 800-AHA-USA1 (800-242-8721). You'll find the latest advice from medical and nutrition experts on the best ways to help keep your levels of blood pressure and cholesterol under control, as well as details on how diet and lifestyle contribute to heart health. You can also keep up with recent developments in the science of weight loss and control and prevention of overweight and obesity.

Use the following chart as a guide to the recommended number of servings from each food group for each day. Remember that in many cases the serving sizes add up easily. For example, if you eat a sandwich with two slices of whole-wheat bread for lunch, you are actually getting two servings' worth of the nutrients from the whole-grain group. If you eat 1 cup of cooked broccoli instead of the normal serving size of $^{1}/_{2}$ cup, you've taken care of two vegetable servings for that day.

recommended servings per day for an average adult

NUMBER OF SERVINGS	WHOLE GRAINS AND LEGUMES	VEGETABLES AND FRUITS	FAT-FREE OR LOW-FAT DAIRY	LEAN MEAT, POULTRY SEAFOOD**, AND VEGETARIAN PROTEIN
6				
5				
4				
3				
2				
1				

* Two or more for children; four or more for teenagers, pregnant or breastfeeding mothers, and older adults.
** Include at least two servings of fish, preferably fatty fish, per week.

how much is one serving?

It is important to become aware of not only what you eat but also how much you eat. To give you a better idea of what we mean by a serving, here are some **one-serving** samples of foods from each food group.

One serving means one of the following:

whole grains, other starches, or legumes
- 1 slice whole-wheat bread
- 1 cup flaked cereal
- $\frac{1}{2}$ cup cooked cereal
- $\frac{1}{2}$ cup cooked rice or whole-grain pasta
- $\frac{1}{2}$ cup cooked starchy vegetables, such as mashed potatoes or corn

vegetables and fruits
- 1 medium piece of fruit
- 1 cup raw leafy greens
- $\frac{3}{4}$ cup fruit or vegetable juice
- $\frac{1}{2}$ cup raw or cooked nonstarchy vegetables, such as asparagus or squash

fat-free or low-fat dairy
- 1 cup fat-free milk
- $\frac{1}{2}$ cup fat-free or low-fat cottage cheese
- 1 ounce fat-free or low-fat cheese

**lean meat, poultry, seafood, or
vegetarian protein**

- 3 ounces cooked (4 ounces raw) lean meat, skinless poultry, or seafood
- 3 ounces canned tuna or salmon
- $\frac{1}{2}$ cup cooked beans (except green beans) or lentils

using the tools in your toolbox: monitor your progress

Once you've chosen a strategy and started to put it in action, stay focused on yourself instead of the food. Ask yourself: What is working? How do I feel? As we

"None of the secrets of success will work unless you do."
—CHINESE FORTUNE COOKIE

mentioned in Chapter 1, it is very important for you to assess your progress. If you find you are not reaching the goals you recorded for your various checkpoints, you probably aren't reducing your calorie intake as much as you think. Are you planning correctly? Try to determine where you may be underestimating your intake. For example, if you've chosen to use the Switch and Swap Approach to cut 500 calories a day by switching five foods, make it a total of eight instead, so you are cutting back even more.

Try a combination of strategies. Find substitutes for your favorite high-calorie foods and cut back on your portion sizes. Perhaps you can prepare some of the suggested menu plans on certain days of the week and then follow the 75% Solution on days when you have less time to cook or when you know you will be eating out. You are the only one who will know which strategies are the right tools for you.

coping with hunger and cravings

Changing your eating habits is not easy and will cause some level of stress. You are not alone if you feel challenged by the food-oriented world around you. In addition to the obvious basic need to feed your body, there are lots of social and cultural reasons to eat. To make things even more challenging, as you take in fewer calories than you're used to, you may feel hungry. Experiment with the various ways to deal with cravings and hunger to see what works best for you.

One technique is to fill up on low-calorie foods (see the following list). You can use these items to snack wisely without sabotaging your diet efforts. You can also use these foods to round out a meal and help you feel full.

Don't underestimate the value of a glass or two of water to fill you up—no calories and lots of benefits. For many people, a hot beverage helps take the edge off hunger. A cup of hot tea or a serving of bouillon might do the trick.

hunger-buster foods

Looking for a low-calorie snack? Try some of these—they all contain 50 calories or less!

4 **animal crackers**	44		½ cup fat-free, sugar-free flavored **gelatin**	10
1 medium **apricot**	17		1 frozen **gelatin pop** (1.5 ounces)	31
1 **Asian pear** (4.3 ounces)	50		1 square **graham cracker** (.24 ounces)	30
1 large **bell pepper**	44		½ medium **grapefruit**	38
½ cup **blackberries**	31		10 **grapes**	35
½ cup **blueberries**	41		1 **ice pop** (2 fluid ounces)	42
1 medium **breadstick** (hard)	41		10 small **jelly beans**	40
½ cup cubed **cantaloupe**	27		1 medium **kiwifruit**	46
1 raw baby **carrot**	6		1 piece **melba toast,** any flavor	20
1 **celery** rib	10		3 large black **olives**	15
1 ounce low-fat **Cheddar cheese**	49		3 extra-large green **olives**	15
10 sweet **cherries**	43		1 medium **peach**	37
1 ounce low-fat **Colby cheese**	49		½-ounce chocolate-covered **peppermint patty**	50
1 medium **cucumber**	46			
1 **fortune cookie**	28			
1 medium **dill pickle** (3¾ inch)	12		2 tablespoons **picante sauce** or tomato-based **salsa**	9
½ cup **fruit cocktail** (packed in water)	40			

1 slice fresh **pineapple**	42	1 1/2 cups mixed **salad greens**	15
1 **plum**	36	1/2 cup **strawberries**	27
1 cup light microwaved **popcorn**	21	1 medium **tomato**	27
10 **pretzel sticks**	10	1/2 cup cubed **watermelon**	23
1 tablespoon seedless **raisins**	27	2 **whole-wheat crackers** (8 g)	36
1 flavored **rice cake** (0.5 ounces)	50	1/2 cup sliced raw **zucchini**	9
3 **saltine crackers**	39		

It's also important to know when to give in! When you're experiencing a strong craving for a certain food and can't think of anything except that food, maybe you should give in—within reason. When you feel denied and frustrated, you may actually overeat as a consequence. If you're really craving chocolate, for example, it might be a good idea to have just one small piece of excellent chocolate. Just write your treat down in your food diary and move on.

Finally, before you put something in your mouth, always ask yourself, "Am I really hungry enough to eat this? If this were something I didn't like very much, am I hungry enough to eat it anyway? Am I truly hungry, or do I just crave the sensation of eating?" If you listen to your answers, it will be easier to make a healthful choice.

get moving to get the weight off

Although the change in your eating habits will have the most dramatic effect on your weight loss, we strongly recommend that you add at least 10 minutes of physical activity to your daily routine—especially if you are not active now. Just two 5-minute segments, such as walking to the end of your block and back or around the parking lot at work, will get you started. No matter which eating plan you choose, the sooner you start to move, the sooner you start to remake your habits and reset your Energy Balance. Being active on a regular basis is a big part of being able to keep the weight off for good. The next chapter, "Move More," will help you find the best ways to add a full schedule of activity to your life.

live your best life

The beauty of knowing that the success of a diet plan stems from your choices is that it frees you to live your own life. You do not need to follow a restricted regimen unless that's what works for you. Instead, make your own decisions, find out what works, and let go of the yo-yo behaviors. It won't always be easy, but the reward is that you gain the control that will enable you to make lifelong changes. Even the smallest steps taken consistently in the right direction will bring you to your destination: a happy, healthy you.

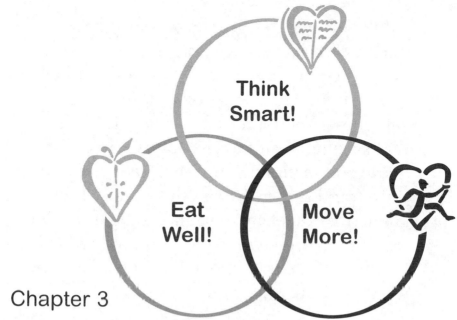

Chapter 3

MOVE MORE: more fit and less fat

Experts agree that diet alone is not enough to keep you fit and trim over time. Healthcare professionals have found that the best predictor of whether people will regain lost weight is whether they make physical activity a regular part of their life. If you are committed to breaking the yo-yo cycles—if you don't ever want to regain the weight you lose—it's important to get used to moving more.

Like many other people, you may have started each January with a shiny new resolution to "get more exercise." Perhaps you joined a gym or bought a series of workout tapes to get you going. You found out quickly, however, that keeping to an exercise routine takes more than good intentions. But you know that being active can bring many health benefits. If you are less active now than you'd like to be, this chapter will help you with some practical, workable solutions to increase the level of physical activity in your busy life.

**Good news: My doctor told me
I have to exercise
only on the days I eat!**

Are you willing to take the steps needed to achieve permanent weight loss? Recent research has shown that you don't need to work as hard as once thought to reap the benefits of physical activity. Prolonged, moderately intense activities such as brisk walking can, like higher-intensity jogs and bike rides, improve health and fitness. Don't feel pressured to join an expensive gym if that very idea makes you uncomfortable. Find something you enjoy and can fit into your life—and get moving!

simple steps to weight control

1. Self-assess: how active are you now?

2. Start to walk for at least 10 minutes each day.

3. Decide on your personal fitness goals: Start at 10 minutes; progress to 30 to 60 minutes a day.

4. Choose the activity strategy that works best for you.
   - The Lifestyle Approach
   - The Walking Program
   - The Organized Activity Option

5. Monitor your progress and reassess at six weeks.

❝ I decided to lose weight and get fit in time for my daughter's wedding by walking regularly every day. After a slow start, I really began to enjoy it. I put on my exercise clothes before I had my coffee, so I didn't have a chance to think about not going out. As my clothes started to fit better, it sure got easier to get up each day and put on my walking shoes! By the time the

wedding came around, I could bend down to tie those shoes without any strain. I'm happy to say that both my daughter and I looked great in those wedding photos! **"**

52-YEAR-OLD MOTHER,
SACRAMENTO,
CALIFORNIA

self-assess: how active are you now?

Before you start exercising your body, exercise your brain. Do an honest (but not brutal) self-assessment of where you are—or aren't—with regard to physical activity. Only you know how active you are and which activities truly appeal to you. Your current weight and your individual health situation both will influence your activity choices and goals.

Your first step is to use the activity diary page in Appendix F to record your daily activities for one week. Write down what you did, for how long, how hard you worked, and how much you enjoyed yourself. In the same way your daily food diary helps you understand your eating habits, this information will help you see how active you are now—and when and why you aren't.

A reliable pedometer is a great tool to help you determine your baseline activity level, no matter which activity strategy you ultimately decide to follow. Pedometers record every step you take, thus giving you a good idea of how everything you do during the day adds up. Wear the pedometer for one week. Add the daily totals and divide by 7 to find your average number of daily steps. The average American who does not exercise takes about 2,500 to 3,500 steps in one day. Your daily average is your current baseline, which will help you determine how active you are now.

gauge your activity level

Not active = 2,000 to 4,000 steps per day on average

Moderately active = 5,000 to 7,000 steps per day on average

Very active = At least 10,000 steps per day on average

do you need a medical exam before you start?

Most authorities feel that healthy people with no history of heart disease, chest pain, chest pressure, or unusual shortness of breath with physical exertion do not need a medical examination or stress test before starting an activity program such as brisk walking. However, if you have a medical condition (such as diabetes, high cholesterol, obesity, or high blood pressure), take prescription medication, are a smoker, are over 65, are at risk for heart disease because of your family history, or have not been physically active in recent months, be sure to talk with your healthcare professional before starting any exercise program. If while exercising you experience any symptoms such as chest pain or pressure, dizziness, unusual shortness of breath, or heart palpitations, stop exercising and get medical attention right away.

if you're not particularly active now

If you are not used to much activity, you may feel a sense of inertia, as if a heavy weight is holding you back. Ask yourself what barriers are keeping you from being more active. Is it lack of time or lack of motivation? Perhaps you keep procrastinating, saying that next week you'll start to exercise more. To get past that feeling of inertia, begin with just 10 minutes a day of some form of light activity—perhaps a walk around the parking lot before you go home from work. Or add five 2-minute walks to your usual workday. Give yourself small goals, and plan how you can fit them into your day. (For more information on setting goals, see page 87.) The first step is the hardest, but every step counts.

The best way to move from being sedentary to living a more active life is to see yourself as a fit person who will continue to get more fit. Your goal for lifelong activity is to work up to being active for 30 to 60 minutes on most (preferably all) days of the week. You can choose whether to exercise once a day or in shorter sessions, about 10 to 15 minutes each, a few times a day.

if you are moderately active

If you are a weekend athlete or a daily neighborhood stroller, just add to your existing activities to complement your weight-loss efforts. If you now walk at a moderate pace for at least 30 minutes a day on most days of the week, you are well on your way to overall fitness. To complement the changes you make to your diet to lose weight, and to best maintain that loss, you should work up to 60 minutes of activity each day.

exercising at the right level

While you're thinking about activity levels, it's good to get an idea of the intensity of an activity. You can use this information when you set your goals (page 87) and when you write entries in your exercise diary (page 705). Here are three ways you can judge the intensity of your activities.

One easy way is to think about how comfortable you are at differing levels of exercise. Imagine how you would feel in the situations below. You are the best judge of how hard you can work. Use these examples of walking as comparisons to get an idea of the intensities of other types of daily activity.

You are on your way to an important meeting:

- Moderately intense—"Unless I walk fast, I will be late for my meeting."
- Intense—"I need to walk faster because I'm already late for my meeting."
- Very intense—"I'm so late now, I'd better really push it!"

You may want to start your exercise program at the moderately intense level and increase when you feel you can.

You can also use the scale below to rate your perception of how hard you are working. The scale is based on the idea that your brain is a good judge of how much work you are doing. Your body provides the information you need in the ways it reacts during physical activity: increased heart rate, increased breathing rate, increased perspiration, and fatigue.

perceived effort scale

0 =	Nothing at all
1 =	Very, very light
2 =	Very light
3 =	Light
4 =	Moderate/brisk
5 =	Somewhat hard
6 =	Hard
7 =	Very hard
8 =	Very, very hard
9 =	Extremely hard
10 =	Absolute maximal effort

The shaded area indicates a safe and effective effort level for most people.

Many experts recommend that you use your heart rate to determine whether you are exercising at an appropriate level. Your heart and lungs will benefit the **most** from physical activity when you exercise strenuously enough to raise your heart rate to your "target zone." Your target heart rate should be 60 to 85 percent of your maximum heart rate, which is the fastest your heart can beat.

target heart rate

AGE	AVERAGE MAXIMUM HEART RATE*	TARGET ZONE: 60% TO 85% OF MAXIMUM*
20 years	200 bpm	120 to 170 bpm
25	195	117 to 166
30	190	114 to 162
35	185	111 to 157
40	180	108 to 153
45	175	105 to 149
50	170	102 to 145
55	165	99 to 140
60	160	96 to 136
65	155	93 to 132
70	150	90 to 128

Note: A few medicines lower the maximum heart rate and, thus, the target zone rate. If you are taking a beta-blocker or a high blood pressure medication, ask your doctor what your target heart rate should be.
*These figures are averages and should be used as general guidelines. bpm indicates beats per minute.

To check whether you're exercising within your target heart rate zone, take your pulse on the inside of your wrist, on the thumb side, for

10 seconds. Use the tips of your first two fingers (not your thumb) to press lightly over the blood vessels on your wrist. Count your pulse for 10 seconds and multiply by 6 for the number of beats per minute. This number should be within your target heart rate zone. If it's too high, you're straining, and you should slow down. If it's too low and the intensity feels "light" or "moderate/brisk" (a rating of 3 or 4 on the Perceived Effort Scale), push yourself to exercise a little harder.

When you start exercising, aim for the lower end of your target zone: 60 percent of your maximum heart rate. As you get stronger, strive for the higher end (85 percent of maximum). Don't try to do too much: Remember that you should always listen to your body.

progress to more daily activity

You can gradually work up to a full hour of exercise by comfortably easing into a weekly routine, as the progression chart shows. If you are currently getting about 20 minutes of exercise on most days of the week, enter the progression at Week 7 at 25 minutes instead of starting at the top at Week 1. Follow the chart for as long as you need to until you reach the goal of 60 minutes of daily activity. Small steps are the key to making long-lasting progress.

progression to 60 minutes of daily activity

	ACTIVITY ON MOST DAYS OF THE WEEK*
Weeks 1 and 2	10 minutes
Weeks 3 and 4	15 minutes
Weeks 5 and 6	20 minutes
Weeks 7 and 8	25 minutes
Weeks 9 and 10	30 minutes
Weeks 11, 12, and 13	35 minutes
Weeks 14, 15, and 16	40 minutes
Weeks 17, 18, and 19	45 minutes
Weeks 20, 21, and 22	50 minutes
Weeks 23, 24, and 25	55 minutes
Weeks 26 on	60 minutes

*Activity does not need to be continuous, but sessions of at least 10 minutes' duration have been shown to increase fitness, modify risk factors, and help maintain weight loss.

66 Fitness is important for everyone, regardless of weight. An active way of life brings health benefits even when you are still overweight. Apart from the weight loss that may result from exercise, being fit at any weight will reduce your risk of cardiovascu-

lar disease, compared with a person of the same weight who is not physically fit.**"**

.... BARRY FRANKLIN, PHD, FAHA
Director of Cardiac Rehabilitation
and Exercise Laboratories
William Beaumont Hospital,
Michigan

decide on your personal fitness goals

What result is most important to you? Is maintaining weight loss the main focus for you, or are you more interested in increasing your stamina? Do you want to be able to play more actively with your children without feeling winded? Maybe you are concerned about your blood pressure or another health factor that exercise can help improve.

Once you know your priorities, establish your short- and long-term goals. A long-term activity goal is something you want to achieve in six months or a year. It can be specific, such as being able to exercise for 60 minutes each day without feeling exhausted or sore the next day, but it should also be flexible enough to accommodate both unforeseen difficulties and opportunities. Long-term goals keep you focused on the end result.

Short-term goals are the smaller steps that lead you to your desired result and help you feel successful along the way. For example, you can decide to buy a new pair of walking shoes by the end of the week, or you can set up a schedule to work out with a videotape for 30 minutes on Mondays, Wednesdays, and Fridays for a week or two. Short-term goals must be specific to be useful: Decide exactly what you want and how you will go about making it happen.

If you are not active now, we recommend that you begin with some form of light activity for just 10 minutes each day. Your ultimate goal is to work up to being active for about 60 minutes on most (preferably all) days of the week.

Use the sample goal-setting "contract" on the following page to organize how you are going to make activity a priority as you lose weight. Write down your long-term goal and three short-term goals. After you've started your program, be sure to reward yourself each time you reach one of your targets. Remember also to record your efforts in your activity log so you can monitor your progress.

Review your short-term goals every two weeks and set new goals when you achieve the current ones. As you progress, adjust both your long-term and short-term goals to help you progress toward your ultimate goal.

my activity goals

Date: _____

My long-term activity goal is to

_____

by _____.

My short-term activity goals are to

1. _____by _____ and

2. _____by _____ and

3. _____by _____

I plan to achieve my goals through these specific actions:

Doing this: _____

This often: _____

At this level: _____

For this long: _____

The rewards for reaching my goals are:

1. _____ and

2. _____ and

3. _____.

Signature: _____

choose the activity strategy that works best for you

You have several options to reach your activity goals: the Lifestyle Approach (or finding ways to integrate fitness into your daily routine), the Walking Program, or the Organized Activity Option. You can also try a combination of two or all three. The important thing is to choose things that you will do on a regular basis **in addition to** your current level of activity.

The questionnaire below will help you identify which approach may work best for you. After you've completed the questionnaire, take a look at the descriptions of the three strategies and choose the one or ones that you think will work best for you.

Which Strategy Will Work Best for You?

1. Do you enjoy regular physical activity?
   A. Not really
   B. Somewhat
   C. Absolutely _____

2. Do you enjoy participating in organized activities and sports?
   A. Hate it
   B. It's okay
   C. Love it _____

3. Can you carve out 30 to 60 minutes a day on most days to do some physical activity?
   A. Not a chance
   B. Maybe
   C. Definitely _____

4. Do you like to learn new activities?
   A. No way
   B. If they aren't too hard
   C. Absolutely _____

5. Do you like to be around others when you participate in physical activity?
   A. Not really
   B. When they help motivate me
   C. Absolutely _____

6. How do you feel about perspiring?
   A. Hate it
   B. It's okay
   C. Like it because it means I'm getting the most out of my workout _____

7. Do you have a place to participate in physical activity?
   A. Not really
   B. Safe walking trail or quiet streets
   C. Home (with exercise equipment, exercise videos, etc.), gym, or sports center _____

8. Have you ever enjoyed playing sports?
   A. Never
   B. Loved it as a kid
   C. Still enjoy it _____

9. How ready are you to get moving?
   A. Not very
   B. Pretty ready
   C. Can't wait to get started   _____

10. How much variety do you want in your physical activity?
    A. Lots
    B. I'd rather stick to one thing
    C. Some   _____

         Total Number of As   _____

         Total Number of Bs   _____

         Total Number of Cs   _____

What Your Score Means

6–10 As   Try the Lifestyle Approach.

6–10 Bs   Try the Walking Program.

6–10 Cs   Try the Organized Activity Option.

What if your scores are fairly evenly split? Choose the strategy that appeals to you most, or try combining the two that have the highest number. For example, if you have mostly As and Bs, try the Lifestyle Approach on some days and the Walking Program on others. For real variety, try some of each activity.

STRATEGY 1:
the lifestyle approach

One of the simplest ways to live a more active lifestyle is what we call the Lifestyle Approach.

Taking the Lifestyle Approach means that you commit to performing enough small activities throughout your day—on top of what you normally do—to add up to an increased amount of total activity.

Review your initial entries in your activity diary. Look carefully at your day to identify ways you can fit in more exercise. Also look for the obstacles that keep you from being more active. Make a plan that will help you remove or lessen those barriers. The idea is to build on your baseline exercise level by adding activities to your daily routine. For instance, if you normally take the elevator, choose to climb the stairs instead. Park your car as far as possible from your office so you will walk farther than you do now. Everyday tasks such as doing housework and raking leaves also count as physical activity if you act with vigor and speed. Instead of finding ways to avoid the physical aspects of these tasks (such as using a leaf blower), embrace the idea of improving fitness by doing more, not less.

Success using the Lifestyle Approach doesn't depend on which activity you choose, but rather on how well you add the activity to your lifestyle.

As part of your self-assessment, we suggested that you use a pedometer to determine your level of activity in terms of a baseline number of daily steps. This baseline value will be a big help in setting your goals using the Lifestyle Approach to become more active. If you're like the average sedentary American, your baseline is about 2,500 to 3,500 daily steps. You should aim to add an average of between 4,000 and 6,000 steps to your baseline over time, which reflects about 30 minutes of additional walking. Ideally, your eventual target for weight loss should be about 60 minutes of daily activity. (If you are already active, be sure to set your personal goal well **above** your baseline number of steps.)

stairstep to increased activity

You can use a gradual approach to reach your goal. Each week, add just 250 steps per day, averaged out over the week. That means that if your baseline daily average is about 2,500 steps, your daily average in week two should be about

2,750 steps. In week three, it should be about 3,000 steps, and so on.

Make a point of wearing your pedometer while walking through the places you go as part of your everyday life. For example, walk around your grocery store twice. How many steps does that take? Or walk around your mall, through your office building, across campus, or to and from your child's school. You can add these segments of steps that you have measured out as you progress toward more and more activity.

did you know . . .

In an enlightening study of an Old Order Amish community of about 100 adults, researchers found that the Amish men and women averaged between 14,000 and 18,000 steps daily. The Amish lifestyle depends on labor-intensive farming methods and discourages the use of modern devices such as automobiles, washing machines, and computers. Interestingly, the study also showed that only 4 percent of these adults could be considered obese, compared with 31 percent of the U.S. adult population.

Over the past decade, several research studies have shown that for adults who were not active at the beginning of the study, the Lifestyle

Approach to physical activity and a traditional structured exercise program resulted in beneficial effects on heart and lung fitness, body fat, and coronary risk factors.

choices, choices

One of the great benefits of the Lifestyle Approach is that you can do what you enjoy and what fits best into your daily routine. It's easy to add measured chunks of activity into your day. Play a pickup game of basketball or get some friends together for a softball game. Go bowling, go dancing, or get working in your garden. The following chart will help you incorporate the things you like to do into a personalized activity routine that fits into your life. Maybe you enjoyed riding a bike when you were a teenager (before you got the keys to the car)—you might like to try bicycling again.

People of different weights burn calories at different rates when doing the same physical activity at the same intensity for the same amount of time, so remember to check your approximate weight level. In general, the heavier you are, the more calories you burn for any given activity. The activities you choose—and how long and energetically you do them—will make a big difference in how you balance your Calories In with your Calories Out.

checkpoints along the way

What type of checkpoints should you use as you implement the Lifestyle Approach? Because this strategy is based on your daily activities, the interim targets are up to you. Each week, check your diary to see how what you are doing every day compares to your initial goals. You can use simple tests to check your progress: How long does it take you to swim a lap at the pool? How far can you walk in 10 minutes? How winded are you after riding your bike around the block? You'll know you're reaching your goal when you can go farther, move faster, or move more easily (with less huffing).

calories burned in 30 minutes of continuous activity by approximate weight

ACTIVITY*	APPROX. 150 LBS.	APPROX. 175 LBS.	APPROX. 200 LBS.	APPROX. 225 LBS.
Badminton (social doubles)	135	158	180	203
Baseball and softball	141	165	188	212
Basketball	282	329	376	423
Bicycling	163	190	217	244
Billiards and bowling	98	114	130	147
Canoeing (at $2^{1}/2$ mph)	98	114	130	147
Cleaning windows	135	158	180	203
Desk work	68	79	90	102
Football	270	315	360	405
Gardening	195	228	260	293

Activity				
Golfing (carrying the clubs)	165	193	220	248
Golfing (riding in a power cart)	98	114	130	147
Gymnastics	135	158	180	203
Hiking and backpacking	204	238	272	306
Horseback riding (walking)	98	114	130	147
Horseshoe pitching	135	158	180	203
Ice and field hockey	273	319	364	410
Ice- and roller-skating	195	228	260	293
Jogging (at 5 mph)	270	315	360	405
Jumping rope	375	438	500	563
Mowing (pushing a light power mower)	135	158	180	203

ACTIVITY*	APPROX. 150 LBS.	APPROX. 175 LBS.	APPROX. 200 LBS.	APPROX. 225 LBS.
Mowing (using a riding lawn mower)	98	114	130	147
Racquetball	375	438	500	563
Raking leaves	165	193	170	248
Running (at 5½ mph)	317	370	422	475
Sailing (handling a small boat)	135	158	180	203
Sewing and knitting	68	79	90	102
Skiing (cross-country)	350	408	467	525
Skiing (light downhill)	225	263	300	338
Soccer	270	315	360	405

Square dancing	225	263	300	338
Swimming	194	227	259	291
Tennis (singles)	234	271	310	349
Tennis (doubles)	165	193	170	248
Touch football	270	315	360	405
Walking (strolling at 1 mph)	68	79	90	102
Walking (at 5 mph)	225	263	300	338
Water-skiing	225	263	300	338

*Note: These figures are for comparison purposes only. Some of the activities are **not** aerobic exercise and burn very few calories.

STRATEGY 2:
the walking program

Walking is one of the most popular forms of physical activity in America today. It's inexpensive, easy, and convenient. That may be why people who walk for exercise tend to stick with it. Join the countless others and walk your way to fitness.

ready, set, go

What do you need to start a walking program? Lightweight clothing that fits loosely is perfect. Dress in layers so you can be warm when you begin and easily remove layers as needed.

Good shoes are very important for fitness walking: For each mile you walk, your feet will hit the ground between 1,500 and 2,000 times. If you have shoes that you haven't worn in a while, check the inside cushioning and the tread to be sure they're in good condition. If not, you probably need new shoes.

Any athletic-type shoe will do, but your best bet is a walking shoe. Walking shoes have a curved sole that helps transfer weight from the back to the front of the foot with each step. Here are some tips for buying walking shoes:

- Choose a shoe that is flexible and has special cushioning.

- Try on shoes at the end of the day when your feet are biggest, wearing the same kind of athletic socks you'll wear on your walks.

- Check to make sure the shoe fits you well in the toe box, the arch, and the heel.

- Walk briskly around the store so you'll know whether the shoe is comfortable. If it isn't, try another style or a different brand.

You need a safe and convenient place to walk. You can walk around your neighborhood, the track at the local school, a trail at a community center, a park trail, a hiking trail, or your local shopping mall. Perhaps you can use a treadmill, walk along with a recorded audio program, or walk with a buddy. Use whatever options, with or without a pedometer, work best in your particular situation.

man's best friend

Have you ever noticed how much dogs enjoy being taken for a walk? Well, in some ways, they are smarter about their bodies than we are. So think about walking that dog at least twice a day—whether you have one or not!

pace yourself

There are different ways to tell what walking pace is right for you. Use the information in "Exercising at the Right Level" on page 81 to gauge the intensity of your effort.

Another indicator of your pace is the talking test. If you find you can't talk comfortably when you are walking, you are probably walking too fast. If you can sing as you walk, you are probably walking too slowly. Try a pace at which you can talk comfortably.

step it up

During the first two weeks that you are actively trying to lose weight, begin walking **in addition to** your current level of activity. For example, if you don't already walk regularly, add at least one 10-minute walk every day. As you begin week three, step things up. Choose three or four days in the week that you can fit in 20-minute walks—either all at one time or in two sessions. Commit to walking 20 minutes on those days, and continue to walk 10 minutes on the other days.

The following table shows you how to add walking time by increments each week. By the sixth week, you should be comfortable walking 30 minutes on most days.

sample walking times for a 6-week jump start to fitness

WEEK 1	WEEK 2	WEEK 3	WEEK 4	WEEK 5	WEEK 6
10 minutes on most days	10 minutes on 7 days	20 minutes on 3 days; 10 minutes on 4 days	20 minutes on 7 days	30 minutes on 3 days; 20 minutes on 4 days	30 minutes on 7 days

Note that each 20- or 30-minute walk can be broken into 10- or 15-minute segments to better fit into your lifestyle.

Each week, review your activity diary. Evaluate whether you've accomplished what you set out to do—for example, walking for 30 minutes on five days each week. Are you walking farther in that 30 minutes after several weeks? Are you continuing to lose weight? If not, you may want to step up your program. On the other hand, you may find that a walking goal that once seemed very hard to achieve has become easy. That's certainly a success!

STRATEGY 3:
the organized activity option

With this strategy, you participate in scheduled classes or play sports to add activity into your life. Besides getting more fit, you'll benefit from the social support of your classmates and teammates. It's a lot harder to skip out of your planned activity if you have ten people waiting for you! You may want to start with something you enjoy and do it twice a week for 30 to 60 minutes. Then add more activity over time. Remember that your ultimate goal is to be active for 60 minutes on most (preferably all) days of the week.

game, set, match

The most challenging part of this approach may be deciding which activity to choose from so many options. It's important to find a good match, something you can enjoy and do regularly. "Organized" doesn't have to mean a team sport, however. You may want to sample a few introductory classes for activities you would like to try. Taking lessons is a good way to hone your skills and increase your activity level.

Check your local newspaper or community newsletter for classes or group activities offered in your area. Try something new! Thousands of people have found dozens of ways to enjoy being physically active—don't hesitate to join them. The activity chart on page 98 lists a number of sports and activities that lend themselves to group participation.

You also can establish a regular routine at home using exercise equipment, such as a treadmill or an exercise bike, or videotapes for aerobics or dance. This works well for lots of people, but it means that you are the one to crack the whip. Be sure to establish a clear schedule for your regimen and record your activity in your diary. When you're exercising at home, turn off the phone, shut the door, and don't let distractions disrupt your workout. Once you get into the routine of scheduling your activity, you will enjoy the time you spend doing something good for yourself.

adding activity to your routine

When you are ready to take on more activity, look at your diary entries and think about what you do and don't like about your routine now. If you enjoy the activity you have chosen, find more days to participate and maybe other groups to join. If you would like more variety, try another sport or organized activity on a different day of the week or a different time of day. If you are going to the gym for racquetball two evenings during the week, you may want to join a swimming program on Saturday mornings. If all of your activities take place indoors but you would love to be outside in good weather, look for an outdoor organized activity.

Only you can choose what is best for you. The important thing is to keep it fun, stay committed, and do more when you're ready. If you need help maintaining that forward momentum, look at some of the strategies in Chapter 4, "Maintaining Momentum."

❝ I had been playing team tennis three days a week for over a year—and enjoying every minute of it. I loved my teammates, the competitiveness of the sport, and being outside. I had lost over 20 pounds, and I believe that my regular tennis games helped keep the weight off. When we started playing only two days a week, I thought I would add a weekly workout at the gym. But without a schedule and without my friends urging me on, I just didn't enjoy being at the gym and started going less and less often. I was worried about

gaining weight back, so my husband and I joined a bicycling group that rides every Saturday afternoon. Now I'm back to my three-times-a-week schedule of physical activity, and I haven't gained a pound. **"**

29-YEAR-OLD MOTHER,
ALBUQUERQUE,
NEW MEXICO

mix and match the strategies

Feel free to combine two or all three strategies for maximum benefit, flexibility, and variety. You could go for a fitness walk on some days, use a pedometer to track lifestyle steps on busy days, and play sports on the weekend or in the summer months. Try incorporating other types of exercise into the Walking Program for variety. For a 20-minute session, try cycling for 10 minutes and then walking for 10 minutes. Be creative: If you love the water, try swimming and then rowing or kayaking. The key is to find the combination that works for you.

Monitor your progress every two weeks. Reassess your long-term goals at six weeks. As you achieve each milestone, reward yourself (but not with food) and continue to add to your program of fitness for life.

assess your success

Over time, you may experience an improvement in your overall fitness or inches lost without much effect on weight loss. Sometimes this means you're building more muscle tissue and developing cardiovascular stamina, which will still help you maintain weight loss in the long run. If your chosen activity doesn't seem to be getting easier, you'll want to find out why. See how your diary entries compare with the following sample.

sample activity diary page

Date: January 11 ☐ Mon. ☒ Tues. ☐ Wed. ☐ Thurs. ☐ Fri. ☐ Sat. ☐ Sun.

TIME OF DAY	ACTIVITY	DURATION	LEVEL OF EXERTION	LEVEL OF ENJOYMENT
6:00 A.M.	Walked around the neighborhood with the dog	15 minutes	4	3
8:25 A.M. & 5:30 P.M.	Walked up and down the stairs in the parking garage	3 minutes	4	2
3:00 P.M.	Walked around the building at work	10 minutes	3	3

TIME OF DAY	ACTIVITY	DURATION	LEVEL OF EXERTION	LEVEL OF ENJOYMENT
6:00 P.M.	Walked from the back of the parking lot into the grocery store	2 minutes	4	2
7:00 P.M.	Took an aerobics class at the local recreation center	30 minutes	5	3

TOTAL Daily Activity Minutes: 60

Notes:
Had a stressful day at work and didn't feel like going to aerobics class. Went anyway and am glad I did—it relieved a lot of my stress!

If you've made honest entries in your diary, you'll have a written record of the times you didn't exercise and the reasons why. What were your thoughts on a day when you decided not to exercise? When you have another chance to make that choice, recognize that you can choose to think **differently** about the importance of activity and weight loss. So what if you blew it this time, you can decide to get back on track at the very next opportunity. You may find ways to fit in fitness that you overlooked at the beginning. If you've reached your goal, congratulations!

Don't Let Barriers Get You Down! Tips on How to Keep Moving

• Recruit a buddy. Find someone who will help motivate you and join you in your activity.

• Create a rainy-day plan. If you normally engage in outdoor physical activity, plan alternative activities you can enjoy inside in case of rain, snow, cold, or heat.

• Carve out time. You can't add more hours to your day for exercise, so you just have to find the time. Try carving out one 30-minute chunk of time on most days—before work, after school, or whenever you can. The trick is to find a time that is right for you and then stick with it.

- Be open to change. When you can't exercise at your chosen time or do your preferred activity, be creative and find an alternative.

- Find a champion who supports your efforts. Tell your friend or loved one how much it means to you to have that support—and relish it.

- Enjoy! Remember to choose something you like to do, not what you think will burn the most calories. Then keep it fun and keep at it.

reality check

Don't get derailed by the many commonly held beliefs about how physical activity affects weight loss. Most are based on misconceptions; some are just not true. We are surrounded by advertisements for miracle products and gadgets that promise quick and easy weight loss. However, if it sounds too good to be true, it probably is. We want to set the record straight and refute just a few of the myths to help you meet those weight-loss goals.

Myth: All I have to do to lose weight is exercise, then I can eat what I like.

Reality: Exercise alone cannot burn away an unlimited amount of excess calories if you are eating too much. When you enjoy an active lifestyle, you benefit both physically and psychologically, but exercising does not mean you can then reward yourself by eating anything you want. The truth is that 20 minutes of moderate-intensity activity burns about 100 calories. That won't have as great an effect on your Energy Balance as will watching what you eat and limiting your calorie intake. Once you've lost weight, however, good eating habits and regular activity go hand in hand to keep you fit and trim.

Myth: Exercise can be targeted to burn fat in certain parts of my body.

Reality: Plainly and simply, the answer is no. All those heavily advertised exercise devices do more to slim down your wallet than your hips or thighs. A classic study from the 1970s was reinforced by more recent evidence that localized exercise does not "burn off" fat from that area. Rather, whenever you exercise, fat is taken from stores throughout your body to supply the energy needed. You can build up specific muscles with specific exercises, but you won't lose more fat in that area of your body than in others.

Myth: I can lose weight with "effortless" exercise.

Reality: The desire to melt away fat effortlessly is not new. The rubberized "sweat suits" and heated belts on the market today are modern versions of the vapor baths of yesteryear. These products create only temporary loss of body water (dehydration), which can be dangerous. Although your body measurements may be less after you wear these garments, the body weight you thought you lost will come right back once your body is rehydrated. Likewise, mechanical vibrating machines and electrical stimulating devices that promise the health benefits of exercise without the effort may make the fat tissue move around, but they do not remove it.

Myth: Exercise increases the appetite.

Reality: Some people believe that exercise will make them feel hungrier and they will eat even more. Most research suggests that moderate exercise doesn't increase appetite at all, especially for people who were previously inactive. In fact, exercise may even make you feel less hungry. You may find it easier to say no to those extra calories as you step into a new image of yourself—one of a fit, confident person who makes healthy choices.

keep the focus on you

Being physically active is vitally important for overall good health and especially to keep off weight that you have lost. It's also important to enjoy what you do to stay active. Having fun in the process makes it much easier to plan with enthusiasm, counteract negative thinking, overcome obstacles, meet your goals, and reap the benefits. Chapter 4, "Maintaining Momentum," will help you stay on track for success and celebrate your accomplishments.

key strategies for fitness success

- Think of yourself as a healthy, fit person.

- Write down your goals, both short and long-term.

- Choose an activity that is fun for you.

- Start out slowly to avoid injury.

- Establish a routine.

- Seek enthusiastic, capable exercise leaders for group activities.

- Get support from your family or friends.

- Keep track of your progress with a diary and regular assessments.

- Vary your activities—enjoy yourself!

- Congratulate yourself for taking better care of your health.

Chapter 4

MAINTAINING MOMENTUM: keep up the good work

We know it's exciting to get started on a new program that you think will work for you. The sticking point, however, is being able to turn that first burst of enthusiasm into the willpower to keep going. That transition takes an essential but sometimes elusive ingredient—momentum.

On any path to losing weight, it is only reasonable to expect pitfalls as well as successes. To keep the downs you encounter from being downers, you need motivation on your side. Motivation comes from the first Circle of Success, Think Smart. Desire is what binds your eating and physical activity strategies into a lifestyle that leads to lifelong weight control.

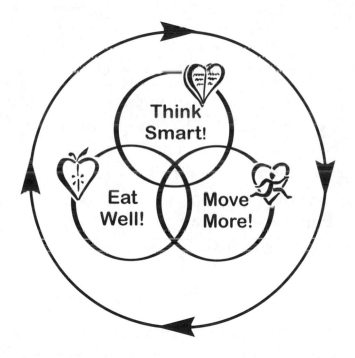

To keep your motivation strong, ask:

- What inspires me and gives me strength to resist temptation?
- How do I get past the plateaus to keep going?
- Can I form new habits that I can live with forever?

The answers to these questions can help you pick yourself up and get back on track when you experience the difficult times that come with making lifestyle changes. Any positive action you take, no matter how little it may seem, will help you overcome feelings of inertia or helplessness. You have the power to find the combination of factors that really works for you.

power up to keep going

Success comes from a progressive movement toward your goal. Small changes on a daily basis can bring big results. When you find your conviction flagging or you run into an obstacle, use the following techniques to keep the momentum going as you move through the different stages of weight loss.

use your power of observation

Don't obsess about the numbers on the scale; pay attention to how you feel and what works over time. Be ready to respond to the cues your body is giving you. Then tune in to the results of your efforts. For example, post a photo of yourself on the refrigerator. As you feel your clothes becoming looser, take a new picture and put it right next to the original. Keep a pair of your old jeans in the closet. Try them on once in a while to demonstrate how many inches you've lost. Choose something that works for you to keep the spotlight on your successes.

use the power of the written word

The pen is mightier than the scale! Writing down goals and keeping a written record of your progress are proven ways to make your weight loss a reality. The act of writing gets you to focus better on your goals and to pay attention to your progress.

❝ I'm only 53, and I felt fine, but I was really surprised to find that I'd put on 15 pounds since my last annual physical. When the doctor said my blood pressure and cholesterol were both borderline high, I was blown away. I've always been the healthy one in my family!

The doctor told me to keep a food and physical activity diary for six weeks, then come in for a follow-up appointment. It seemed hokey, but I did it. I already knew that I wasn't getting much exercise, but the diary was a shocker. It made me realize how often I was snacking. I was eating something sugary almost every afternoon

or while I watched TV at night—sometimes both. What an eye-opener!

Once I realized what I was doing, I cut out all those snacks. I also started using the stairs at work, and I made a point of parking as far from the office as I could. When I had my six-week follow-up, I had lost 5 pounds! The doctor said I'd probably get my numbers back in the normal range just by watching what I ate and moving around a bit more. It's been another six weeks, and I'm still eating more carefully and walking at the mall after work.

I have lost all 15 pounds, my blood pressure is normal, and my blood cholesterol has dropped 20 points. It hasn't always been real easy, but you know what? It's been worth the effort! **"**

SALESMAN, PORTLAND, OREGON

Monitoring your progress is an important key to turning a short-term weight-loss plan into a lifetime of fitness and healthy weight maintenance. Take a look at your diary. Are you making progress toward your goals? If not, perhaps your goals are less realistic than you thought. What unexpected barriers did you encounter? What specific action can you take to remove the problem?

For example, instead of committing to eating salads for lunch every day for two weeks, you can commit to eating three salads for lunches next week. If that works for you, set the same goal for the following week, or try a new goal that pushes you a little further. Did you plan to walk every day for a month but found that rainy days kept you indoors? Seek practical ways to overcome that barrier—by finding a place to walk indoors or trying an indoor activity instead.

Your diary is the best way to keep track of how you're doing and what barriers you've encountered. Remember to record your successes too. Documenting the first time someone says, "You've lost weight" will be a great motivator.

use the power of choice

You can choose among the several options available to create your personal eating and activity programs. Are you happy with your results? If so, celebrate being a successful loser. If not, reassess whether you're using the right tools. Go back to the options to see whether you need a new approach to your eating and activity strategies.

use the power of imagination

Set reasonable goals and have reasonable expectations. Then imagine yourself as the person who makes those goals a reality. Remember to Think Smart by using the visualization, self-talk, and other strategies in Chapter 1. See in your mind's eye the possibilities of the future—a fit and healthier you. Imagine yourself as a thinner person doing the things you love—playing with your kids, walking on the beach, or playing softball. Whenever you have the urge to stray from your plan, think of one of these images.

use your people power

Studies show that people who seek social support as they work toward their weight-loss goals are more likely to reach those goals. Ask family members, friends, and coworkers to be your champions.

Spouses in particular can make or break a weight-loss plan. The supportive ones will encourage you and help you maintain your momentum without hovering. Sometimes, however, spouses and other people who are overweight themselves are threatened by your success. Being aware of this possibility makes it easier for you to disarm or ignore those who might subconsciously (or even consciously) sabotage your efforts. Try to get them involved in small ways, such as cooking with you or going with you for a short walk. If you find that doesn't work, just remember to try to spend time with people who will support you and celebrate your successes with you.

Consider also joining a weight-loss group—either an established one with a trained leader or one you form yourself among friends with similar weight-loss goals and approaches.

> **❝My husband has been very supportive of my efforts to lose weight right from the start. He helped me to avoid my first pitfall after I started my diet. My daughter lovingly presented me with a sizable bowl of chocolate mousse that she'd made. Seeing the look of mingled fear and longing on my face, my husband immediately, but gently, intervened. "Honey, Mommy will have just a taste. She can't really eat more than that because of her diet, remember? She's trying to do something very important." The mousse certainly did taste wonderful, but I had the strength to stop after one spoonful because of my husband's reminder. Many times he has encouraged me by saying, 'You look great!' It's true what they say about support. It makes all the difference to have someone who stands by you. ❞**
>
> 38-YEAR-OLD WORKING
> MOTHER, DALLAS, TEXAS

use the power of reward!

As you meet your goals and expectations, remember to pat yourself on the back. As they say, if you don't value yourself, no one else will. When you set each of your short-term goals, make a note of a special reward that isn't a food. Perhaps it's an evening soak in a luxurious bath, a new DVD, or tickets to a concert or special game. Promise yourself that you'll buy a new pair of jeans when you've lost 10 pounds, or take yourself to the spa for a day of pampering— whatever will make you feel that your efforts are well rewarded. After all, you are worth it.

Success depends on your backbone, not your wishbone.

what to celebrate and what to watch for

Is there any better feeling than noticing that your clothes are getting a little loose? Talk about momentum! The wonderful thing about truly feeling motivated is that each time you take one step forward, you will feel buoyed by the payback, no matter how small it may seem. Life can throw some curves into the road, though, so it's good to know what's ahead and how to handle potential obstacles.

preparing for plateaus

Don't waste your energy on guilt about the downs: Losing weight is difficult. Remember, the research shows that once you've gained weight, the body works hard to maintain it. After making great progress, you may go for two weeks without losing another pound, even though you're following your eating strategy faithfully. An occasional slowdown of weight loss is a normal part of the process, and you will be much better off if you are mentally prepared for these plateaus.

When you hit a plateau—and sooner or later you will—don't give up. Stick to your plan and refocus. Look at your diary entries. Try to find out what may no longer be working or may have changed. Look for new ways to cut back on calories or be more active. What changes can you make to get back on track? See that plateau for what it is: a momentary stall, not a total breakdown. Hitting a plateau does not mean you've failed, and it does not mean you won't lose weight again.

disarming the time bomb

Family, work, and social obligations all claim large portions of the precious hours in a day.

Lack of time is a constant threat to the momentum of your weight-loss efforts. But the time crunch doesn't have to derail you completely. Whatever type of calendar you use to keep track of what's going on in your life—whether computerized or hanging on your wall—can be used to schedule time for your weight-loss efforts.

- **Plan your meals.** Think through how eating fits into your schedule. When will you be eating each day? If you work outside the home, plan to pack a healthful lunch so you don't have to eat out. If your son has a baseball game on Thursday, prepare Thursday's dinner on Wednesday night, when things may be less hectic. You can't plan everything in advance, but planning what you can will make your life a lot easier.

- **Fit in physical activity.** Schedule fitness time just as you would a doctor's appointment, a meeting, or any other must-do event. Once you write it down, you're more likely to follow through. After all, you wouldn't cancel a "regular" appointment without a good reason. Don't cancel out on yourself either.

Different things work better for different people, so establish a healthful routine that works for you. For example, everyone needs to eat something for breakfast every morning. But you can let your schedule determine whether you choose a quick smoothie on the go or prepare a full meal for your family.

The information in the appendixes on shopping and cooking (pages 672 to 687) should help you juggle your time while keeping your commitment to eat well. We've also provided a guide to making eating out an enjoyable, more healthful, and less fattening experience (Appendix C, page 688).

practicing crisis management

If you have learned to reach for food whenever you feel stress, it's important to think through an alternate plan before you hit a bad patch. Imagine the different scenarios that would calm you after a stressful day or divert your attention from comfort foods.

- To restore your inner resolve, try isolating yourself for a few of minutes of peace and quiet so you can reflect on your successes.

- Maybe you need to sit down and plan your meals for the next few days. A good meal plan can be a big help to keep you from eating without thinking during a period of stress.

- Try bumping up your exercise routine. Working your body can help relieve stress and boost your confidence.

You should base your crisis action plan on your own habits and needs—you know what they are. Then, when the unexpected happens, you will be prepared.

managing expectations

One of the greatest challenges to maintaining momentum is managing expectations. Because weight gain doesn't happen overnight, weight loss won't happen quickly either. Compared to an initial quick weight loss, the idea of slow and steady weight control can seem pretty dull. Try not to be tempted to set your goals too high in the first place. If you find you need to adjust your goals to a more realistic level, just keep going and choose another strategy that will work for you.

> **66** My twenty-fifth high-school reunion was only three months away, and I was psyched! I was determined to lose those 30 pounds I'd gained since graduation and get back my high-school figure. I joined an exercise class and banished everything fattening from my house. I lost 10 pounds in the first four weeks! I just knew the other 20 pounds would come off as easily as the first 10. Boy, was I wrong.

Over the next week, I didn't lose a single pound. I'd heard that most dieters get bogged down at some point, but I didn't think it would happen to me. I switched to a 1,000-calorie-a-day liquid diet, but I had no energy for exercise, and I didn't feel as well. I just wanted to give in and forget the reunion.

In the next week, I heard from an old high school friend I hadn't seen in ages. Hey . . . she had put on a few extra pounds too! When I confided my frustration, she laughed and told me she also was trying to lose weight. I realized that I was just trying to go too far, too fast. We decided to go to the reunion together, no matter how much we weighed. Once I let go of my great expectations, I decided to get back on track and went back to my original diet plan. By the time we were pinning on the reunion name tags, I'd lost 18 pounds and felt better than I had in a very long time. **99**

42-YEAR-OLD REAL ESTATE AGENT, COLUMBUS, OHIO

a final word

As healthcare professionals, we want to help you succeed. We can give you sound advice and recommendations on how to eat well and keep your body fit. We can give you the tools you need to live a no-fad lifestyle. And from years of experience in working with real people like you who are trying to reach a healthful weight, we also can offer our observations on how to turn your hopes into reality.

The freedom to choose for yourself is the best thing you have going. You don't have to rely on an outside source for a magic formula or a miracle diet to reach your goals. The keys to creating the best eating and activity plans for your good health lie in **you**. The desire and momentum to keep those new habits in place for a lifetime come from **you**. You have the power to take control, use the tools available, and see the results of your commitment. In the end, that is all you need to be a successful loser!

Chapter 5

PASS IT ON: food, fitness, and the family

You now have the tools to become a healthier and more fit you. It's time to pass along what you've learned to the ones you love. If you consider obesity a problem just for adults, think again. Children in the United States today are gaining weight faster than adults. The statistics are downright scary: The most recent data show that about 15 percent of children and adolescents from 6 to 19 years old are overweight, with another 15 percent considered at risk of becoming overweight. It's also true that overweight children are much more likely than their thinner counterparts to grow up to be overweight or obese adults.

To reverse this trend, we have to recognize the challenges and make a commitment to change the statistics. Our world of abundant high-calorie foods and computerization is moving us away from a healthful diet and an active lifestyle. These changes in environment and technology are affecting the lives of our children, too. Kids are also bombarded with advertising encouraging them to eat "fun," but not necessarily healthful, foods.

an alarming development

In 2002, more than 10 percent of American children aged 2 to 5 years were overweight. This represents a 43 percent increase from 1994. The situation is probably even worse today.

The good news is that you **can** help your children develop good habits for eating well and staying physically active. We encourage you to use the strategies in this book—and advice from your physician and other reliable resources—to take the steps needed to raise kids who are healthy for life.

> **❝ For successful weight management in children, everyone in the house should be involved. Parents have control over what foods are offered in the home environment, but ultimately it is the child who decides what to eat. Those parents who consistently praise their child's good choices and do not give in to inappropriate ones will be able to develop their child's eating and activity habits into healthful behaviors over time. ❞**
>
> Stephen R. Daniels, MD, PhD, FAHA
> Professor of Pediatrics
> University of Cincinnati

when should i start?

Right now! If possible, start at the beginning of your child's life. Studies indicate that early eating experiences—even in the first year—may be very important in helping establish a lifetime of healthful eating. For infants, breastfeeding provides the best nutrition for your baby. Some studies have shown that breastfeeding may protect against later obesity. As your children grow, choose healthful options as soon as you introduce solid foods.

Playing is a wonderful way for children to use their imaginations and their bodies. From the time an infant begins to move around, it's important to create a safe environment to explore. Check with your child's pediatrician to help determine what type of activity is best for each stage of your child's life. Then be sure to encourage and create ample age-appropriate opportunities for active play.

how do i know if my child is overweight?

Because of how a child's body changes during growth, the calculation of his or her body mass index (BMI) is more complicated than that for an adult. Talk with your healthcare professional about your child's situation. Find out how his or her weight fits into an age-appropriate growth chart, and keep track of your child's weight at each visit.

Plotting height and weight numbers on a growth chart can point out the early signs of potential weight problems. You should expect to see occasional shifts up or down; that's a normal part of the growth process. If your pediatrician thinks your child is gaining weight too quickly, however, you can make small changes in your family's diet and physical activity levels.

health effects and social consequences

The health risk of being overweight starts early. More than 60 percent of overweight children between the ages of 5 and 10 already have at least one risk factor for heart disease. High blood pressure, cholesterol abnormalities, diabetes, and sleep apnea are just some of the complications that come with extra pounds. These illnesses used to be considered adult diseases, yet sadly they are becoming more and more prevalent in children.

Being overweight also can affect a child's self-esteem and emotional well-being. Poor self-image can create problems in making friends and doing schoolwork. Kids usually know if they are pudgy, but they may not know what to do about it. Usually they also have to deal with teasing and rejection from their peers. Often, parents aren't sure what to do either. Each family deals with the issue differently. Some focus on it too much, and others ignore it completely, hoping it will just go away. Unfortunately, it usually doesn't: Of the overweight teenagers in the United States today, about 80 percent will be overweight or obese as adults. If you have an overweight child in your family, try to emphasize a healthy lifestyle and practice what you preach.

take part in family fitness friday!

Set aside some time on Fridays to enjoy some physical activity with your children. Planning a fun event for the family each week will make it clear to your kids that you value them and a healthful, active lifestyle.

parenting and weight control

Parents **do** have the ability to influence their children's food choices and activities—more than any other individuals in a child's life. Kids are overweight for the same reasons adults are: too much food, too little activity. If parents embrace good eating habits and enjoy physical activity, they establish a home environment that leads children in the right direction. Families establish life habits together, and they can find a healthful solution to weight control together as well.

Early on, listen to your children's hunger signals. Don't worry if your kids don't eat as much as you think they should. Don't encourage them to clean their plates. Let your children respond to internal hunger cues rather than to learned social cues.

Have fun with your children and find ways to fit more physical activity in their lives. On long car rides, stop for run-and-fun breaks—for you and your children. Make play dates for younger children to get together for active playtime, and let your child have some say in the action.

For older children, remember that not all physical activity is competitive, and not all children are destined to be jocks. Many children who choose not to participate in organized or team sports still enjoy being physically active, and the benefits are the same without so much stress. All they need is the opportunity and a little encouragement.

should children diet?

It is best to avoid the idea of restrictive "dieting" for children. It's far better to teach your children to make the same healthful food choices you want to make for yourself. You want them to take an understanding of good eating habits into adulthood. Overweight children need to overhaul their eating patterns so they are not setting themselves up for a lifelong struggle with weight gain. Encourage them to take small, manageable steps so they will feel good about their progress. Children under 10 years of age have little control over when and what they eat, and their activities are frequently dictated by the schedules of school and parents. Instead of focusing on what a child should not eat, replace the high-calorie, low-nutrient foods with better choices. Don't make a big deal of food, and don't focus on any one child. The whole family, even the thin kids, will benefit from a more healthful diet.

too much of a good thing?

Orange juice is a favorite way for millions of American children to start the day. That's great—unless your 6-year-old gulps down 8 ounces with breakfast, another 8 ounces on the way out the door, and another 8 ounces when he gets home from school. That's over 300 calories! Try offering water to quench early-morning thirst. Serve 6 ounces of orange juice, which counts as one fruit serving, as something to be savored.

Strategies to Introduce Healthful Habits for Life

- Even though you're not always with your children, be aware of their environment. What is the school cafeteria serving for lunch? What snacks do your children grab at home or at friends' houses? If you know what you're dealing with, you may be able to have more influence on your kids' food choices.

- Serve meals at home as much as possible. Sitting down together at the table is the best chance you have to help your child establish good eating habits. You can see what your kids are eating, show off your own good choices, and talk about things that may be troubling your child, perhaps situations that may trigger overeating.

- Practice portion control. Of course, a preschooler and a teenage athlete need different amounts of food. Encourage what is appropriate for each stage of your child's development.

- Keep plenty of nutritious snacks on hand. Fruits and veggies make great snacks for everyone.

- Promote as much physical activity as you can. Limit time spent in front of the television and computer. Don't put a television in your child's room.

- Encourage outdoor and unstructured play activities. Keep equipment such as bikes and basketball hoops in good working order.

- Share: Make it a point to enjoy many kinds of physical activities **together** with your children.

- Finally, be a good role model. Get up, be active, and take your kids with you as you fit in fitness.

kids have choices, too

One of the best ways to teach your kids to make healthful food and activity choices is to get them involved. Let them be part of the whole process of choosing recipes, shopping for ingredients, preparing food, and enjoying great meals. The more they participate, the more they will learn to appreciate the variety of flavor and textures in different foods.

Make food fun. Have your kids choose something that's new to them from the grocery store. Even if they don't like the new food at first, it's important to encourage them to keep trying different things. Did you know it may take ten to fifteen tries over time before a child will decide he or she likes a new food? Kids' taste buds change and develop as they grow. And just because you didn't like spinach as a child, don't avoid it now. Adults' tastes evolve with time also.

did you know . . .

that sports drinks often have 1 tablespoon of sugar in each cup? Along with the electrolytes in these heavily promoted drinks, you're getting a hefty dose of calories. Water is inexpensive, readily available, and quenches thirst well—without one unnecessary calorie. Teach your children to respond to thirst first with a natural thirst-quencher—water.

new fast-food options

Would you like fries with that? Maybe not! More and more fast-food restaurants are offering better alternatives to the french fries and soft drinks that usually accompany so many children's meals. Some places offer salads instead of fries, applesauce or fruit for dessert, and fat-free milk or juice instead of soda. This trend is sure to continue as long as consumers ask for more healthful ways to enjoy eating out with their kids. So when you're ordering fast food, encourage your kids to ask for what's good for them.

just a teaspoon of sugar . . .

You might be surprised to learn that a 20-ounce bottle of cola contains over $1/6$ cup of sugar. You may have a hard time visualizing the amount of sugar in processed foods because most food labels list sugar in grams. Converting grams to teaspoons is easy: Just divide the grams of sugar by 5. So, if the label indicates 10 grams of sugar, that's 2 teaspoons. If it indicates 60 grams of sugar, that's 12 teaspoons, or $1/4$ cup.

pack up a lunch for good

When you send your child to school with a lunch from home, make sure it packs nutrition and taste. Put together a meal from all the food groups, including servings of a grain (preferably whole), vegetable or fruit, dairy product, and protein source. Instead of the usual sandwich, try 2 ounces of turkey breast and 1 ounce of low-fat cheese wrapped up in a tortilla with any favorite vegetables that won't get too soggy, such as lettuce, shredded carrots, or cucumber. Avoid the high-sugar drinks, even if the packaging is temptingly convenient.

Healthful School Lunch Ideas

- Spread peanut butter or all-fruit spread on a toasted fat-free whole-grain waffle. Top it off with a second toasted waffle to make a sandwich.

- Cut light deli turkey or ham into bite-size pieces and put them in a plastic container. Send a plastic fork and a packet of mustard or hot sauce for dipping.

- Include vegetables in your child's lunch. Grill some asparagus spears and cut them into 1-inch pieces. Steam broccoli florets and slice them into smaller "trees." Send along a packet or separate container of light vinaigrette dressing.

- Homemade trail mix is a filling snack. A good combination is pretzels, rice or wheat cereal squares, raisins, unsalted sunflower seeds, and a few candy-coated chocolate pieces. Let your child choose his or her favorite ingredients.

- "Ants on a log" is still a favorite snack for younger children. Fill a celery stick with peanut butter and press raisins (the ants) into the peanut butter.

- Send a small container of salad. Use the darker greens or at least mix them in with iceberg lettuce. Include a packet of reduced-fat ranch or light vinaigrette dressing.

- Pack fruit for dessert. For a treat that is low in calories and fat, send a slice of angelfood cake or a small bag of caramel popcorn.

- If your child just won't or can't drink milk, be sure to pack a calcium-fortified beverage such as soy milk, rice milk, or juice.

holiday hints

Sugary treats abound from Valentine's Day to Halloween and beyond. Limiting your child's choices during those times can be daunting. Don't fret too much. Offer healthful options, such as fruit, light popcorn, and trail mix, and allow your child to choose a few favorites to have at snack time. Encourage reasonable restraint. Then turn to other options for enjoying the holiday. Read a book, do a craft project, play a board game, or have some active playtime—all around the holiday theme. Those quality times together will become lifelong memories that will mean more to your child than any amount of candy.

steps to success

Kids who make small, progressive changes in their behavior are likely to stick with new habits for good. Even more important, they will be better equipped to make the right choices when they are on their own. Just like adults, when kids feel good about themselves, when they feel valued, they flourish. Encourage your children to find activities that develop their unique strengths. If they are busy with new pursuits and hobbies, they won't rely so much on passive entertainment. Rather, their time will be filled with the personal rewards of an active life.

prevention is the key

Finally, the best way to avoid excessive weight gain is to prevent it in the first place. Teach your children good eating habits and the joy of an active lifestyle. These are the gifts that will last a lifetime.

Part II

MENU PLANNING AND RECIPES

getting started

The first step in creating a low-calorie and healthful diet is good planning. It's important, when possible, to plan your meals for the week. If you plan for a week, you can, for example, be sure to include at least two fish-based meals and at least one vegetarian meal. You can also even out your sodium intake for the week.

There's no right or wrong way to build a menu plan, so it's best to start where it makes most sense for you. You could begin with the foods that you know you will eat during the week. Think about what you enjoy having on a regular basis, perhaps a roll or a glass of wine with dinner. Or if you always eat cereal for breakfast, start there. Once these foods are accounted for, find out how many calories and saturated fat grams and other nutritional values they include. You can find that information on labels of prepared food, with the recipes in this and in many other cookbooks, or from a fat, calorie, and sodium counter book or website. Once you know those details, you'll know what is left over so you can add the remaining meals and snacks to complete your customized meal plan.

Similarly, take your eating patterns into consideration. That will help ensure that you'll stick to your plan. If you know that you get hungriest at breakfast, start there with the heaviest meal. If you bring a sandwich to work for lunch every day, try to make it as healthful as possible. Likewise, if you know that you come home hungry and grab a snack before fixing dinner, plan accordingly. In addition, as you plan for the week, think about any meals that you may not be preparing. For example, if you know that you're having pizza for lunch at work on Friday, plan to have a lighter dinner that evening.

creating your own healthful meal plans

Providing balance and variety in your diet is important as you craft your meal plans. Each food group makes an important contribution to healthful weight loss. Our menu plans were created using the following American Heart Association dietary guidelines. (See pages 66–68 in Chapter 2, "Eating Well.") We recommend referring to them when creating your own menu plans. Think, too, of how foods will look together on the plate. Aim for a mixture of colors, sizes, shapes, and textures.

FRUITS AND VEGETABLES

- Include a minimum of five $\frac{1}{2}$-cup servings of veggies and fruit each day.

- Use a variety of fruits and veggies, including lots of dark leafy greens; other green, red, orange, and yellow veggies; and dark (red, orange, and blue) fruits.

- Remember that however foods are used in a meal, they count toward your goal. For example, $^{1}/_{2}$ cup of marinara sauce for your pasta counts as a serving, and the chopped veggies in the casserole count. If you choose frozen vegetables and you want to have a sauce with them, make your own so you can control the fats, cholesterol, and sodium.

- If choosing canned vegetables, rinse them to reduce the sodium. Better yet, buy vegetables with no salt added when they are available.

- Try to limit juices since the actual fruits and veggies themselves provide more fiber.

DAIRY

- Include at least three fat-free or low-fat dairy products per day. An example of a dairy serving is 8 ounces of milk, 1 ounce of cheese, or $^{1}/_{2}$ cup of ice cream.

- If you put milk in your coffee, it counts toward your dairy intake. So does the milk you included in a cream sauce and other prepared foods.

- Vary your dairy intake by using different cheeses, adding fruits or vegetables to cottage cheese, making fat-free or low-fat milkshakes or hot chocolate, and adding fruit and nuts to yogurt.

MEAT, POULTRY, AND SEAFOOD

- Include no more than 6 ounces of cooked weight (8 ounces raw weight) of lean meat, poultry, and seafood daily. The rule of thumb is that these foods lose about 25 percent of their weight in cooking.
- If you want a big steak for dinner, balance it out with a vegetarian lunch so you don't each too much protein.
- Remember that the cheese you sprinkle over your salad counts as part of your dairy servings as well as part of your protein.
- Include at least two meals per week that feature fish, preferably fatty fish, such as salmon, tuna, and halibut.

VEGETARIAN

- Include at least one vegetarian meal per week. Tofu, quinoa, meatless "hamburgers," cheese, and beans and rice are a few options. Don't overlook the chapter of vegetarian entrées, which begins on page 514.

GRAINS

- Aim for 6 or more servings of breads, cereals, pasta, and starchy veggies (white potatoes and corn, for example) each day.
- Try to have at least half of those servings be whole grains, such as whole-wheat pasta and brown rice.
- Starchy vegetables include all potatoes, corn and corn products (such as hominy and corn tortillas), green peas (sugar snap peas and snow peas count as nonstarchy vegetables), and beans except green beans (for example, lima beans).
- Quinoa, couscous, barley, and lentils are among other foods you can choose from in this category.

FATS

- Try to consume no more than 30 percent of calories from fat per day, with no more than 10 percent of your daily calories from saturated fat.

SODIUM

- Keep your sodium intake to less than 2,300 mg daily. If you are following a lower-calorie plan, you may need to average your sodium intake over a week. Sodium includes salt added at the table and salt in foods at restaurants as well as salt used when making food at home.

CHOLESTEROL

- Try to keep your cholesterol intake to a maximum of 300 mg daily.

FIBER

- If you are consuming 1,600 calories a day or more, try to consume 25 to 30 g of fiber per day. If you're consuming 1,200 to 1,599 calories a day, be sure to consume at least 15 g.

using the menus

The menus on the following pages, based on the American Heart Association dietary guidelines, are a starting point for your commitment to a healthful lifestyle. Each day's meal plans—at all three calorie levels—give you the protein, dairy, fruits and vegetables, and grains that the American Heart Association recommends for all healthy Americans over two years old. The week's menus also include at least two servings of fatty fish, which are high in omega-3 fatty acids, and at least one vegetarian meal. Also, the amount of sodium averaged over the week is under the recommended 2,300 mg per day.

The menus are designed so that certain foods, especially entrées, are used for the same meal at 1,200, 1,600, and 2,000 calories. That's so everyone at the table can eat many of the same foods, regardless of each person's calorie intake goal. This approach not only lets you reduce food preparation time but also shows you how easy it is to adapt menus for various calorie levels.

Because it is often quicker to make a sandwich than cook an entrée from scratch, the menus offer many meals and snacks that do not require you to follow a recipe. However, we've included almost 200 healthful recipes (pages 244–669) for you to use in your customized meal plans when you wish. We've included a handy calorie bar with every recipe. That tool lets you know at a glance how many calories that recipe contains. We've also provided a list of recipes grouped by calorie count. Both of these tools will make your planning easier. If you don't want the sandwich shown for lunch on Wednesday of the first week (216 calories), perhaps you'd prefer a hearty soup, such as Bayou Andouille and Chicken Chowder (206 calories; pages 292–293). Just keep in mind the guidelines you learned (pages 66–68), so you get all the nutrients you need without too many calories and too much saturated fat, cholesterol, and sodium.

Feel free to experiment as you plan delicious, healthful meals. As you go through the provided menus (pages 158–229), you may make changes to suit your tastes and/or to accommodate the seasons. Keep those marked-up menus and your changes to them as a record of what you liked. Spend the time to make up another two weeks' worth of menus. Keep those menus as well. Now you have a month's worth of menus that you can rotate, thus saving time. You could even make and keep a list of the ingredients needed for the week. Enjoy the creativity and control—as well as the many health benefits—that come with making wise choices and eating well.

By design, some of the provided menus don't include the maximum allowed calories. That allows you to amass an emergency stash of calories in case you splurge unexpectedly or have an extra snack.

week one • 1,200 calories

Some of the following meals use the two-for-one concept, allowing you to cook once and eat twice. For example, if you grill extra Honey-Lime Flank Steak (Tuesday's dinner entrée; page 464), you can transform what's left into Flank Steak Salad with Sesame-Lime Dressing (Thursday's lunch; page 334).

monday

breakfast:	1 cup whole-grain cereal with	134
	8 ounces fat-free milk,	90
	1 cup sliced strawberries, and	53
	1 teaspoon sugar	16
	total breakfast calories	**293**
snack:	1 medium tangerine	**43**
lunch:	Sandwich of 2 slices light	
	whole-wheat bread,	80
	1 ounce Neufchâtel cheese,	70
	6 thin slices cucumber, and	5
	1 tablespoon minced watercress	0
	½ cup Broccoli and Edamame Salad	
	with Dill (page 310)	86
	½ cup fat-free, sugar-free instant	
	pudding, made with fat-free milk	67
	total lunch calories	**308**
snack:	3 cups light microwave popcorn	**63**

dinner: 3 ounces grilled (4 ounces raw)	
halibut, basted with	119
1 teaspoon olive or canola oil	
and herbs of choice	40
½ cup Italian Barley and Mushrooms	
(page 574)	133
Salad of 2 cups torn lettuce leaves,	11
1 medium tomato,	27
½ cup sliced jícama,	23
¼ large bell pepper, sliced,	8
½ cup grated carrot, and	23
2 tablespoons green onions with	5
2 tablespoons light salad dressing	45
total dinner calories	**434**
total daily calories:	**1,141**

tuesday

breakfast:	1 slice Apple and Dried Cherry Quick Bread (page 613)	77
	6-ounce container fat-free, sugar-free yogurt, plain or any flavor, with	111
	½ cup blueberries	41
	total breakfast calories	**229**
snack:	4 low-salt whole-wheat crackers	71
	1 ounce light Swiss cheese	81
	total snack calories	**152**
lunch:	6-inch fast-food ham submarine sandwich	290
	8 ounces fat-free milk	90
	½ cup cubed pineapple	37
	total lunch calories	**417**
snack:	1 cup button mushrooms	21
	3 tablespoons Dilled Yogurt Dipping Sauce (page 259)	21
	total snack calories	**42**
dinner:	3 ounces Honey-Lime Flank Steak (page 464)	162
	½ cup cooked brown rice with	108
	1 teaspoon light tub margarine	13
	½ cup cooked broccoli, cooked in	22
	1 teaspoon olive or canola oil	40
	total dinner calories	**345**
	total daily calories:	**1,185**

wednesday

breakfast: 1 cup sliced strawberries with   53
         1 teaspoon sugar   16
         ¾ cup bran flakes with   90
         8 ounces fat-free milk   90

         total breakfast calories   **249**

snack: 10 sweet cherries   **43**

lunch: Sandwich of 4-inch whole-wheat pita with   120
         2 ounces 97% fat-free beef pastrami,   54
         2 lettuce leaves,   3
         4 tomato slices, and   14
         2 teaspoons reduced-calorie mayonnaise dressing   25
         ½ cup raw baby carrots   27
         8 ounces fat-free milk   90

         total lunch calories   **333**

snack: 10 grapes   **35**

dinner: 3 ounces Black-Pepper Chicken (make extra for Friday lunch if desired) (page 411)   155
         ½ cup cooked whole-wheat pasta with   87
         1 teaspoon light tub margarine   13
         ½ cup cooked green peas, cooked in   67
         1 teaspoon olive or canola oil   41
         ½ cup fat-free or light ice cream with   100
         1½ tablespoons chopped pecans   77

         total dinner calories   **540**

         total daily calories: **1,200**

thursday

breakfast:	1 slice Apple and Dried Cherry Quick Bread (page 613)	77
	¼ large cantaloupe	69
	8 ounces fat-free milk	90
	total breakfast calories	**236**
snack:	1 ounce low-fat Cheddar cheese	49
	4 low-salt whole-wheat crackers	71
	total snack calories	**120**
lunch:	1½ cups Flank Steak Salad with Sesame-Lime Dressing (page 334)	271
	1 medium orange	70
	½ cup fat-free or light ice cream	100
	total lunch calories	**441**
snack:	3 cups light microwave popcorn	**63**
dinner:	1 Veggie Burger with Gorgonzola (page 565)	175
	1 large tomato, sliced	33
	1 cup cucumber slices	16
	½ cup Smashed Potatoes with Aromatic Herbs (page 598)	100
	total dinner calories	**324**
	total daily calories:	**1,184**

friday

breakfast:	8 ounces Banana-Blueberry Smoothie (page 269)	207

snack:	½ whole-wheat English muffin with	67
	1 teaspoon light tub margarine	13
	total snack calories	**80**

lunch:	2 ounces Black-Pepper Chicken (page 411) on	104
	2 cups torn salad greens with	18
	½ small cucumber,	10
	4 cherry tomatoes, and	10
	½ cup canned no-salt-added whole-kernel corn, drained, with	91
	2 tablespoons low-fat salad dressing	45
	½ cup fat-free or light ice cream	100
	total lunch calories	**378**

snack:	1 large rectangle low-fat graham crackers	54
	½ cup cubed watermelon	23
	total snack calories	**77**

dinner:	1 serving Saucy Minute Steak (page 473)	169
	½ cup cooked whole-wheat pasta with	87
	2 teaspoons olive oil and fresh basil	80
	½ cup cubed mango	54
	½ cup fat-free, sugar-free pudding, made with fat-free milk	67
	total dinner calories	**457**

total daily calories:	**1,199**

saturday

breakfast:	1 1/4 cups cornflakes with	110
	1/2 cup blueberries,	41
	1 teaspoon sugar, and	16
	8 ounces fat-free milk	90
	3/4 cup low-sodium tomato or mixed vegetable juice	40
	total breakfast calories	**297**
snack:	6-ounce container fat-free, sugar-free yogurt, any flavor	**111**
lunch:	1/2 cup low-fat (2%) cottage cheese with	102
	4 cherry tomatoes, chopped, and	10
	4 medium green olives, sliced	17
	2 slices melba toast	39
	1/2 cup cubed watermelon	23
	total lunch calories	**191**
snack:	2 medium apricots	**34**
dinner:	3 ounces Bistro Chicken with Fresh Asparagus (page 398)	261
	1 cup cooked whole-wheat spaghetti with	174
	1 teaspoon olive or canola oil and herbs of choice	40
	1/2 cup peach slices with	33
	1 tablespoon chopped pecans	51
	total dinner calories	**559**
	total daily calories:	**1,192**

sunday

breakfast:	8 ounces fat-free milk	90
	2 Pumpkin-Cranberry Pancakes	
	(page 620) with	225
	2 teaspoons light tub margarine	27
	total breakfast calories	**342**

snack:	6-ounce container fat-free, sugar-free yogurt,	
	plain or any flavor, with	111
	1/2 cup blackberries	31
	total snack calories	**142**

lunch:	Cheese toast made of 1 ounce low-fat	
	shredded Cheddar cheese and	49
	2 slices light whole-wheat bread	80
	3/4 cup Chilled Tomato-Basil Soup	
	(page 278)	84
	1/2 cup canned fruit, such as fruit	
	cocktail, packed in extra-light syrup	60
	total lunch calories	**273**

snack:	7 unsalted mini rice cakes	54
	1 medium apricot	17
	total snack calories	**71**

dinner:	3 ounces Salmon with Creamy	
	Caper Sauce (page 350)	160
	½ cup cooked green beans, cooked in	22
	1 teaspoon olive or canola oil	40
	½ cup Lemon-Herb Brown Rice	
	(page 600)	89
	½ cup Vegetable Salad Vinaigrette	
	(page 308)	51
	total dinner calories	**362**
	total daily calories:	**1,190**

week two • 1,200 calories

Did you follow last week's menus according to plan? Review this week's menus and make modifications to best suit your lifestyle. Be sure to refer to "Recipes by Calorie Count" (pages 232–243) and "Common Foods by Calorie Count" (page 695–701) for easy substitutions.

monday

breakfast:	¾ cup cooked oatmeal, made with water, with	111
	1 teaspoon sugar,	16
	1 teaspoon light tub margarine,	13
	1 tablespoon chopped pecans, and	51
	½ medium banana	53
	8 ounces fat-free milk	90
	total breakfast calories	**334**
snack:	¾ cup Chilled Tomato-Basil Soup (page 278)	**84**
lunch:	1 ounce Neufchâtel cheese	71
	4 slices melba toast	78
	½ cup cubed watermelon	23
	8 ounces fat-free milk	90
	total lunch calories	**262**
snack:	2 cups light microwave popcorn	**42**

dinner:	2 slices Barbeque Chicken Pizza (page 441)	346
	Salad of 2 cups torn salad greens with	18
	¼ cup chopped tomatoes,	8
	¼ cup sliced celery,	4
	¼ cup sliced carrots, and	13
	¼ cup chopped cauliflower with	6
	2 tablespoons light salad dressing	45
	total dinner calories	**440**
	total daily calories:	**1,162**

tuesday

breakfast: 8 ounces Banana-Blueberry Smoothie
(page 269)   207

snack: 1 whole-wheat English muffin with   134
2 teaspoons light tub margarine   27

total snack calories   161

lunch: 2 cups Fruit and Spinach Salad
with Fresh Mint (page 304) with   126
2 ounces boneless, skinless cooked
chicken breast   94
4 low-salt whole-wheat crackers   71

total lunch calories   291

snack: 8 ounces fat-free milk   **90**

dinner: 1 1/2 cups Tuna and Broccoli with
Lemon Caper Brown Rice
(page 379)   257
1/2 cup cooked carrots with fat-free
spray margarine   34
1/2 cup fat-free or light ice cream with   100
1 tablespoon chopped pecans   51

total dinner calories   442

total daily calories   1,191

wednesday

breakfast:	1 glazed doughnut (fast food)	160
	8 ounces fat-free milk	90
	total breakfast calories	**250**

snack:	6-ounce container fat-free, sugar-free yogurt, any flavor	**111**

lunch:	Salad of 2 cups torn lettuce leaves,	11
	1 ounce part-skim mozzarella cheese,	72
	1 medium tomato,	27
	1/4 medium red bell pepper, sliced, and	8
	1 tablespoon chopped green onions with	3
	2 tablespoons light salad dressing	45
	1 crusty French roll	130
	total lunch calories	**296**

snack:	7 unsalted mini rice cakes	**54**

dinner:	1 1/2 cups Soba Noodles in Peanut Sauce (page 528)	377
	1/2 cup cooked pea pods, cooked in	35
	1 teaspoon olive or canola oil	40
	1 medium peach, sliced	37
	total dinner calories	**489**

total daily calories	**1,200**

thursday

breakfast:	1 cup sliced strawberries with	53
	1 teaspoon sugar	16
	2 slices light whole-wheat toast with	80
	2 teaspoons light tub margarine	27
	6-ounce container fat-free, sugar-free	
	yogurt, any flavor	111
	total breakfast calories	**287**

snack:	4 Crunchy Cinnamon Chips	
	(page 256)	73
	10 grapes	35
	total snack calories	**108**

lunch:	Cheese toast made of 1 ounce low-fat	
	shredded Cheddar cheese and	49
	1 whole-wheat English muffin	134
	½ cup baby carrots	27
	½ cup fat-free or light ice cream	100
	total lunch calories	**310**

| **snack:** | ½ medium banana, sliced | **53** |

dinner:	1 serving Pork Tenderloin with	
	Cranberry Salsa (3 ounces pork	
	and ½ cup salsa) (page 497)	222
	1 medium baked sweet potato with	130
	2 teaspoons light tub margarine	27
	½ cup cooked green beans, cooked in	22
	1 teaspoon olive or canola oil	40
	total dinner calories	**441**

| | **total daily calories** | **1,199** |

friday

breakfast: 8 ounces Banana-Blueberry
Smoothie (page 269) **207**

snack: 1 whole-wheat English muffin with 134
2 teaspoons light tub margarine 27
total snack calories **161**

lunch: 1 ounce low-fat Colby cheese 49
4 low-salt whole-wheat crackers 71
10 dried apricot halves 84
1/2 cup fat-free, sugar-free gelatin 10
8 ounces fat-free milk 90
total lunch calories **304**

snack: 1/2 cup fat-free, sugar-free instant
pudding, made with fat-free milk **67**

dinner: 1 slice Meat Loaf with a Twist
(page 483) 209
1/2 cup Asparagus and Cucumber
Salad with Lemon and Mint
(page 178) 39
1/2 cup cooked yellow summer squash,
cooked in 18
1 teaspoon olive or canola oil 40
1 Pan-Style Whole-Wheat Dinner
Roll (page 617) with 109
1 teaspoon light tub margarine 13
total dinner calories **428**

total daily calories **1,167**

saturday

breakfast: 1 Peach Cornmeal Waffle (page 622)
with 192
2 teaspoons light tub margarine 27
8 ounces fat-free milk 90

total breakfast calories **309**

snack: 4 Crunchy Cinnamon Chips
(page 256) **73**

lunch: 1 ounce part-skim mozzarella cheese,
cubed 72
4 slices melba toast 78
6 cherry tomatoes 15
¼ cup sliced zucchini 5
½ cup fat-free sugar-free, instant
pudding, made with fat-free milk 67

total lunch calories **237**

snack: 1 medium apple, sliced **72**

dinner: 1 serving Salmon Florentine
(3 ounces salmon and
½ cup spinach) (page 348) 199
Salad of 2 cups torn salad greens, 18
¼ cup sliced red bell pepper, 6
¼ cup chopped button mushrooms, 4
¼ cup sliced carrots, and 13
¼ cup chopped cauliflower with 6
2 tablespoons light salad dressing 45
½ cup Orzo with Tomato and
Capers (page 594) 107
1 Dinner Biscuit (page 615) with 81
1 teaspoon light tub margarine 13

total dinner calories **492**

total daily calories: **1,183**

sunday

breakfast: ¼ large cantaloupe, sliced   69

1½ slices Crisp French Toast
(page 624) with   168

1 tablespoon light, sugar-free
pancake syrup   25

total breakfast calories   262

snack: 4 low-salt whole-wheat crackers   71

8 ounces fat-free milk   90

total snack calories   161

lunch: Sandwich of 1 ounce Neufchâtel
cheese,   71

6 thin slices cucumber,   5

1 tablespoon minced watercress, and   0

2 slices light whole-wheat bread,
toasted   80

½ cup celery sticks   8

1 medium pear   97

total lunch calories   261

snack: ½ cup fat-free or light ice cream with   100

¼ ounce chopped walnuts   46

dinner:	3 ounces Sunday-Best Roast Chicken	
	Breasts (page 394)	127
	2 cups Greek Salad with Sun-Dried	
	Tomato Vinaigrette (page 300)	84
	½ cup cooked zucchini, cooked in	14
	1 teaspoon olive or canola oil	40
	½ cup cooked couscous, with fat-free	
	spray margarine	88
	total dinner calories	**353**
	total daily calories:	**1,183**

week one • 1,600 calories

If you see a food in this week's menu that doesn't appeal to you, simply refer to the "Recipes by Calorie Count" (pages 232–243) and the "Common Foods by Calorie Count" (pages 695–701) charts to find alternate choices.

monday

breakfast:	1 cup Fruit-and-Cinnamon Oatmeal (page 626)	289
	1 cup sliced strawberries with	53
	1 teaspoon sugar	16
	8 ounces fat-free milk	90
	total breakfast calories	**448**
snack:	4 reduced-fat vanilla-flavored afer-type cookies	60
	1 cup hot chocolate, made with	
	8 ounces fat-free milk and	90
	2 tablespoons light chocolate syrup	50
	total snack calories	**200**
lunch:	¾ cup Quick Mexican-Style Soup (page 280)	35
	Sandwich of 2 slices whole-wheat bread,	138
	2 ounces oven-roasted deli turkey breast,	45
	2 lettuce leaves,	3
	4 tomato slices, and	14

2 teaspoons reduced-calorie
   mayonnaise dressing   25
1/2 cup fat-free, sugar-free instant
   pudding, made with fat-free milk   67

total lunch calories   327

snack: 3 cups light microwave popcorn   63
        3/4 cup Orange Froth (page 265)   102

total snack calories   165

dinner: 3 ounces grilled (4 ounces raw)
      halibut, basted with   119
      1 teaspoon olive or canola oil
      and herbs of choice   40
      1/2 cup cooked spinach, cooked in   21
      1 teaspoon olive or canola oil,
      lemon juice, and oregano   40
      1/2 cup Italian Barley and Mushrooms
      (page 574)   133
      Salad of 2 cups torn lettuce leaves,   11
      1 medium tomato,   27
      1/4 cup grated carrot, and   11
      1 tablespoon green onions with   3
      2 tablespoons light salad dressing   45

total dinner calories   450

total daily calories: 1,590

tuesday

breakfast:	2 slices Apple and Dried Cherry Quick Bread (page 613)	154
	6-ounce container fat-free, sugar-free yogurt, plain or any flavor, with	111
	½ cup blueberries	41
	6 ounces orange juice	84
	total breakfast calories	**390**
snack:	1 ounce light Swiss cheese	81
	4 low-salt whole-wheat crackers	71
	total snack calories	**152**
lunch:	6-inch fast-food ham submarine sandwich	290
	2 medium apricots	34
	8 ounces fat-free milk	90
	total lunch calories	**414**
snack:	1 medium banana	**105**
dinner:	3 ounces Honey-Lime Flank Steak (page 464)	162
	½ cup cooked brown rice, cooked in salt-free beef bouillon	108
	1 cup cooked broccoli (2 servings), cooked in	44
	2 teaspoons olive or canola oil	80
	1 Pan-Style Whole-Wheat Dinner Roll (page 617) with	109
	1 teaspoon light tub margarine	13
	total dinner calories	**516**
	total daily calories:	**1,577**

wednesday

breakfast:	1 cup sliced strawberries with	53
	1 teaspoon sugar	16
	¼ cup egg substitute, scrambled with	30
	1 tablespoon fat-free milk, cooked in	5
	2 teaspoons light tub margarine	27
	½ 3½-inch plain bagel with	98
	1 tablespoon light cream cheese	35
	total breakfast calories	**264**
snack:	1 large rectangle low-fat graham crackers	54
	½ cup canned fruit, such as fruit cocktail, packed in extra-light syrup	60
	total snack calories	**114**
lunch:	Sandwich of 2 slices light whole-wheat bread with	80
	2 ounces 96% fat-free, low-sodium ham,	61
	2 lettuce leaves,	3
	4 tomato slices, and	14
	2 teaspoons mustard	7
	½ cup Black-Eyed Pea Salad (page 319)	75
	8 ounces fat-free milk	90
	1 medium pear	97
	total lunch calories	**427**
snack:	½ cup fat-free or light ice cream with	100
	2 tablespoons chopped pecans	103
	total snack calories	**203**

dinner: 1 cup Curried Pumpkin Soup
(page 276) 110
3 ounces Black-Pepper Chicken
(make extra for Friday lunch
if desired) (page 411) 155
½ cup cooked whole-wheat pasta with 87
1 teaspoon light tub margarine 13
½ cup cooked green peas, cooked in 67
1 teaspoon olive or canola oil 40
½ cup fat-free, sugar-free instant
pudding, made with fat-free milk 67

total dinner calories 539

total daily calories: 1,547

thursday

breakfast:	2 slices Apple and Dried Cherry Quick Bread (page 613)	154
	1/4 large cantaloupe	69
	8 ounces fat-free milk	90
	total breakfast calories	**313**
snack:	1 ounce low-fat Cheddar cheese	49
	4 low-salt whole-wheat crackers	71
	total snack calories	**120**
lunch:	1 1/2 cups Flank Steak Salad with Sesame-Lime Dressing (page 334)	271
	4 slices melba toast	78
	1 medium orange	70
	1/2 cup fat-free or light ice cream with	100
	1 tablespoon light chocolate syrup	25
	total lunch calories	**544**
snack:	3 cups light microwave popcorn	**63**
dinner:	1 Veggie Burger with Gorgonzola (page 565)	175
	1 large tomato, sliced, and	33
	1 cup cucumber slices, drizzled with	16
	1 teaspoon olive oil and chopped fresh herbs	40
	1/2 cup Smashed Potatoes with Aromatic Herbs (page 598)	100
	1 slice Pear and Apricot Cake (page 630)	195
	total dinner calories	**559**
	total daily calories:	**1,599**

friday

breakfast: 8 ounces Banana-Blueberry Smoothie
(page 269)   207
½ whole-wheat English muffin with   67
1 tablespoon low-sugar preserves   25
total breakfast calories   299

snack: 2 large rectangles low-fat graham
crackers   108
8 ounces fat-free milk   90
total snack calories   198

lunch: 1 cup Cream of Triple-Mushroom
Soup (page 273)   105
3 ounces Black-Pepper Chicken
(page 411) on   155
1 cup torn salad greens with   9
¼ medium avocado, sliced,   80
1 medium rib of celery,   10
½ small cucumber, and   10
4 cherry tomatoes with   10
2 tablespoons vinaigrette,
made with
1½ tablespoons olive oil and   179
1½ teaspoons vinegar   1
total lunch calories   559

snack: 2 tablespoons Creamy Cannellini
Dip (page 250)   31
4 baby carrots   14
total snack calories   45

dinner: 1 serving Saucy Minute Steak
(page 473)   169
½ cup cooked whole-wheat pasta with   87
¼ cup spaghetti sauce   21
½ cup Broccoli Bake with Three
Cheeses (page 576)   101
1 medium kiwifruit, sliced, with   46
½ cup cubed mango and   54
5 grapes   18

total dinner calories   **496**

total daily calories: **1,597**

saturday

breakfast:	¼ cup egg substitute, scrambled with	30
	1 tablespoon fat-free milk, cooked in	6
	2 teaspoons light tub margarine	27
	1 whole-wheat English muffin with	134
	1 teaspoon honey	22
	¾ cup low-sodium tomato or	
	mixed-vegetable juice	40
	total breakfast calories	**259**
snack:	6-ounce container fat-free, sugar-free yogurt, any flavor	**111**
lunch:	Sandwich of 2 ounces 97% fat-free,	
	reduced-sodium deli roast beef,	70
	2 lettuce leaves,	3
	4 tomato slices, and	14
	1 teaspoon mustard on	3
	3½-inch plain bagel	195
	1 ounce baked potato chips	110
	8 ounces fat-free milk	90
	total lunch calories	**485**
snack:	1 large tangerine	**43**

dinner:	1½ cups Chicken and Bow-Ties with Green Beans (page 426)	295
	½ cup cooked carrots with	34
	1 teaspoon light tub margarine	13
	1 Pan-Style Whole-Wheat Dinner Roll (page 617) with	109
	1 teaspoon light tub margarine	13
	½ cup fat-free or light ice cream with	100
	½ cup sliced strawberries and	27
	2 tablespoons chopped pecans	103
	total dinner calories	**694**
	total daily calories:	**1,592**

sunday

breakfast:	6 ounces orange juice	84
	2 Pumpkin-Cranberry Pancakes	
	(page 620) with	225
	2 teaspoons light tub margarine	27
	total breakfast calories	**336**

snack:	8 ounces fat-free milk	90
	½ cup blackberries with	31
	1 teaspoon sugar	16
	total snack calories	**137**

lunch:	Cheese toast made of 1 ounce low-fat	
	shredded Cheddar cheese and	49
	2 slices whole-wheat bread	138
	¾ cup Chilled Tomato-Basil Soup	
	(page 278)	84
	½ cup cubed cantaloupe	27
	½ cup fat-free or light ice cream	100
	total lunch calories	**398**

snack:	2 tablespoons Creamy Cannellini	
	Dip (page 250)	31
	4 low-salt whole-wheat crackers	71
	total snack calories	**102**

dinner:	1 cup Cream of Triple-Mushroom	
	Soup (page 273)	105
	3 ounces Salmon with Creamy	
	Caper Sauce (page 350)	160
	½ cup cooked brown rice, cooked	
	in salt-free beef bouillon	
	with herbs of choice	108
	½ cup Vegetable Salad Vinaigrette	
	(page 308)	51
	1 slice Pear and Apricot Cake	
	(page 630)	195
	total dinner calories	**619**
	total daily calories:	**1,592**

week two • 1,600 calories

Are you ready for seven more days of mouthwatering and healthful meals? See what delicious recipes we've suggested for you this week!

monday

breakfast:	1 cup Fruit-and-Cinnamon Oatmeal (page 626)	289
	8 ounces fat-free milk	90
	total breakfast calories	**379**
snack:	1 medium nectarine	60
	2 large rectangles low-fat graham crackers	108
	total snack calories	**168**
lunch:	¾ cup Chilled Tomato-Basil Soup (page 278)	84
	1 ounce Neufchâtel cheese	71
	4 slices melba toast	78
	½ cup cubed watermelon mixed with	23
	½ cup cantaloupe	27
	total lunch calories	**283**
snack:	¼ cup Creamy Cannellini Dip (page 250)	62
	6 baby carrots	21
	total snack calories	**83**

dinner: 2 slices Barbeque Chicken Pizza	
(page 441)	346
Salad of 2 cups torn salad greens,	18
¼ cup chopped tomatoes,	8
¼ cup sliced celery,	4
¼ cup sliced carrots, and	13
¼ cup chopped cauliflower with	6
2 tablespoons vinaigrette, made with	
1½ tablespoons olive oil and	179
1½ teaspoons vinegar	1
½ cup fat-free, sugar-free instant pudding, made with	
fat-free milk, and	67
¼ medium banana	26
total dinner calories	**668**
total daily calories:	**1,581**

tuesday

breakfast: 8 ounces Banana-Blueberry Smoothie
(page 269)   207
½ whole-wheat English muffin with   67
1 teaspoon light tub margarine and   13
1 teaspoon low-sugar preserves   8
total breakfast calories 295

snack: 1 ounce walnuts   185
1 medium orange   70
total snack calories 255

lunch: 2 cups Fruit and Spinach Salad
with Fresh Mint (page 304) with   126
2 ounces boneless, skinless cooked
chicken breast   94
4 low-salt whole-wheat crackers   71
½ cup fat-free, sugar-free instant
pudding, made with fat-free milk   67
total lunch calories 358

snack: 1 cup hot chocolate, made with
8 ounces fat-free milk and   90
2 tablespoons light chocolate syrup 50
5 unsalted mini rice cakes   39
total snack calories 179

dinner:	1½ cups Tuna and Broccoli with Lemon-Caper Brown Rice (page 379)	257
	2 cups Greek Salad with Sun-Dried Tomato Vinaigrette (page 300)	84
	1 cup cooked carrots with spray margarine	67
	1 Dinner Biscuit (page 615) with	81
	1 teaspoon light tub margarine	13
	total dinner calories	**502**
	total daily calories	**1,589**

wednesday

breakfast:	1 glazed doughnut (fast food)	160
	6-ounce container fat-free,	
	sugar-free yogurt, any flavor	111
	total breakfast calories	**271**

snack:	1 ounce part-skim mozzarella cheese	72
	4 low-salt whole-wheat crackers	71
	1/2 cup blueberries with	41
	1 teaspoon sugar	16
total snack calories		**200**

lunch:	3/4 cup Quick Mexican-Style Soup	
	(page 280)	35
	Salad of 2 cups torn lettuce leaves,	11
	1 medium tomato,	27
	1/2 cup mushroom slices,	8
	1/4 medium red bell pepper,	8
	1 tablespoon green onions, and	3
	3-ounce can white tuna in distilled	
	or spring water, drained, with	109
	2 tablespoons light salad dressing	45
	1 crusty French roll with	130
	2 teaspoons light tub margarine	27
	total lunch calories	**403**

snack:	1 cup hot chocolate, made with	
	8 ounces fat-free milk and	90
	2 tablespoons light chocolate syrup	50
	total snack calories	**140**

dinner:	1½ cups Soba Noodles in Peanut Sauce (page 528)	377
	½ cup cooked pea pods, cooked in	35
	1 teaspoon olive or canola oil	40
	½ cup mandarin oranges canned in light syrup	77
	2 fortune cookies	56
	total dinner calories	**585**
	total daily calories:	**1,599**

thursday

breakfast: 1 cup sliced strawberries with   53
   1 teaspoon sugar   16
¼ cup egg substitute, scrambled with   30
   1 tablespoon fat-free milk, cooked in   6
   2 teaspoons light tub margarine   27
2 slices rye toast with   166
   2 teaspoons light tub margarine and   27
   1 tablespoon low-sugar preserves   25

total breakfast calories   350

snack: 4 Crunchy Cinnamon Chips
(page 256) with   73
   ¼ cup Kiwi-Banana Dip (page 258)   50

total snack calories   123

lunch: Cheese toast made of 1 ounce
   low-fat shredded Cheddar
   cheese and   49
   1 whole-wheat English muffin   134
4 cherry tomatoes   10
1 cup sliced button mushrooms   15
½ cup baby carrots   27
½ cup fat-free or light ice cream   100

total lunch calories   335

snack: 2 Applesauce Oatmeal Cookies
(page 648)   105
8 ounces fat-free milk   90

total snack calories   195

dinner:	1 serving Pork Tenderloin with Cranberry Salsa (3 ounces pork and ½ cup salsa) (page 497)	222
	1 medium baked sweet potato with	130
	2 teaspoons light tub margarine	27
	½ cup cooked green beans, cooked in	22
	1 teaspoon olive or canola oil	40
	1 Pan-Style Whole-Wheat Dinner Roll (page 617) with	109
	1 teaspoon light tub margarine	13
	total dinner calories	**563**
	total daily calories:	**1,566**

friday

breakfast:	8 ounces Banana-Blueberry Smoothie (page 269)	207
	1 whole-wheat English muffin with	134
	2 teaspoons light tub margarine	27
	total breakfast calories	**368**

snack:	½ cup canned pineapple tidbits in their own juice	**54**

lunch:	¾ cup Chilled Tomato-Basil Soup (page 278)	84
	½ cup Chicken and Toasted Walnut Salad (page 330) on	231
	⅛ large cantaloupe, sliced	35
	4 low-salt whole-wheat crackers	71
	total lunch calories	**421**

snack:	1 ounce part-skim mozzarella cheese, cubed	72
	4 slices melba toast	78
	8 ounces fat-free milk	90
	total snack calories	**240**

dinner:	1 slice Meat Loaf with a Twist (page 483)	209
	1 cup Asparagus and Cucumber Salad with Lemon and Mint (page 306)	78
	½ cup cooked brown rice, cooked in salt-free beef bouillon	108
	1 Pan-Style Whole-Wheat Dinner Roll (page 617) with	109
	1 teaspoon light tub margarine	13
	total dinner calories	**517**
	total daily calories:	**1,600**

saturday

breakfast: 1 Peach Cornmeal Waffle
(page 622) with   192
2 teaspoons light tub margarine   27
6 ounces orange juice   84

total breakfast calories   303

snack: Milkshake made of 8 ounces
fat-free milk,   90
1/2 cup fat-free or light vanilla
or chocolate ice cream, and   100
2 tablespoons light chocolate syrup   50

total snack calories   240

lunch: 1 medium baked potato with   100
2 tablespoons fat-free or light
sour cream and   35
2 tablespoons salsa or picante sauce   10
1 cup Cream of Triple-Mushroom
Soup (page 273)   105
1/2 cup fat-free, sugar-free instant
pudding, made with fat-free milk   67

total lunch calories   317

snack: 4 Crunchy Cinnamon Chips
(page 256) with   73
1/4 cup Kiwi-Banana Dip (page 258)   50

total snack calories   123

dinner:	1 serving Salmon Florentine (3 ounces salmon and ½ cup spinach) (page 348)	199
	Salad of 2 cups torn salad greens,	18
	¼ cup sliced button mushrooms,	4
	¼ cup sliced celery,	4
	¼ cup sliced carrots, and	13
	¼ cup chopped cauliflower with	6
	2 tablespoons light salad dressing	45
	½ cup Orzo with Tomato and Capers (page 594)	107
	1 slice Pear and Apricot Cake (page 630)	195
	total dinner calories	**591**
	total daily calories:	**1,574**

sunday

breakfast:	⅛ large cantaloupe, sliced	35
	1½ slices Crisp French Toast	
	(page 624) with	168
	2 tablespoons light, sugar-free	
	pancake syrup	50
	8 ounces fat-free milk	90
	total breakfast calories	**343**
snack:	1 ounce Neufchâtel cheese	71
	5 unsalted mini rice cakes	39
	total snack calories	**110**
lunch:	Sandwich of 1 slice Meat Loaf	
	with a Twist (page 483),	209
	1 tablespoon no-salt-added	
	ketchup, and	16
	2 slices whole-wheat bread	138
	1 medium ear corn on the cob with	77
	2 teaspoons light tub margarine	27
	1 cup Peach Blush (page 268)	119
	total lunch calories	**586**
snack:	½ cup fat-free or light ice cream with	100
	1 medium apricot, sliced	17
	total snack calories	**117**

dinner: 3 ounces Sunday-Best Roast
Chicken Breasts (page 394)   127
2 cups Greek Salad with Sun-Dried
Tomato Vinaigrette (page 300)   84
$\frac{1}{2}$ cup cooked zucchini, cooked in   14
1 teaspoon olive or canola oil   40
$\frac{1}{2}$ cup cooked whole-wheat pasta,
cooked in 98% fat-free,
reduced-sodium chicken broth   87
1 Fruit Kebab with choice of
2 tablespoons dipping sauce
(page 252)   92

total dinner calories   444

total daily calories: 1,600

week one • 2,000 calories

For some of the nonrecipe items, such as fat-free or light ice cream, the actual calories of the product you purchase may differ from the amount listed on the menus. That's because manufacturers' products—and even flavors from the same manufacturer—may differ. Watch for these discrepancies and make modifications as necessary.

monday

breakfast:	1 cup Fruit-and-Cinnamon Oatmeal (page 626)	289
	1 cup sliced strawberries with	53
	1 teaspoon sugar	16
	8 ounces fat-free milk	90
	total breakfast calories	**448**
snack:	6-ounce container fat-free, sugar-free yogurt, plain or any flavor, with	111
	1/2 cup blueberries	41
	total snack calories	**152**
lunch:	Sandwich of 2 slices whole-wheat bread with	138
	1 ounce oven-roasted deli turkey breast,	23
	1 ounce soft goat cheese,	76
	2 lettuce leaves,	3
	4 tomato slices, and	14
	1/4 medium avocado, sliced	80

½ cup Multicolored Marinated Slaw
(page 314) 82

total lunch calories 416

snack: 4 reduced-fat vanilla-flavored
wafer-type cookies 60
1 cup Peach Blush (page 268) 119

total snack calories 179

dinner: 3 ounces grilled (4 ounces raw)
halibut, basted with 119
1 teaspoon olive or canola oil
and herbs of choice 40
½ cup cooked spinach, cooked in 21
1 teaspoon olive or canola oil,
lemon juice, and oregano 40
½ cup Italian Barley and Mushrooms
(page 574) 133
Salad of 2 cups torn lettuce leaves, 11
1 medium tomato, 27
½ cup grated carrot, and 23
1 tablespoon green onions with 3
2 tablespoons light salad dressing 45
1 Dinner Biscuit (page 615) with 81
2 teaspoons light tub margarine 27
½ cup Pumpkin Praline Mousse
(page 655) 188

total dinner calories 758

total daily calories: 1,953

tuesday

breakfast: 1 cup Fruit-and-Cinnamon
           Oatmeal (page 626)   289
           1 medium orange   70
           8 ounces fat-free milk   90

           total breakfast calories   **449**

snack: 6-ounce container fat-free, sugar-free
           yogurt, plain or any flavor   111
           1 ounce walnuts   185

           total snack calories   **296**

lunch: 6-inch fast-food ham submarine
           sandwich   290
           1/2 cup mixed fresh fruit   50
           8 ounces fat-free milk   90

           total lunch calories   **430**

snack: 1 medium banana   105

dinner: 3 ounces Honey-Lime Flank Steak
           (page 464)   162
           1/2 cup cooked brown rice, cooked
           in salt-free beef broth   108
           1 cup cooked broccoli, cooked in   44
           2 teaspoons olive or canola oil   80
           1 Pan-Style Whole Wheat Dinner
           Roll (page 617) with   109
           1 teaspoon light tub margarine   13
           1/2 cup Pumpkin Praline Mousse
           (page 655)   188

           total dinner calories   **704**

           total daily calories: **1,984**

wednesday

breakfast: 1 omelet made with
$\frac{1}{2}$ cup egg substitute, scrambled
with   60
2 tablespoons fat-free milk, with   11
$\frac{1}{4}$ cup sliced button mushrooms and 4
$\frac{1}{2}$ cup fresh spinach leaves cooked in 3
1 teaspoon olive or canola oil,
then omelet cooked in   40
2 teaspoons light tub margarine   27
$\frac{1}{2}$ whole-wheat English muffin with 67
1 teaspoon light tub margarine and 13
1 tablespoon low-sugar preserves   25
6 ounces low-sodium tomato
or mixed-vegetable juice   40

| | **total breakfast calories** | **290** |

snack: 6-ounce container fat-free,
sugar-free yogurt,
plain or any flavor, with   111
$\frac{1}{2}$ cup raspberries   32

| | **total snack calories** | **143** |

lunch: Sandwich of 3 ounces 97% fat-free, reduced-sodium deli roast beef with	105
2 lettuce leaves,	3
4 slices tomato, and	14
2 teaspoons mustard on	7
2 slices whole-wheat bread	138
1 ounce baked potato chips	110
½ cup blueberries with	41
1 teaspoon sugar	16
8 ounces fat-free milk	90
total lunch calories	**524**
snack: 1 medium banana	**105**
dinner: 3 ounces Bistro Chicken with Fresh Asparagus (page 398)	261
1 cup cooked yellow summer squash with	36
2 teaspoons light tub margarine	27
½ cup cooked couscous, cooked in 98% fat-free, reduced-sodium chicken broth with herbs of choice	88
1 Pan-Style Whole-Wheat Dinner Roll (page 617) with	109
1 teaspoon diet tub margarine	13
½ cup fat-free or light ice cream with	100
½ cup peach slices and	33
¼ cup sliced almonds	206
total dinner calories	**873**
total daily calories:	**1,935**

thursday

breakfast:
1 slice Apple and Dried Cherry
Quick Bread (page 613)   77
1/4 large cantaloupe   69
8 ounces fat-free milk   90

total breakfast calories   236

snack:
1 ounce low-fat Cheddar cheese   49
4 low-salt whole-wheat crackers   71
1 medium apple   72

total snack calories   192

lunch:
1 1/2 cups Flank Steak Salad
with Sesame-Lime Dressing
(page 334)   271
1 crusty French roll with   130
2 teaspoons light tub margarine   27
1 medium tangerine   37
8 ounces fat-free milk   90

total lunch calories   555

snack:
4 Crunchy Cinnamon Chips
(page 256) with   73
1/4 cup Kiwi-Banana Dip (page 258)   50
1 ounce pecans   196

total snack calories   319

dinner: ½ cup Multicolored Marinated
Slaw (page 314)   82
1 Veggie Burger with Gorgonzola
(page 565) with   175
1 multigrain hamburger bun,   150
½ medium tomato, sliced, and   13
2 lettuce leaves   3
½ cup cooked broccoli, cooked in   22
1 teaspoon olive or canola oil   40
1 slice Pear and Apricot Cake
(page 630)   195

total dinner calories	**680**
total daily calories:	**1,982**

friday

breakfast: 8 ounces Banana-Blueberry Smoothie
(page 269)   207
1 whole-wheat English muffin with   134
   2 teaspoons light tub margarine and   27
2 tablespoons low-sugar preserves   50

                    total breakfast calories   418

snack: 2 large rectangles low-fat graham
crackers   108
8 ounces fat-free milk   90
1 cup sliced strawberries with   53
   1 teaspoon sugar   16

                       total snack calories   267

lunch: 1 cup Cream of Triple-Mushroom
Soup (page 273)   105
3 ounces Black-Pepper Chicken
(page 411) (or cooked
skinless chicken) on   155
2 cups torn salad greens with   18
1 medium rib of celery,   10
$\frac{1}{2}$ small cucumber, and   10
4 cherry tomatoes with   10
2 tablespoons vinaigrette, made with
   1$\frac{1}{2}$ tablespoons olive or
   canola oil and   179
   1$\frac{1}{2}$ teaspoons vinegar   1
6-ounce container fat-free, sugar-free
yogurt, any flavor   111

                         total lunch calories   599

snack:	2 tablespoons Creamy Cannellini Dip (page 250)	31
	4 low-salt whole-wheat crackers	71
	total snack calories	**102**
dinner:	$^{1}/_{2}$ cup cubed mango	54
	1 serving Saucy Minute Steak (page 473)	169
	$^{1}/_{2}$ cup cooked whole-wheat pasta with	87
	$^{1}/_{4}$ cup spaghetti sauce	21
	$^{1}/_{2}$ cup Broccoli Bake with Three Cheeses (page 576)	101
	1 wedge Clafouti (page 637)	155
	total dinner calories	**587**
	total daily calories:	**1,973**

saturday

breakfast:	1 cup sliced strawberries with	53
	1 teaspoon sugar	16
	¼ cup egg substitute, scrambled with	30
	1 tablespoon fat-free milk, cooked in	6
	2 teaspoons light tub margarine	27
	2 slices reduced-calorie oat bran toast with	93
	2 teaspoons light tub margarine and	27
	1 tablespoon low-sugar preserves	25
	8 ounces fat-free milk	90
	total breakfast calories	**367**
snack:	10 grapes	35
	2 large rectangles low-fat graham crackers	108
	total snack calories	**143**
lunch:	Sandwich of 2 slices whole-wheat bread with	138
	3 ounces 96% fat-free, low-sodium ham,	92
	2 lettuce leaves,	3
	4 tomato slices, and	14
	2 teaspoons mustard	7
	1 cup Carrot-Pineapple Slaw with Ginger (page 313)	194
	8 ounces fat-free milk	90
	total lunch calories	**538**

snack:	½ cup fat-free or light ice cream with	100
	1 medium banana, sliced, and	105
	2 tablespoons chopped pecans	103
	total snack calories	**308**
dinner:	½ cup Mango-Avocado Salad (page 316)	89
	1½ cups Chicken and Bow-Ties with Green Beans (page 426)	295
	1 cup cooked carrots with	67
	2 teaspoons light tub margarine	27
	1 wedge Clafouti (page 637)	155
	total dinner calories	**633**
	total daily calories:	**1,989**

sunday

breakfast: 2 Pumpkin-Cranberry Pancakes
(page 620) with   225
2 teaspoons diet tub margarine   27
1 medium orange   70
8 ounces fat-free milk   90

total breakfast calories   412

snack: 6-ounce container fat-free,
sugar-free yogurt,
plain or any flavor, with   111
1/2 cup blackberries   31
1 large rectangle low-fat graham
crackers   54

total snack calories   196

lunch: 1 cup Cream of Triple-Mushroom
Soup (page 273)   105
1/2 cup Chicken and Toasted
Walnut Salad (page 330) on   231
1/3 large cantaloupe, sliced   104
1/2 cup cubed pineapple   37

total lunch calories   477

snack: 1 ounce Neufchâtel cheese with   71
1/2 ounce chopped walnuts on   93
4 slices melba toast   78

total snack calories   242

dinner: 3 ounces Salmon with Creamy
Caper Sauce (page 350)   160
½ cup cooked green beans, cooked
in   22
1 teaspoon olive or canola oil   40
6.5-ounce baked potato with skin
with   139
2 teaspoons light tub margarine
and   27
2 teaspoons chopped green onion   2
½ cup Vegetable Salad Vinaigrette
(page 308)   51
1 cup Vanilla Soufflé with B
randy-Plum Sauce (page 651)   191

total dinner calories   632

total daily calories: 1,959

week two • 2,000 calories

You can enjoy a variety of tasty and healthful foods and still keep within your daily calorie allowance. This week's menus offer you plenty of textures and flavors to suit your taste buds while you work toward achieving your weight-loss goals.

monday

breakfast:	6-ounce container fat-free, sugar-free yogurt, any flavor	111
	1/4 cup egg substitute, scrambled with	30
	1 tablespoon fat-free milk, cooked in	6
	2 teaspoons light tub margarine	27
	6 ounces orange juice	84
	1 slice Apple and Dried Cherry Quick Bread (page 613)	77
	total breakfast calories	**335**
snack:	1 medium nectarine	60
	2 large rectangles low-fat graham crackers	108
	8 ounces fat-free milk	90
	total snack calories	**258**

lunch:	1 1/2 cups Tuna Pasta Provençal (page 325)	300
	1 cup cooked asparagus, drizzled with	40
	1 teaspoon olive or canola oil	40
	2 slices melba toast	39
	total lunch calories	**419**
snack:	3 cups light microwave popcorn	63
	1 cup hot chocolate, made with	
	8 ounces fat-free milk and	90
	2 tablespoons light chocolate syrup	50
	total snack calories	**203**
dinner:	2 slices Barbeque Chicken Pizza (page 441)	346
	Salad of 2 cups torn salad greens,	18
	1/4 cup chopped tomatoes,	8
	1/4 cup sliced celery,	4
	1/4 cup sliced carrots, and	13
	1/4 chopped cauliflower with	6
	2 tablespoons vinaigrette, made with	
	1 1/2 tablespoons olive or canola oil and	179
	1 1/2 teaspoons vinegar	1
	1 slice Pear and Apricot Cake (page 630)	195
	total dinner calories	**770**
	total daily calories:	**1,985**

tuesday

breakfast: 1 biscuit with bacon (fast food)   360
6 ounces orange juice   84

      total breakfast calories   **444**

snack: 1 ounce Neufchâtel cheese   71
4 low-salt whole-wheat crackers   71
8 ounces fat-free milk   90

      total snack calories   **232**

lunch: 2 cups Fruit and Spinach Salad
with Fresh Mint (page 304) with   126
2 ounces boneless, skinless cooked
chicken breast   94
5 saltines with unsalted tops   63
½ cup fat-free or light ice cream with   100
1 tablespoon pecans   47

      total lunch calories   **430**

snack: 10 dried apricot halves   84
4 Crunchy Cinnamon Chips
(page 256)   73

      total snack calories   **157**

dinner: 1½ cups Tuna and Broccoli
with Lemon-Caper Brown Rice
(page 379)   257
2 cups Greek Salad with Sun-Dried
Tomato Vinaigrette (page 300)   84
1 cup cooked carrots with fat-free
spray margarine   67
1 slice Garlic Bread (page 611)   103
½ cup Pumpkin Praline Mousse
(page 655)   188

total dinner calories   699

total daily calories: 1,962

wednesday

breakfast: 1 cup Fruit-and-Cinnamon
Oatmeal (page 626) · · · · · · · · · · · · 289
1 cup hot chocolate, made with
8 ounces fat-free milk and · · · · · · · · 90
2 tablespoons light chocolate syrup · · 50

total breakfast calories · · · **429**

snack: 6-ounce container fat-free,
sugar-free yogurt,
plain or any flavor, with · · · · · · · · · 111
½ cup blueberries · · · · · · · · · · · · · · 41

total snack calories · · · **152**

lunch: Salad of 2 cups torn lettuce leaves, · · · 11
1 medium tomato, sliced, · · · · · · · · · 27
½ cup sliced button mushrooms, · · · · 8
¼ medium red bell pepper, sliced, · · · 8
1 tablespoon sliced green onion, and · · 3
3-ounce can white tuna in distilled
or spring water, drained, with · · · · · · 109
2 tablespoons vinaigrette, made with
1½ tablespoons olive or
canola oil and · · · · · · · · · · · · · · · 179
1½ teaspoons vinegar · · · · · · · · · · · 1
1 crusty French roll with · · · · · · · · · 130
2 teaspoons light tub margarine · · · · · 27
8 ounces fat-free milk · · · · · · · · · · · 90

total lunch calories · · · **593**

snack:	1 ounce part-skim mozzarella cheese	72
	4 low-salt whole-wheat crackers	71
	total snack calories	**143**

dinner:	1¹¹/₂ cups Soba Noodles in Peanut Sauce (page 528)	377
	¹/₂ cup cooked pea pods, cooked in	35
	1 teaspoon olive or canola oil	40
	¹/₂ cup mandarin oranges canned in light syrup with	77
	¹/₂ medium banana	53
	¹/₂ cup fat-free or light ice cream	100
	total dinner calories	**682**
	total daily calories:	**1,999**

thursday

breakfast:	8 ounces Banana-Blueberry Smoothie (page 269)	207
	1 3-inch fat-free or low-fat frozen waffle with	60
	1 teaspoon light tub margarine	13
	total breakfast calories	**280**
snack:	2 medium apricots	34
	4 Crunchy Cinnamon Chips (page 256)	73
	total snack calories	**107**
lunch:	1½ cups Easy Two-Bean Chili, without sour cream and cheese (page 541)	249
	½ cup Mango-Avocado Salad (page 316)	89
	2 6-inch corn tortillas with	62
	2 teaspoons light tub margarine	27
	2 ginger snaps	58
	8 ounces fat-free milk	90
	total lunch calories	**575**
snack:	1 cup Peach Blush (page 268)	119
	1 ounce almonds	169
	total snack calories	**288**

dinner: 1 serving Pork Tenderloin
with Cranberry Salsa
(3 ounces pork with ½ cup salsa)
(page 497)   222
1 medium baked sweet potato with   130
2 teaspoons light tub margarine   27
1 cup cooked green beans, cooked in   44
2 teaspoons olive or canola oil   80
1 Pan-Style Whole-Wheat Dinner
Roll (page 617) with   109
1 teaspoon light tub margarine   13
½ cup fat-free or light ice cream   100
total dinner calories   **725**

total daily calories: **1,975**

friday

breakfast:	1 cup Fruit-and-Cinnamon Oatmeal (page 626)	289
	³⁄4 ounce sliced almonds	126
	8 ounces fat-free milk	90
	total breakfast calories	**505**
snack:	½ cup canned pineapple tidbits in their own juice	**54**
lunch:	1½ cups Chilled Tomato-Basil Soup (page 278)	84
	½ cup Chicken and Toasted Walnut Salad (page 330) on	231
	1 whole-wheat English muffin	134
	½ cup cubed cantaloupe and	27
	½ cup cubed watermelon	23
	total lunch calories	**499**
snack:	Milkshake made of 8 ounces fat-free milk,	90
	½ cup fat-free or light vanilla or chocolate ice cream, and	100
	2 tablespoons light chocolate syrup	50
	total snack calories	**240**

dinner: 1 slice Meat Loaf with a Twist
(page 483) 209
½ cup Asparagus and Cucumber
Salad with Lemon and Mint
(page 306) 39
1 cup cooked yellow summer
squash with 36
2 teaspoons light tub margarine 27
½ cup cooked brown rice, cooked
in salt-free beef broth 108
1 Pan-Style Whole-Wheat Dinner
Roll (page 617) with 109
1 teaspoon light tub margarine 13
½12 angel food cake from mix 140
total dinner calories **681**

total daily calories: **1,979**

saturday

breakfast:	1 Peach Cornmeal Waffle (page 622) with	192
	2 teaspoons light tub margarine	27
	6 ounces orange juice	84
	total breakfast calories	**303**

snack:	2 Applesauce Oatmeal Cookies (page 648)	105
	8 ounces fat-free milk	90
	total snack calories	**195**

lunch:	1 cup Cream of Triple-Mushroom Soup (page 273)	105
	1 medium baked potato with	100
	1 tablespoon light tub margarine,	40
	½ ounce reduced-fat Cheddar cheese, and	41
	1 tablespoon chopped green onion	3
	8 ounces fat-free milk	90
	6-ounce container fat-free, sugar-free yogurt, plain or any flavor, with	111
	½ cup raspberries	32
	total lunch calories	**522**

snack:	1 Frozen Chocolate Banana Pop (page 261)	120
	2 large rectangles low-fat graham crackers	108
	total snack calories	**228**

dinner:	1 serving Salmon Florentine (3 ounces salmon and ½ cup spinach) (page 348)	199
	2 cups Chopped Salad with Gorgonzola (page 298)	116
	½ cup Orzo with Tomato and Capers (page 594)	107
	1 Pan-Style Whole-Wheat Dinner Roll (page 617) with	109
	1 teaspoons light tub margarine	13
	1 slice Pear and Apricot Cake (page 630)	195
	total dinner calories	**739**
	total daily calories:	**1,987**

sunday

breakfast:	¼ large cantaloupe, sliced	69
	1½ slices Crisp French Toast (page 624) with	168
	2 tablespoons light, sugar-free pancake syrup	50
	8 ounces fat-free milk	90
	total breakfast calories	**377**
snack:	1 ounce Neufchâtel cheese	71
	4 low-salt whole-wheat crackers	71
	total snack calories	**142**
lunch:	Sandwich of 1 slice Meat Loaf with a Twist (page 483) with	209
	1 tablespoon no-salt-added ketchup and	16
	2 slices whole-wheat bread	138
	1 medium ear corn on the cob with fat-free spray margarine	77
	½ cup Carrot-Pineapple Slaw with Ginger (page 313)	97
	total lunch calories	**537**
snack:	½ cup fat-free or light ice cream	**100**

dinner: 1 serving Chicken Breasts
with Spinach, Apricots,
and Pine Nuts (page 407)   310

2 cups Greek Salad with Sun-Dried
Tomato Vinaigrette (page 300)   84

1/2 cup cooked whole-wheat pasta,
cooked in
98% fat-free, reduced-sodium
chicken broth, with   87

1 teaspoon olive or canola oil   40

1 Pan-Style Whole-Wheat Dinner
Roll (page 617) with   109

1 teaspoon light tub margarine   13

2 pieces Chocolate Chocolate
Biscotti (page 643)   198

total dinner calories   **841**

total daily calories: **1,997**

about the recipes

When you need delectable recipes for a healthful meal for yourself and your family or friends, look no further. The following pages provide almost 200 recipes, each designed to help you meet the American Heart Association dietary guidelines deliciously. Choose just an entrée or create a whole meal from soup to dessert. You'll find many winning recipes that will satisfy any successful loser's palette and meet your daily calorie-intake level. You'll be tempted to try them all!

To help keep track of your calorie intake, look for the handy calorie bar at the end of each recipe. At a glance, you'll be able to see the number of calories for each recipe and determine how it will fit into your daily eating plan. (Each recipe has been rounded to the nearest 50.)

Also, look for "Recipes by Calorie Count," opposite. This chart will help you easily identify groups of recipes that fall within a certain calorie range. Use this chart if you need to replace a recipe on our sample menu plans with another recipe that has a similar amount of calories.

using the recipes

To help you with meal planning, we have carefully analyzed each recipe in this book to provide useful nutrition information. Each recipe includes a nutrition analysis that lists the number of calories and the amount of total fat, saturated fat, polyunsaturated fat, monounsaturated fat, cholesterol, sodium, carbohydrate, fiber, and protein in one serving. Here are some other important things you should know about the analyses.

- When ingredient options are listed, the first one is analyzed.
- When a range of ingredients is given, the average is analyzed.
- Values for saturated, monounsaturated, and polyunsaturated fats are rounded and may not

add up to the amount listed for total fat. Total fat also includes other fatty substances and glycerol.

- The reduced-fat cheese we use for analysis has no more than 3 grams of fat per serving.

- When meat, poultry, or seafood is marinated and the marinade is discarded, we calculate only the amount of marinade absorbed, using data from the U.S. Department of Agriculture.

- Meat statistics are based on cooked lean meat with all visible fat removed.

- Values for ground beef are used on meat that is 90 percent fat free.

- We use the abbreviations "g" for gram and "mg" for milligram.

- If a recipe calls for alcohol, we estimate that most of the alcohol calories evaporate during the cooking process.

recipes by calorie count

appetizers, snacks, and beverages

RECIPE TITLE	CALORIES
Dilled Yogurt Dipping Sauce	21
Cucumber and Avocado Dip	23
Artichoke and Spinach Dip	25

soups

RECIPE TITLE	CALORIES
Artichoke and Spinach Soup	198
Bayou Andouille and Chicken Chowder	206
Wild Rice and Chicken Chowder	245
Vegetable Beef Soup	245
Market-Fresh Fish and Vegetable Soup	269
Chicken Minestrone	278

salads

RECIPE TITLE	CALORIES
Asparagus and Cucumber Salad with Lemon and Mint	39
Vegetable Salad Vinaigrette	51
Zingy Carrot Salad	60
Black-Eyed Pea Salad	75
Greek Potato and Artichoke Salad	82
Multicolored Marinated Slaw	82
Greek Salad with Sun-Dried Tomato Vinaigrette	84
Broccoli and Edamame Salad with Dill	86
Mango-Avocado Salad	89
Asian Citrus Salad	90
Carrot-Pineapple Slaw with Ginger	97
Baby Greens with Spiced Cranberry Vinaigrette	106

seafood

RECIPE TITLE	CALORIES
Skillet-Poached Salmon with Wasabi and Soy Sauce	205
Cajun-Creole Stuffed Sole	226
Cumin Shrimp and Rice Toss	247
Fish Tacos with Tomato and Avocado Salsa	252
Tuna and Broccoli with Lemon-Caper Brown Rice	257
Hazelnut-Crusted Trout with Balsamic Glaze	267
Jambalaya	282
Tomato-Caper Shrimp with Herbed Feta	294
Lime-Cilantro Swordfish with Mixed Bean and Pineapple Salsa	295
Pasta with Salmon, Roasted Mushrooms, and Asparagus	299
Baked Almond-Crunch Sea Bass	306
Gourmet Tuna-Noodle Casserole	321
Tropical Tuna Hero Sandwiches	358
Shrimp and Lemon-Basil Pasta	381

poultry

RECIPE TITLE	CALORIES
Slow-Roasted Sage Turkey Breast	122
Sunday-Best Roast Chicken Breasts	127

RECIPE TITLE	CALORIES
Chicken Enchiladas	331
Barbecue Chicken Pizza	346
Risotto with Porcini Mushrooms and Chicken	388
Chicken Parmesan Supreme	395
Chicken with Penne Pasta and Mixed Greens	421

meats

RECIPE TITLE	CALORIES
Honey-Lime Flank Steak	162
Pork Tenderloin with Orange-Ginger Sweet Potatoes	167
Saucy Minute Steaks	169
Lamb Kebabs with Apricot-Rosemary Dipping Sauce	190
Beef Tenderloin with Horseradish Cream	200
Meat Loaf with a Twist	209
Satay-Style Sirloin with Peanut Dipping Sauce	217
Pork Tenderloin with Cranberry Salsa	222
Orange Beef Stir-Fry	235
Filet Mignon with Balsamic Berry Sauce	238

vegetarian entrées

RECIPE TITLE	CALORIES
Veggie Burgers with Gorgonzola	175
Garden Veggie Tostadas	191
Fried Rice with Snow Peas, Bell Pepper, and Water Chestnuts	201
Creole Ratatouille	203
One-Pot Vegetable and Grain Medley	239
Easy Two-Bean Chili (without sour cream and cheese)	247
Penne with Matchstick Zucchini and Mozzarella Cubes	247
Pesto Florentine Pasta	256
Mediterranean Vegetable Stew	267
Stuffed Shells with Arugula and Four Cheeses	273
Make-Ahead Manicotti	274
Cajun Red Beans and Brown Rice	284
Spinach and Bean Quesadillas with Homemade Salsa (without sour cream)	284
Easy Two-Bean Chili (with sour cream and cheese)	284
Braised Edamame with Bok Choy	293
Couscous with Bell Pepper and Pine Nuts	295
Mushroom and Artichoke Gnocchi with Capers	297
Spinach and Bean Quesadillas with Homemade Salsa (with sour cream)	319

vegetables and side dishes

RECIPE TITLE	CALORIES
Orzo with Tomato and Capers	107
Red Cabbage Braised with Balsamic Vinegar	112
Oven-Fried Eggplant	124
Pesto and Pecan Rice	126
Italian Barley and Mushrooms	133
Creole Lentils	139

breads and breakfast dishes

RECIPE TITLE	CALORIES
Apple and Dried Cherry Quick Bread	77
Dinner Biscuits	81
Garlic Bread	103
Pan-Style Whole-Wheat Dinner Rolls	109
Crisp French Toast	168
Peach Cornmeal Waffles	192
Pumpkin-Cranberry Pancakes	225
Fruit-and-Cinnamon Oatmeal	289

desserts

RECIPE TITLE	CALORIES
Fruit and Yogurt Sauce	31
Fruit Sauce	33

appetizers, snacks, and beverages

Cucumber and Avocado Dip

Artichoke and Spinach Dip

Creamy Cannellini Dip

Fruit Kebabs with Dipping Sauces

Crunchy Cinnamon Chips

Kiwi-Banana Dip

Dilled Yogurt Dipping Sauce

Frozen Chocolate Banana Pops

Wrapped Asparagus Spears
   with Tarragon Aïoli

Orange Froth

Green Tea Latte

Peach Blush

Banana-Blueberry Smoothie

cucumber and avocado dip
Serves 12; 2 tablespoons per serving

So cool and creamy, this jade-green dip is the perfect accompaniment to a platter of raw or grilled vegetables. You also can use it to top a baked potato for an interesting side dish.

1 medium cucumber

1 small avocado (about 4 ounces)

¼ cup fat-free or light sour cream

2 teaspoons snipped fresh dillweed or ½ teaspoon dried, crumbled

1 teaspoon grated lime zest

1 tablespoon fresh lime juice

¼ teaspoon salt

Peel the cucumber and cut in half lengthwise. Using a spoon, remove and discard the seeds. Cut the cucumber into 1-inch slices. Peel and dice the avocado.

In a food processor or blender, process all the ingredients until smooth.

Serve immediately, or cover and refrigerate for up to two days.

PER SERVING ··

calories 23
total fat 1.5 g
 saturated 0.0 g
 polyunsaturated 0.0 g
 monounsaturated 1.0 g
cholesterol 1 mg

sodium 54 mg
carbohydrates 2 g
 fiber 1 g
 sugar 1 g
protein 1 g

100   200   300   400   **DIETARY EXCHANGES**
½ fat

artichoke and spinach dip
Serves 30; 2 tablespoons per serving

Serve this robust dip with raw bell pepper strips of assorted colors, carrot and celery sticks, and broccoli or cauliflower florets. It also partners well with steamed vegetables or toasted wedges of pita bread.

15- to 16-ounce can no-salt-added cannellini beans, rinsed and drained

4 medium green onions (green and white parts), chopped

2 medium garlic cloves, minced

14-ounce can quartered artichoke hearts, rinsed and drained, or 10-ounce package frozen artichoke hearts, thawed and drained

10 ounces frozen chopped spinach, thawed and squeezed dry

1 cup fat-free or low-fat plain yogurt or fat-free or light sour cream

1 teaspoon grated lemon zest

3 tablespoons fresh lemon juice

1/2 teaspoon ground cumin

1/4 teaspoon crushed red pepper flakes

1/4 teaspoon salt

1/4 teaspoon pepper

In a food processor or blender, process the beans, green onions, and garlic until smooth, scraping the side several times.

Add the remaining ingredients. Process until smooth.

Transfer the dip to a container with a tight-fitting lid. Refrigerate for 2 hours to 4 days before serving.

PER SERVING

calories 25
total fat 0.0 g
  saturated 0.0 g
  polyunsaturated 0.0 g
  monounsaturated 0.0 g
cholesterol 0 mg

sodium 56 mg
carbohydrates 5 g
fiber 1 g
sugar 1 g
protein 2 g

100 200 300 400

DIETARY EXCHANGES
1 vegetable

creamy cannellini dip

Serves 16; 2 tablespoons per serving

Bits of roasted red bell pepper add texture and color to this tantalizing dip.

15- to 16-ounce can no-salt-added cannellini beans, rinsed and drained

1/4 cup fat-free or light sour cream

2 tablespoons snipped fresh parsley

1 tablespoon fresh lemon juice

1 large garlic clove, minced

1/2 teaspoon red hot-pepper sauce, or to taste

1/4 teaspoon salt

7-ounce jar roasted red bell peppers, rinsed and drained

In a food processor or blender, process all the ingredients except the bell peppers for 15 to 20 seconds, or until almost smooth.

Add the peppers. Pulse until the peppers are distributed throughout the dip but are still large enough to add texture. Cover and refrigerate for 2 to 48 hours.

Stir before serving.

COOK'S TIP ON SNIPPING PARSLEY:
To easily cut parsley down to size, put a small amount in a custard cup. Point kitchen shears or small, sharp scissors down into the cup. Snip until the parsley reaches the desired fineness.

PER SERVING

calories 31
total fat 0.0 g
  saturated 0.0 g
  polyunsaturated 0.0 g
  monounsaturated 0.0 g
cholesterol 1 mg

sodium 87 mg
carbohydrates 6 g
fiber 1 g
sugar 1 g
protein 2 g

100 200 300 400

DIETARY EXCHANGES
$^{1}/_{2}$ starch

fruit kebabs with dipping sauces

Serves 4; ½ cup fruit and 2 tablespoons sauce per serving

Serve these attractive kebabs with your choice of three yogurt dipping sauces, all of which are great dressings for fruit salad. Substitute in-season fruits when making the kebabs, if you wish.

Yucatán, Maple-Peanut, or Poppy Seed Dipping Sauce (recipes follow)

4 1-inch pineapple cubes

12 seedless red grapes

4 large strawberries, hulled

2 medium green kiwifruit, peeled and cut in half vertically

In a small bowl, stir together the ingredients for your choice of sauce. Cover and refrigerate for at least 1 hour.

Slide the fruit onto four 6-inch bamboo skewers, in the following order: pineapple, grape, strawberry, grape, kiwifruit, grape. (The grapes keep the strawberries from discoloring the other fruits.)

Serve the kebabs with the chilled dipping sauce.

yucatán dipping sauce

½ cup fat-free or low-fat vanilla yogurt
½ tablespoon fresh lime juice
¼ teaspoon cayenne, or to taste
Pinch of salt

maple-peanut dipping sauce

½ cup fat-free or low-fat plain yogurt
1 tablespoon reduced-fat smooth peanut butter
1 teaspoon maple syrup
Pinch of salt

poppy seed dipping sauce

½ cup fat-free or low-fat vanilla yogurt
1 teaspoon poppy seeds
½ teaspoon very finely grated onion, or to taste
¼ to ½ teaspoon raspberry vinegar
⅛ to ¼ teaspoon dry mustard
Pinch of salt

COOK'S TIP: To prepare in advance, wrap each kebab in wax paper or plastic wrap and refrigerate. Bananas, apples, and pears aren't recommended for this recipe because they turn brown once exposed to the air. (Brushing with pineapple or citrus juice won't prevent browning long enough for use on a buffet.) For a beautiful buffet presentation, wipe the leaves of a whole pineapple with vegetable oil so they shine. Cut off the bottom of the pineapple to create a flat, stable base. Place the pineapple on a serving plate. Triple or quadruple the amount of fruit to make more skewers. Stick the skewers into the pineapple. Make additional sauce or serve more than one of the sauces.

YUCATÁN DIPPING SAUCE

PER SERVING

calories 76

total fat 0.5 g

 saturated 0.0 g

 polyunsaturated 0.0 g

 monounsaturated 0.0 g

cholesterol 1 mg

sodium 60 mg

carbohydrates 17 g

fiber 2 g

sugar 14 g

protein 2 g

100 200 300 400

DIETARY EXCHANGES
1 fruit; $^1/_2$ very lean meat

MAPLE-PEANUT DIPPING SAUCE

PER SERVING

calories 92
total fat 2.0 g
 saturated 0.5 g
 polyunsaturated 0.0 g
 monounsaturated 0.0 g
cholesterol 1 mg

sodium 94 mg
carbohydrates 17 g
fiber 2 g
sugar 12 g
protein 4 g

100 200 300 400

DIETARY EXCHANGES
1 fruit; ½ lean meat

POPPY SEED DIPPING SAUCE

PER SERVING

calories 79
total fat 0.5 g
 saturated 0.0 g
 polyunsaturated 0.5 g
 monounsaturated 0.0 g
cholesterol 1 mg

sodium 60 mg
carbohydrates 17 g
fiber 2 g
sugar 14 g
protein 3 g

100 200 300 400

DIETARY EXCHANGES
1 fruit; ½ very lean meat

crunchy cinnamon chips

Serves 4; 4 cinnamon chips per serving

These tasty chips are perfect for a snack, or serve them with Kiwi-Banana Dip on the facing page for a light dessert.

$\frac{1}{2}$ tablespoon sugar

$\frac{1}{2}$ tablespoon firmly packed light brown sugar

$\frac{1}{4}$ teaspoon ground cinnamon

2 8-inch fat-free or low-fat flour tortillas
  Vegetable oil spray

Preheat the oven to 375°F.

In a small bowl, stir together the sugars and cinnamon.

Stack the tortillas and cut them into 8 equal triangles (16 total). Put the triangles in a single layer on an ungreased baking sheet. Lightly spray with vegetable oil spray. Sprinkle with the sugar mixture.

Bake for 6 to 8 minutes, or until the chips are light brown and beginning to crisp. Transfer to a serving plate to cool. (As the chips cool, they will become crisper.)

PER SERVING

calories 73
total fat 0.5 g
 saturated 0.0 g
 polyunsaturated 0.0 g
 monounsaturated 0.0 g
cholesterol 0 mg

sodium 171 mg
carbohydrates 15 g
fiber 1 g
sugar 4 g
protein 2 g

100 200 300 400 **DIETARY EXCHANGES**
1 starch

kiwi-banana dip

Serves 4; $\frac{1}{4}$ cup per serving

Be adventurous with this dip by using a variety of fruit.

$\frac{1}{4}$ cup fat-free or low-fat plain yogurt
1 tablespoon dried cherries or dried sweetened cranberries
1 tablespoon all-fruit orange marmalade (optional)
1 small banana, sliced or quartered
1 green kiwifruit, peeled and chopped

In a small bowl, stir together the ingredients.

PER SERVING

calories 50
total fat 0.0 g
  saturated 0.0 g
  polyunsaturated 0.0 g
  monounsaturated 0.0 g
cholesterol 0 mg

sodium 13 mg
carbohydrates 11 g
fiber 1 g
sugar 7 g
protein 2 g

100   200   300   400   **DIETARY EXCHANGES**
1 fruit

dilled yogurt dipping sauce

Serves 4; 2 tablespoons per serving

This zingy dill dip is refreshing and delightful with raw, broiled, or grilled vegetables.

¼ cup plus 2 tablespoons fat-free or low-fat plain yogurt

2 tablespoons fat-free or light mayonnaise dressing

½ to ¾ teaspoon dried dillweed, crumbled

¼ teaspoon salt

In a small bowl, stir together the ingredients. Cover with plastic wrap and refrigerate until needed.

COOK'S TIP ON BROILED VEGETABLES:
When you broil vegetables to use as dippers, let them cool to room temperature, about 10 minutes. They will have a firmer texture and therefore be better for dipping.

PER SERVING

calories 21

total fat 0.0 g
  saturated 0.0 g
  polyunsaturated 0.0 g
  monounsaturated 0.0 g
cholesterol 1 mg

sodium 226 mg
carbohydrates 3 g
fiber 0 g
sugar 3 g
protein 1 g

100   200   300   400   **DIETARY EXCHANGES**
Free

frozen chocolate banana pops

Serves 4; 1 pop per serving

Young children will enjoy helping you prepare this fun after-school snack. Keep a supply handy in the freezer for a quick, filling nibble—for you and for them.

1 cup fat-free or low-fat plain yogurt

1 very ripe medium banana, mashed ($1/3$ to $1/2$ cup)

$1/2$ teaspoon vanilla extract

1 tablespoon mini semisweet chocolate chips

2 tablespoons fat-free chocolate syrup

2 teaspoons mini semisweet chocolate chips

2 teaspoons fat-free chocolate syrup

In small bowl, stir together the yogurt, banana, and vanilla.

Stir in 1 tablespoon chocolate chips and 2 tablespoons chocolate syrup.

To assemble, divide the remaining 2 teaspoons chocolate chips into four 4- to 7-ounce paper or plastic juice cups. Spoon 3 tablespoons yogurt mixture over the chips in each cup. Spoon the remaining 2 teaspoons chocolate syrup over the banana mixture. Top with the remaining banana mixture.

Insert a wooden craft or Popsicle stick into the center of each filled cup. Cover with plastic wrap or aluminum foil, poking the stick through the covering. Place the cups with the stick side up on a flat surface in the freezer. Freeze for 2 hours, or until frozen.

To serve, uncover and peel the frozen pops, or gently squeeze them out of the cups.

PER SERVING

calories 120

total fat 1.5 g

  saturated 1.0 g

  polyunsaturated 0.0 g

  monounsaturated 0.5 g

cholesterol 1 mg

sodium 56 mg

carbohydrates 23 g

fiber 1 g

sugar 16 g

protein 4 g

100 200 300 400

DIETARY EXCHANGES

$\frac{1}{2}$ skim milk; $\frac{1}{2}$ fruit; $\frac{1}{2}$ other carbohydrate

wrapped asparagus spears with tarragon aïoli

Serves 6; 2 wrapped asparagus spears per serving

Aïoli (**ay-OH-lee**), which is mayonnaise flavored with garlic, adds an elegant touch to this super-easy-to-make finger food.

½ cup fat-free or light mayonnaise dressing

1 teaspoon chopped fresh tarragon or ¼ teaspoon dried, crumbled

⅛ teaspoon garlic powder

⅛ teaspoon grated lemon zest

Dash of cayenne

12 asparagus spears

12 thin slices skinless deli turkey or chicken (about 5 ounces), all visible fat discarded

For the aïoli, stir together the mayonnaise, tarragon, garlic powder, lemon zest, and cayenne. Cover and refrigerate for at least 3 hours to allow the flavors to blend.

Trim the asparagus, removing 1 inch or more but still leaving the spears long enough so that at least ¼ inch of the tip will extend beyond the turkey once wrapped.

Fill a Dutch oven with about 4 inches of water. Bring to a boil over high heat. Cook the asparagus for 3 minutes. Remove the asparagus immediately and plunge it into a bowl of ice water. This stops the cooking process and locks in the bright green color of the asparagus. Drain well and pat dry thoroughly.

To assemble, place a slice of turkey with a long edge toward you. Spread 1 tablespoon aïoli on the turkey, leaving a ¼-inch border uncovered. Place an asparagus spear at one short end of the turkey with the bottom of the spear aligned with the lower edge of the turkey. The asparagus will extend above the top edge of the turkey. Roll up jelly-roll style and place with the seam side down on a platter. Repeat with the remaining ingredients. Refrigerate until ready to serve.

COOK'S TIP ON AÏOLI: You can add any herbs of your choice—such as basil, oregano, cilantro, or dillweed—to flavor aïoli, or try sun-dried tomatoes or chipotle peppers. If you have any leftover aïoli, mix it with tuna canned in distilled or spring water for a quick and delicious lunch or dinner entrée.

PER SERVING

calories 55
total fat 0.5 g
  saturated 0.0 g
  polyunsaturated 0.0 g
  monounsaturated 0.0 g
cholesterol 10 mg

sodium 457 mg
carbohydrates 5 g
fiber 1 g
sugar 4 g
protein 5 g

100 200 300 400 **DIETARY EXCHANGES**
1 vegetable;
½ very lean meat

orange froth

Serves 4; $^1/_2$ cup per serving

For a refreshing lift, try this easy way to enjoy one of your daily fruit servings.

2 cups crushed ice
6-ounce can frozen orange juice concentrate
6 ounces lime-flavored sparkling water

Put the crushed ice and orange juice concentrate in a blender or food processor. Process until smooth.

Pour in the sparkling water. Process just long enough to combine.

PER SERVING

calories 68
total fat 0.0 g
  saturated 0.0 g
  polyunsaturated 0.0 g
  monounsaturated 0.0 g
cholesterol 0 mg

sodium 4 mg
carbohydrates 16 g
fiber 0 g
sugar 16 g
protein 1 g

100 200 300 400   **DIETARY EXCHANGES**
1 fruit

green tea latte

Serves 4; 1 cup per serving

This frothy beverage—garnished with festive fruit—is a great conversation piece at parties. Keep chilled green tea and a variety of fruit juices, such as apricot, mango, guava, and tropical blends, on hand so you can make it anytime.

1 cup water
4 bags green tea
1 cup fruit nectar or fruit juice, such as apricot, mango, guava, or tropical blend
1 cup fat-free milk or vanilla soy milk
1 cup ice cubes
1/2 star fruit, cut crosswise into 4 slices (optional)

In a small saucepan, bring the water to a boil over high heat. Remove from the heat. Put the tea bags in the water and let steep, covered, for 5 minutes. Discard the tea bags.

In a blender, process the tea and the remaining ingredients except the star fruit until smooth. Pour the mixture into tall glasses.

Cut a small slit in each of the star fruit slices. Place a slice over the rim of each glass.

COOK'S TIP ON STAR FRUIT:

Also called carambola, star fruit looks like a star when cut crosswise. Do not peel it before slicing. Look for star fruit from August through February. If it is not available, you can substitute 4 large strawberries or orange, lemon, or lime slices.

PER SERVING

calories 59
total fat 0.0 g
 saturated 0.0 g
 polyunsaturated 0.0 g
 monounsaturated 0.0 g
cholesterol 1 mg

sodium 36 mg
carbohydrates 13 g
fiber 1 g
sugar 12 g
protein 2 g

100   200   300   400   DIETARY EXCHANGES
1 fruit

peach blush

Serves 4; 1 cup per serving

Served as a slush in chilled wine glasses or with straws in tall, skinny glasses, this beverage is great as is or with a splash of rum or vodka.

12 ounces unsweetened frozen peach slices
1½ cups sweetened cranberry juice
  12-ounce can diet ginger ale
¼ cup frozen orange juice concentrate

In a blender or food processor, process all the ingredients until smooth. Serve immediately.

PER SERVING

calories 119
total fat 0.5 g
  saturated 0.0 g
  polyunsaturated 0.5 g
  monounsaturated 0.5 g
cholesterol 0 mg

sodium 25 mg
carbohydrates 28 g
fiber 2 g
sugar 23 g
protein 1 g

100	200	300	400	DIETARY EXCHANGES
■■				2 fruit

banana-blueberry smoothie

Serves 2; 1 cup per serving

Here's an easy and satisfying breakfast that gets you going—and keeps you going.

8 ounces fat-free milk

6 or 8 ounces fat-free, sugar-free plain yogurt

1 cup fresh or frozen blueberries

1 medium banana

Put all the ingredients in a blender or food processor. Process until smooth.

PER SERVING

calories 207
total fat 0.5 g
  saturated 0.0 g
  polyunsaturated 0.0 g
  monounsaturated 0.0 g
cholesterol 4 mg

sodium 161 mg
carbohydrates 40 g
fiber 3 g
sugar 30 g
protein 13 g

100	200	300	400

DIETARY EXCHANGES
1½ fruit; 1½ skim milk

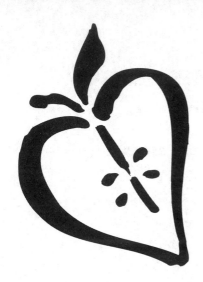

soups

Artichoke and Spinach Soup

Cream of Triple-Mushroom Soup

Curried Pumpkin Soup

Chilled Tomato-Basil Soup

Quick Mexican-Style Soup

Egg Drop Soup with Crabmeat
and Vegetables

Market-Fresh Fish
and Vegetable Soup

Chicken Minestrone

Wild Rice and Chicken Chowder

Vegetable Beef Soup

Bayou Andouille and Chicken
Chowder

Lima Bean Soup

artichoke and spinach soup
Serves 4; 1 cup per serving

Baby spinach leaves provide the vibrant green color of this thick, smooth soup, and artichokes and navy beans give it a mellow flavor. Serve with crusty multigrain rolls.

1 teaspoon olive oil

8 cups baby spinach leaves

4 medium green onions (green and white parts), chopped

15-ounce can no-salt-added navy beans, rinsed and drained

9 ounces frozen artichoke hearts, thawed and drained

1 cup fat-free, low-sodium chicken broth

1/2 cup fat-free half-and-half

1 teaspoon dried dillweed, crumbled

1/4 teaspoon salt

1/4 teaspoon pepper

1/4 cup crumbled fat-free or reduced-fat feta cheese

2 tablespoons shredded or grated Parmesan cheese

Heat a medium saucepan over medium heat. Pour the oil into the pan and swirl to coat the bottom. Cook the spinach and green onions for 1 to 2 minutes, or until the spinach is wilted, stirring occasionally.

In a food processor or blender, process the spinach mixture with the beans, artichokes, and broth until smooth. Pour the mixture back into the saucepan.

Stir in the half-and-half, dillweed, salt, and pepper. Cook over medium heat for 6 to 8 minutes, or until the mixture is warmed through, stirring occasionally.

Stir in the feta and Parmesan. Cook for 1 minute, or until the cheese is melted, stirring occasionally.

PER SERVING

calories 198
total fat 2.0 g
  saturated 0.5 g
  polyunsaturated 0.0 g
  monounsaturated 1.0 g
cholesterol 2 mg

sodium 474 mg
carbohydrates 32 g
  fiber 11 g
  sugar 7 g
protein 15 g

100   200   300   400

DIETARY EXCHANGES
$1\frac{1}{2}$ starch;
$1\frac{1}{2}$ vegetable;
1 very lean meat

cream of triple-mushroom soup

Serves 6; 1 cup per serving

This impressive soup combines dried and fresh mushrooms in a very rich tasting starter for family or guests.

1/2 ounce dried morel mushrooms

1/2 ounce dried chanterelle mushrooms

3/4 cup chopped button mushrooms

2 cups Vegetable Broth (recipe follows) or commercial fat-free, low-sodium vegetable broth

1 cup chopped onions

2 tablespoons low-salt soy sauce

1/2 cup whole-wheat flour

1/2 cup water

1 teaspoon sugar

1 cup fat-free or low-fat buttermilk

1/2 cup fat-free evaporated milk

Paprika to taste

In a small bowl, soak the dried mushrooms in warm water for 20 to 30 minutes, or until soft. Drain the mushrooms. Chop.

In a large saucepan, stir together the rehydrated mushrooms, button mushrooms, broth, onions, and soy sauce. Bring to a boil over high heat. Reduce the heat and simmer, covered, while you proceed.

In a small bowl, whisk the flour, water, and sugar into a smooth paste. Stir in 1 tablespoon soup. Whisk until blended. Add 2 tablespoons soup. Whisk until blended. Pour the flour mixture through a sieve into the soup, stirring until blended. Simmer, uncovered, for 3 minutes, stirring occasionally.

Pour in the buttermilk and evaporated milk. Return to a simmer and remove from the heat. Let cool for 5 to 10 minutes.

In a food processor or blender, process the soup in batches until smooth.

Return the soup to the saucepan. Cook over medium heat until the soup just begins to simmer, stirring constantly.

To serve, ladle into soup bowls. Sprinkle with paprika.

vegetable broth

 3 medium parsnips

 2 large carrots

 1 large onion

 2 medium tomatoes

¼ medium head green cabbage

 1 medium rib of celery

 6 medium garlic cloves

½ bunch fresh parsley

 2 tablespoons fresh thyme leaves or 1 teaspoon dried, crumbled

 2 tablespoons fresh basil leaves or 1 teaspoon dried, crumbled

 2 bay leaves

1 teaspoon whole black peppercorns

12 cups water

Coarsely chop the parsnips, carrots, onion, tomatoes, cabbage, celery, and garlic. Place in a large pot. Add the parsley, thyme, basil, bay leaves, and peppercorns. Pour in the water. Bring to a boil over high heat. Reduce the heat and simmer, uncovered, for 1 hour 30 minutes, stirring constantly. Let cool slightly for at least 30 minutes for easier handling. Strain through a sieve, discarding the vegetables and seasonings.

COOK'S TIP ON FREEZING BROTH OR STOCK: Freeze larger quantities of broth or stock (vegetable, chicken, beef, or seafood) in covered plastic containers for future use. Freeze by the tablespoonful in ice-cube trays, pop the frozen broth from the container, and store it in a reusable plastic freezer bag. Use the frozen broth (thaw larger amounts first) to cook vegetables, replace oil in stir-fries, or flavor a wide variety of foods.

PER SERVING

calories 105
total fat 1.0 g
 saturated 0.5 g
 polyunsaturated 0.0 g
 monounsaturated 0.0 g
cholesterol 3 mg

sodium 217 mg
carbohydrates 19 g
 fiber 2 g
 sugar 7 g
 protein 7 g

100 200 300 400   **DIETARY EXCHANGES**
½ starch; 2 vegetable

curried pumpkin soup

Serves 4; 1 cup per serving

This interesting soup is great as a first course for an elegant dinner or with sandwiches while watching the big game.

    1 teaspoon olive oil
  1/2 cup minced onion
      15-ounce can solid-pack pumpkin
      (not pie filling)
1 1/2 cups water
    1 teaspoon curry powder
  1/2 teaspoon salt
  1/8 teaspoon cayenne
    1 cup fat-free half-and-half
    1 tablespoon light tub margarine
    1 teaspoon sugar

Heat a medium saucepan over medium heat. Pour the oil into the pan and swirl to coat the bottom. Cook the onion for 4 minutes, stirring frequently.

Stir in the pumpkin, water, curry powder, salt, and cayenne. Increase the heat to high and bring to a boil. Reduce the heat and simmer, uncovered, for 10 minutes. Remove from the heat.

Stir in the half-and-half, margarine, and sugar. Cover and let stand for 3 minutes to allow the flavors to blend before serving.

COOK'S TIP ON CANNED PUMPKIN: Check the label on the can when you shop for pumpkin. For this recipe, the only ingredient that should be listed is 100 percent pure pumpkin puree.

PER SERVING

calories 110
total fat 2.5 g
  saturated 0.5 g
  polyunsaturated 0.5 g
  monounsaturated 1.5 g
cholesterol 0 mg

sodium 381 mg
carbohydrates 20 g
  fiber 4 g
  sugar 9 g
protein 5 g

100 200 300 400

DIETARY EXCHANGES
$2\frac{1}{2}$ vegetable;
$\frac{1}{2}$ skim milk; $\frac{1}{2}$ fat

chilled tomato-basil soup

Serves 4; ¾ cup per serving

If you are a fan of gazpacho, a refreshing Spanish soup, you have to try this version with an Italian twist!

½ 14.5-ounce can artichokes, rinsed and drained
8 kalamata olives
2 medium tomatoes, quartered
1 cup low-sodium mixed-vegetable juice
4 medium green onions (green and white parts), cut into big pieces
2 to 3 tablespoons cider vinegar
2 teaspoons paprika
½ medium garlic clove
¼ cup finely chopped fresh basil leaves, or 2 tablespoons dried basil, crumbled, and 2 tablespoons finely snipped fresh parsley
¾ teaspoon olive oil (extra-virgin preferred)
¼ teaspoon crushed red pepper flakes
¼ teaspoon salt

In a food processor or blender, coarsely chop the artichokes. Add the olives. Finely chop. Transfer to a medium bowl.

Process the tomatoes, vegetable juice, green onions, vinegar, paprika, and garlic until smooth. Add to the artichoke mixture.

Stir in the remaining ingredients. Cover with plastic

wrap and refrigerate for 30 minutes to allow the flavors to blend.

COOK'S TIP: It's important to include the paprika in this soup. It imparts a deep, rich color.

PER SERVING

calories 84
total fat 3.0 g
  saturated 0.5 g
  polyunsaturated 0.5 g
  monounsaturated 2.0 g
cholesterol 0 mg

sodium 393 mg
carbohydrates 12 g
  fiber 3 g
  sugar 6 g
protein 2 g

100 200 300 400

DIETARY EXCHANGES
2$\frac{1}{2}$ vegetable; $\frac{1}{2}$ fat

quick mexican-style soup
Serves 4; $^3/4$ cup per serving

A perfect last-minute side dish, this super-fast soup abounds in south-of-the-border flavors. It weighs in at only 35 calories per serving.

14-ounce can fat-free, low-sodium chicken broth
1 large tomato, seeded and diced
4-ounce can chopped mild green chiles
$^1/4$ cup snipped fresh cilantro
1 to 2 tablespoons fresh lime juice
$^1/2$ tablespoon olive oil (extra-virgin preferred)
$^3/4$ teaspoon ground cumin

In a medium saucepan, bring the broth to a boil over high heat. Stir in the tomato and green chiles. Return to a boil. Remove from the heat.

Stir in the remaining ingredients. Let stand, covered, for 5 minutes to allow the flavors to blend.

PER SERVING

calories 35
total fat 2.0 g
 saturated 0.0 g
 polyunsaturated 0.0 g
 monounsaturated 1.5 g
cholesterol 0 mg

sodium 132 mg
carbohydrates 4 g
 fiber 2 g
 sugar 1 g
 protein 1 g

100 200 300 400 **DIETARY EXCHANGES**
1 vegetable; $^1/2$ fat

egg drop soup with crabmeat and vegetables

Serves 4; 1 cup per serving

Egg drop soup reaches ethereal heights with the addition of shredded carrots, julienned snow peas, and flaked crabmeat, all simmered in broth flavored with toasted sesame oil. Gently stirring the egg substitute in the hot broth produces the egg threads (sometimes called egg flowers) that are prized in this classic Asian soup.

3 cups fat-free, low-sodium chicken broth

2 tablespoons cornstarch

2 medium carrots, shredded

4 ounces snow peas, trimmed and cut into matchstick-size strips

2 medium green onions (green and white parts), chopped

1 teaspoon toasted sesame oil

1/8 teaspoon pepper

4 ounces canned crabmeat, rinsed and drained

Egg substitute equivalent to 2 eggs, or 4 egg whites, lightly beaten

In a medium saucepan, whisk together the broth and cornstarch. Bring to a simmer over medium-high heat. Adjusting the heat as needed, simmer for 2 to 3 minutes, or until thickened, stirring occasionally.

Stir in the carrots, snow peas, green onions, sesame oil, and pepper. Simmer for 1 to 2 minutes, or until the vegetables are tender-crisp, stirring occasionally.

Stir in the crabmeat. Simmer for 1 minute, or until the crabmeat is warmed through.

Pour the egg substitute in a thin stream and circular pattern into the simmering soup. Wait for 10 seconds, then gently stir until the egg substitute is cooked (it will appear shredded or resemble egg threads).

To serve, ladle into soup bowls.

PER SERVING

calories 108

total fat 1.5 g

  saturated 0.5 g

  polyunsaturated 0.5 g

  monounsaturated 0.5 g

cholesterol 25 mg

sodium 160 mg

carbohydrates 11 g

  fiber 2 g

  sugar 4 g

protein 12 g

100 200 300 400

DIETARY EXCHANGES
2 vegetable; $1\frac{1}{2}$ very lean meat

market-fresh fish and vegetable soup

Serves 4; 1½ cups per serving

Stroll through your local market and select the freshest available seafood and seasonal vegetables for this versatile soup. See the Cook's Tip on the facing page for some substitution ideas.

- 1 teaspoon olive oil
- 4 ounces shiitake mushrooms, stems discarded, halved
- 4 medium green onions (green part only), chopped
- 1 medium garlic clove, minced
- 3 cups fat-free, low-sodium chicken broth
- 2 medium Italian plum tomatoes, diced
- ½ cup dried whole-wheat macaroni or small shell pasta (about 3 ounces)
- ¼ teaspoon salt
- ⅛ teaspoon pepper
- ½ pound salmon fillets
- ½ pound halibut fillets
- 8 ounces fresh asparagus, trimmed, cut into 1-inch pieces (8 to 10 medium spears)
- 4 ounces baby broccoli, cut into 1-inch pieces (about 1 cup)
- 1 tablespoon chopped fresh oregano leaves or 1 teaspoon dried, crumbled

Heat a large saucepan over medium-high heat. Pour the oil into the pan and swirl to coat the bottom. Cook the mushrooms, green onions, and garlic for 3 to 4 minutes, or until tender, stirring occasionally.

Stir in the broth and tomatoes. Bring to a simmer, stirring occasionally. Stir in the macaroni, salt, and pepper. Adjusting the heat as necessary, simmer for 5 to 6 minutes, or until the pasta is almost tender, stirring occasionally.

Rinse the fish and pat dry with paper towels. Cut the fish into 1-inch cubes. Stir the fish, asparagus, broccoli, and oregano into the soup. Simmer for 5 to 6 minutes, or until the pasta is tender and the fish flakes easily when tested with a fork, gently stirring occasionally. (Be careful to not break up the fish too much.)

COOK'S TIP: For variety, try some of these tasty substitutions:
- Vegetables: shredded carrots, bok choy, snow peas, sugar snap peas, celery, zucchini, yellow summer squash, baby corn
- Herbs: rosemary, basil, marjoram, thyme, dill, tarragon
- Fish: tuna, cod, tilapia, haddock, red snapper

PER SERVING

calories 269

total fat 5.0 g

  saturated 0.5 g

  polyunsaturated 1.5 g

  monounsaturated 2.0 g

cholesterol 48 mg

sodium 278 mg

carbohydrates 25 g

  fiber 6 g

  sugar 5 g

protein 31 g

100   200   300   400   **DIETARY EXCHANGES**
1 starch; 2 vegetable;
3 lean meat

chicken minestrone

Serves 8; 1¼ cups per serving

Bring a bit of Italian restaurant dining, minus most of the calories and saturated fat, into your own home with this flavorful soup. It's perfect for lunch or dinner. For a side dish, leave out the chicken.

	Vegetable oil spray
1	small onion, chopped
4	medium garlic cloves, minced
2	cups fat-free, low-sodium chicken broth
2	cups low-sodium tomato juice
	15-ounce can no-salt-added chick-peas, rinsed and drained
	14.5-ounce can no-salt-added stewed tomatoes, undrained
½	cup frozen green peas and carrots
½	cup dry red wine (regular or nonalcoholic)
1	medium rib of celery, chopped
½	tablespoon dried basil, crumbled
¼	teaspoon dried oregano, crumbled
	Dash of pepper
2	cups diced cooked skinless chicken breasts, cooked without salt
1	cup dried whole-wheat rotini or pasta shells

1 cup fresh baby spinach leaves

3 tablespoons shredded or grated Parmesan cheese

Heat a Dutch oven over medium heat. Remove from the heat and lightly spray with vegetable oil spray (being careful not to spray near a gas flame). Cook the onion and garlic for 2 minutes, or until the onion is soft, stirring frequently.

Stir in the broth, tomato juice, chick-peas, undrained tomatoes, green peas and carrots, wine, celery, basil, oregano, and pepper. Break the tomatoes into smaller pieces with a spoon. Increase the heat to medium high and bring to a boil. Reduce the heat and simmer, covered, for 45 minutes, stirring occasionally.

Stir in the chicken, pasta, and spinach. Increase the heat to medium high and bring to a boil. Reduce the heat and simmer, uncovered, for 10 to 15 minutes, or until the pasta is tender, stirring occasionally.

To serve, ladle into bowls. Sprinkle with the Parmesan.

COOK'S TIP: This soup will thicken as it cools. You can thin it with water if needed.

PER SERVING

calories 278

total fat 4.0 g
  saturated 1.0 g
  polyunsaturated 1.0 g
  monounsaturated 1.5 g
cholesterol 31 mg

sodium 143 mg
carbohydrates 36 g
  fiber 8 g
  sugar 9 g
protein 21 g

100   200   300   400

DIETARY EXCHANGES
2 starch; 1 vegetable;
2 very lean meat

wild rice and chicken chowder

Serves 4; 1½ cups per serving

This soothing soup is welcome on cold winter days by the fire.

- 1 teaspoon canola or corn oil
- 8 ounces chicken tenders or boneless, skinless chicken breasts, all visible fat discarded, cut into ½-inch cubes
- 1 medium carrot, sliced
- ½ medium onion, thinly sliced
- 3 cups fat-free, low-sodium chicken broth
- ½ 6- to 7-ounce box quick-cooking white and wild rice, seasoning packet discarded
- ½ teaspoon dried thyme, crumbled
- ¼ teaspoon dried sage
- ¼ teaspoon salt
- ⅛ teaspoon pepper
- 8 ounces fresh broccoli florets (about 2 cups)
- ½ cup fat-free half-and-half
- ¼ cup shredded or grated Parmesan cheese

Heat a large saucepan over medium-high heat. Pour the oil into the pan and swirl to coat the bottom. Cook the chicken for 3 to 4 minutes, or until browned, stirring occasionally.

Stir in the carrot and onion. Cook for 2 to 3 minutes, or until the vegetables are tender-crisp, stirring occasionally.

Pour in the broth. Bring to a simmer.

Stir in the rice, thyme, sage, salt, and pepper. Return to a simmer. Simmer, covered, for 20 minutes, stirring occasionally.

Stir in the broccoli. Simmer, covered, for 5 minutes, or until the broccoli and rice are tender.

Stir in the half-and-half and Parmesan. Cook over low heat for 1 to 2 minutes, or until the cheese is melted, stirring occasionally.

PER SERVING

calories 245

total fat 3.5 g
  saturated 1.0 g
  polyunsaturated 0.5 g
  monounsaturated 1.5 g
cholesterol 37 mg

sodium 377 mg

carbohydrates 31 g
  fiber 3 g
  sugar 5 g
protein 23 g

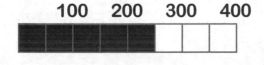

100   200   300   400

DIETARY EXCHANGES
1½ starch; 1½ vegetable; 2 very lean meat

vegetable beef soup

Serves 4; 1^1/2 cups per serving

Yukon gold potatoes and exotic mushrooms update this classic.

Vegetable oil spray

1 pound eye-of-round steak, all visible fat discarded, cut into 1/2-inch cubes

4 ounces shiitake mushrooms, stems discarded, halved

1 medium carrot, cut crosswise into 1/2-inch slices

3 cups fat-free, no-salt-added beef broth

2 medium Yukon gold or other yellow-skinned potatoes (about 8 ounces), cut into 1-inch cubes

4 ounces baby portobello mushrooms, halved

1/4 cup no-salt-added tomato paste

1 teaspoon dried marjoram, crumbled

1 teaspoon dried thyme, crumbled

1 teaspoon onion powder

1/4 teaspoon salt

1/4 teaspoon pepper

1/2 cup frozen green peas

Heat a nonstick Dutch oven or large saucepan over medium-high heat. Remove from the heat and lightly spray with vegetable oil spray (being careful not to spray near a gas flame). Cook the beef for 3 to 4 minutes, or until browned, stirring occasionally.

Stir in the shiitake mushrooms and carrot. Cook for 3 to 4 minutes, or until the mushrooms are tender and the carrot is tender-crisp, stirring occasionally.

Stir in the remaining ingredients except the peas. Bring to a simmer. Reduce the heat and simmer, covered, for 30 to 40 minutes, or until the beef and vegetables are tender (no stirring needed).

Stir in the peas. Simmer, covered, for 4 minutes.

PER SERVING

calories 245

total fat 4.5 g

  saturated 1.5 g

  polyunsaturated 0.5 g

  monounsaturated 1.5 g

cholesterol 59 mg

sodium 305 mg

carbohydrates 21 g

  fiber 4 g

  sugar 6 g

protein 33 g

100	200	300	400

DIETARY EXCHANGES
1 starch; $1\frac{1}{2}$ vegetable; 3 very lean meat

bayou andouille and chicken chowder

Serves 4; 1½ cups per serving

Andouille sausage is a southern favorite with deep, smoky flavors and a nice bit of heat. A little goes a long way!

Vegetable oil spray

2 ounces andouille sausage, cut into ½-inch pieces

2 ounces boneless, skinless chicken breasts, all visible fat discarded, cut into ½-inch pieces

14-ounce can fat-free, low-sodium chicken broth

1½ medium green bell peppers, chopped

1 large onion, chopped

8 ounces baking potatoes (russet preferred), cut into ½-inch pieces

¾ cup frozen whole-kernel corn

½ teaspoon dried thyme, crumbled

½ cup fat-free half-and-half

4-ounce jar diced pimientos, drained

½ cup finely snipped fresh parsley

¼ teaspoon salt

¼ teaspoon pepper

2 ounces shredded fat-free or low-fat sharp Cheddar cheese

Heat a Dutch oven over medium-high heat. Remove from the heat and lightly spray with vegetable oil spray (being careful not to spray near a gas flame). Cook the sausage for 3 minutes, or until beginning to richly brown on the edges, stirring constantly. Transfer to a plate.

Lightly spray the Dutch oven with vegetable oil spray. Add the chicken. Cook for 3 minutes, stirring frequently. Stir in the broth, bell peppers, onion, potatoes, corn, and thyme. Bring to a boil. Reduce the heat and simmer, covered, for 20 minutes, or until the potatoes are tender. Remove from the heat.

Stir in the sausage, half-and-half, pimientos, parsley, salt, and pepper. Let stand, covered, for 15 minutes to allow the flavors to blend and the liquid to thicken slightly.

To serve, ladle into bowls. Sprinkle with the Cheddar.

COOK'S TIP: Be sure to allow the chowder to stand for a full 15 minutes for peak flavor. You can reheat the chowder over medium heat for 2 to 3 minutes if needed.

PER SERVING

calories 206
total fat 4.5 g
  saturated 1.5 g
  polyunsaturated 0.0 g
  monounsaturated 0.0 g
cholesterol 19 mg

sodium 440 mg
carbohydrates 30 g
  fiber 5 g
  sugar 9 g
protein 16 g

100 200 300 400

DIETARY EXCHANGES
1$\frac{1}{2}$ starch; 1$\frac{1}{2}$ vegetable; 1 lean meat

lima bean soup

Serves 4; 1 cup soup and 1 tablespoon sour cream per serving

A little mustard is added to this mild and creamy main-dish soup to give it just a bit of zing.

Vegetable oil spray

1 large onion, chopped

14-ounce can fat-free, low-sodium chicken broth

10 ounces frozen lima beans

3/4 cup fat-free milk

3/4 cup fat-free or light sour cream

1/2 tablespoon prepared mustard

1/2 teaspoon salt

1/4 teaspoon pepper

1/8 teaspoon cayenne

1/4 cup fat-free or light sour cream

1/4 cup snipped fresh cilantro (optional)

Heat a large saucepan over medium heat. Remove from the heat and lightly spray with vegetable oil spray (being careful not to spray near a gas flame). Cook the onion for 4 minutes, or until soft, stirring frequently.

Stir in the broth and lima beans. Increase the heat to high. Bring to a boil. Reduce the heat and simmer, covered, for 20 minutes, or until the beans are tender.

In a food processor or blender, process 1 cup bean mixture until smooth. Transfer to a medium bowl. Process the remaining bean mixture 1 cup at a time.

Return the soup to the saucepan. Stir in the milk. Heat over medium heat for 4 to 5 minutes, or until heated through, stirring frequently. Remove from the heat.

Whisk in ¾ cup sour cream, mustard, salt, pepper, and cayenne.

To serve, ladle the soup into soup bowls. Top each serving with a dollop of sour cream and the cilantro.

COOK'S TIP: To avoid an overflow, be sure to process the bean mixture in 1-cup batches. If using a blender, hold the lid down tightly before and during the pureeing.

PER SERVING

calories 188
total fat 0.0 g
  saturated 0.0 g
  polyunsaturated 0.0 g
  monounsaturated 0.0 g
cholesterol 11 mg

sodium 533 mg
carbohydrates 33 g
  fiber 5 g
  sugar 10 g
protein 11 g

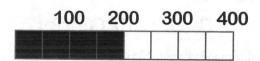

DIETARY EXCHANGES
2 starch; 1 vegetable;
½ very lean meat

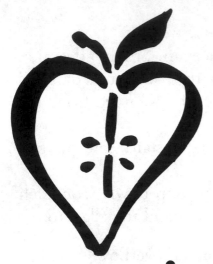

salads

Chopped Salad with Gorgonzola

Greek Salad with Sun-Dried Tomato
Vinaigrette

Baby Greens with Spiced Cranberry
Vinaigrette

Fruit and Spinach Salad
with Fresh Mint

Asparagus and Cucumber Salad
with Lemon and Mint

Vegetable Salad Vinaigrette

Broccoli and Edamame Salad
with Dill

Zingy Carrot Salad

Carrot-Pineapple Slaw with Ginger

Multicolored Marinated Slaw

Mango-Avocado Salad

Asian Citrus Salad

Black-Eyed Pea Salad

Greek Potato and Artichoke Salad

Lemony Rice and Bean Salad
with Feta

Tuna Pasta Provençal

Herbed Chicken and Roasted Beet
Salad

Chicken and Toasted Walnut Salad

Mexican Beef Salad

Flank Steak Salad with Sesame-Lime
Dressing

Cannellini and Black Bean Salad

chopped salad with gorgonzola

Serves 4; 2 cups per serving

Chopped salad seems to be on a lot of menus these days. You can make it at home for a fraction of the price—and a fraction of the calories, saturated fat, and sodium.

6 cups chopped iceberg lettuce (about 9 ounces)
1 cup frozen green peas, thawed
2 medium carrots, thinly sliced
1 medium cucumber, peeled and chopped
½ cup finely chopped red onion
½ cup fat-free or light ranch salad dressing
1 tablespoon plus 1 teaspoon crumbled Gorgonzola cheese

In a large bowl, combine the lettuce, peas, carrots, cucumber, onion, and salad dressing. Toss gently to coat.

Add the Gorgonzola. Toss gently.

PER SERVING

calories 116
total fat 1.0 g
  saturated 0.5 g
  polyunsaturated 0.0 g
  monounsaturated 0.0 g
cholesterol 2 mg

sodium 432 mg
carbohydrates 24 g
  fiber 5 g
  sugar 8 g
protein 4 g

100 200 300 400

DIETARY EXCHANGES
1 starch; 2 vegetable

greek salad with
sun-dried tomato vinaigrette

Serves 4; scant 2 cups salad and 2 table-spoons salad dressing per serving

Jam-packed with assertive ingredients, this is a salad to remember.

sun-dried tomato vinaigrette

- 4 dry-packed sun-dried tomato halves (about ½ ounce)
- ½ cup boiling water
- ¼ cup dry white wine (regular or nonalcoholic)
- 2 tablespoons finely snipped fresh parsley
- 2 tablespoons fresh lemon juice
- 1 tablespoon cider vinegar
- 1 tablespoon olive oil (extra-virgin preferred)
- ½ tablespoon dried oregano, crumbled
- 1 medium garlic clove, minced
- ¼ teaspoon ground cumin
- ¼ teaspoon salt
- ¼ teaspoon pepper

- 7 cups torn lettuce leaves, any variety
- ¼ to ½ cup thinly sliced red onion
- ½ ounce reduced-fat feta cheese with sun-dried tomatoes and basil

Put the tomatoes in a small bowl. Pour in the water. Let stand for 15 minutes, or until very soft. Discard the water.

Meanwhile, put the remaining vinaigrette ingredients in a small jar with a tight-fitting lid.

In a serving bowl, combine the lettuce and onion.

Finely chop the rehydrated tomatoes. Add to the vinaigrette. Shake vigorously until well blended. Pour over the salad. Toss gently to coat.

Crumble the feta. Toss gently into the salad.

PER SERVING

calories 84
total fat 4.0 g
  saturated 0.5 g
  polyunsaturated 0.5 g
  monosaturated 2.5 g
cholesterol 1 mg

sodium 230 mg
carbohydrates 10 g
  fiber 3 g
  sugar 4 g
protein 3 g

100 200 300 400

DIETARY EXCHANGES
2 vegetable; 1 fat

baby greens with spiced cranberry vinaigrette
Serves 4; 2 cups per serving

You don't have to wait until the winter holidays to enjoy cranberries. Cool and refreshing, this salad with cranberry vinaigrette is just right with grilled foods in the heat of summer.

8 cups mixed baby greens or spring greens (about 5 ounces)

1/2 cup thinly sliced onion

1/2 medium Gala or Jonathan apple, unpeeled and sliced

cranberry vinaigrette

1/4 cup sweetened cranberry juice

2 tablespoons red wine vinegar

1 1/2 tablespoons honey

1 teaspoon grated peeled gingerroot

1/2 teaspoon ground cinnamon

1/8 teaspoon ground cloves

1/8 teaspoon salt

2 ounces soft goat cheese, crumbled

Place the greens on plates. Arrange the onion and apple on the greens.

Put the vinaigrette ingredients in a small jar with a tight-fitting lid and shake to combine. Pour the dressing over the salad.

Sprinkle with the goat cheese.

COOK'S TIP ON SALAD DRESSING: Salad dressing clings better to thoroughly dried greens, allowing you to use less dressing.

PER SERVING

calories 106
total fat 3.5 g
  saturated 2.0 g
  polyunsaturated 0.0 g
  monounsaturated 0.5 g
cholesterol 7 mg

sodium 154 mg
carbohydrates 16 g
  fiber 3 g
  sugar 12 g
  protein 5 g

100   200   300   400

DIETARY EXCHANGES
1 vegetable;
$1/2$ other carbohydrate;
$1/2$ very lean meat;
$1/2$ fat

fruit and spinach salad with fresh mint

Serves 6; 1½ cups spinach, ½ cup fruit, and 2½ tablespoons dressing per serving

Enjoy this jewel-toned salad as a side dish or top it with grilled chicken, salmon, or tuna to turn it into a light meal.

8 ounces fresh baby spinach leaves
2 cups fresh strawberries, halved
4 medium green kiwifruit, peeled and sliced
1 medium mango, cubed

dressing

1 cup fat-free or low-fat plain yogurt
¼ cup finely snipped fresh mint
2 tablespoons honey
1 tablespoon fresh orange juice
1 tablespoon fresh lemon juice

6 sprigs of mint (optional)

Place the spinach on plates. Arrange the fruit on top.
In a small bowl, whisk together the dressing ingredients. Spoon the dressing over the salad. Garnish with the mint.

COOK'S TIP ON CHOPPING MANGOES:

Here's one good way to chop a mango. Place an unpeeled mango on its side. Slicing lengthwise, cut about one-third from each side. The pit will be in the middle third. Without cutting through the skin, score the outer two-thirds lengthwise. Give the scored pieces a one-quarter turn and, again without cutting through the skin, score to create small squares. Turn the mango inside out and cut the small squares from the skin.

PER SERVING

calories 126
total fat 1.0 g
  saturated 0.0 g
  polyunsaturated 0.5 g
  monounsaturated 0.0 g
cholesterol 1 mg

sodium 66 mg
carbohydrates 28 g
  fiber 4 g
  sugar 21 g
  protein 5 g

100 200 300 400

DIETARY EXCHANGES
1½ fruit;
½ other carbohydrate

asparagus and cucumber salad with lemon and mint

Serves 4; $^{1}/_{2}$ cup per serving

You'll be tempted to eat this unusual salad with a spoon so you can catch all the great flavors!

4 ounces asparagus spears (4 to 5 medium), trimmed and cut into $^{1}/_{2}$-inch pieces

1 medium cucumber, peeled, seeded, and diced (about 1 cup)

$^{1}/_{2}$ cup finely chopped red onion

$^{1}/_{4}$ cup chopped fresh mint or snipped fresh cilantro

1 tablespoon sugar

$^{1}/_{2}$ tablespoon grated lemon zest

2 tablespoons fresh lemon juice

$^{1}/_{8}$ teaspoon salt

Steam the asparagus for 1½ to 2 minutes, or until just tender-crisp. Immediately drain in a colander and run under cold water to cool completely. Drain well; pat dry with paper towels.

In a medium bowl, combine all the ingredients. Toss gently. Let stand for 10 minutes before serving to allow the flavors to blend.

PER SERVING

calories 39

total fat 0.0 g

  saturated 0.0 g

  polyunsaturated 0.0 g

  monounsaturated 0.0 g

cholesterol 0 mg

sodium 77 mg

carbohydrates 9 g

  fiber 2 g

  sugar 6 g

  protein 1 g

100   200   300   400

DIETARY EXCHANGES

1½ vegetable

vegetable salad vinaigrette
Serves 4; ^{1}/2 cup per serving

If you need a new and refreshing angle on salads, this crunchy combination is it.

1/2 medium cucumber, peeled and diced

1 medium rib of celery, sliced crosswise

3 ounces button mushrooms, coarsely chopped

1/4 cup chopped red onion

1/4 cup snipped fresh parsley

1 tablespoon olive oil (extra-virgin preferred)

1 tablespoon red wine vinegar

1 teaspoon sugar

1/2 teaspoon Dijon mustard (stone-ground preferred)

1/4 teaspoon salt

1/8 teaspoon crushed red pepper flakes

In a medium bowl, toss together all the ingredients. Serve immediately for peak flavors.

COOK'S TIP: To prepare this salad in advance, combine the cucumber, celery, mushrooms, onion, and parsley in a medium bowl. In a small bowl, combine the remaining ingredients. Cover with plastic wrap and refrigerate for up to 8 hours. When ready to serve, stir the dressing. Pour it over the vegetable mixture. Toss.

PER SERVING

calories 51
total fat 3.5 g
  saturated 0.5 g
  polyunsaturated 0.5 g
  monounsaturated 2.5 g
cholesterol 0 mg

sodium 175 mg
carbohydrates 4 g
  fiber 1 g
  sugar 2 g
protein 1 g

100   200   300   400

DIETARY EXCHANGES
1 vegetable; $\frac{1}{2}$ fat

broccoli and edamame salad with dill

Serves 6; $\frac{1}{2}$ cup per serving

Buy some fresh baby dillweed and make this salad when you want something unusual to perk up your dinner menu. You can turn it into an entrée by adding slices of skinless cooked chicken breast.

salad

  1 cup frozen shelled edamame (soybeans)

  2 cups fresh broccoli florets, cut into bite-size pieces

  $\frac{1}{3}$ cup chopped sweet onion (red preferred)

  $\frac{1}{4}$ cup dried sweetened cranberries

  2 tablespoons finely snipped dillweed (baby dillweed preferred)

dressing

  $\frac{1}{3}$ cup plain rice vinegar

  1 tablespoon honey

  1 teaspoon olive oil (extra-virgin preferred)

Cook the edamame according to the package directions, omitting the salt. Drain well.

Meanwhile, in a large bowl, combine the remaining salad ingredients.

In a small bowl, whisk together the dressing ingredients.

To assemble, add the edamame to the broccoli mixture. Pour the dressing over the salad. Cover and refrigerate for about 1 hour, stirring occasionally, to allow the flavors to blend.

COOK'S TIP ON EDAMAME, OR SOYBEANS: Edamame has a slightly sweet taste, similar to that of sweet peas. You can sometimes buy fresh edamame, but it is much more widely available frozen, in the pod or shelled. Although higher in calories and fat (most of the fat is unsaturated) than other legumes, edamame contains more protein and calcium than the others. In fact, edamame is the only vegetable food whose protein is complete.

PER SERVING

calories 86
total fat 2.5 g
 saturated 0.5 g
 polyunsaturated 1.0 g
 monounsaturated 1.0 g
cholesterol 0 mg

sodium 12 mg
carbohydrates 12 g
 fiber 3 g
 sugar 8 g
 protein 4 g

100   200   300   400

DIETARY EXCHANGES
1/2 fruit; 1 vegetable; 1/2 fat

zingy carrot salad

Serves 4; $^1/_2$ cup per serving

Double or triple this quick and easy dish to serve a group or to ensure having leftovers.

2 medium carrots, cut crosswise into $^1/_8$-inch slices
$^1/_2$ medium green bell pepper, cut into thin strips
$^1/_2$ cup thinly sliced onion
2 tablespoons firmly packed dark brown sugar
3 tablespoons balsamic vinegar
$^1/_8$ teaspoon salt

Steam the carrots for 3 to 4 minutes, or until just tender. Drain well in a colander.

In a medium bowl, toss together all the ingredients. Cover and refrigerate for 1 hour to allow the flavors to blend.

PER SERVING

calories 60
total fat 0.0 g
  saturated 0.0 g
  polyunsaturated 0.0 g
  monounsaturated 0.0 g
cholesterol 0 mg

sodium 104 mg
carbohydrates 15 g
  fiber 2 g
  sugar 12 g
protein 1 g

100   200   300   400   DIETARY EXCHANGES
1$^1/_2$ vegetable;
$^1/_2$ other carbohydrate

carrot-pineapple slaw with ginger

Serves 4; $^1/_2$ cup per serving

Definitely not the 1950s carrot-raisin salad, this modernized version is bursting with fresh citrus and ginger.

1 $^1/_2$ cups shredded carrots (about 5 ounces)

    8-ounce can crushed pineapple in its own juice, drained

$^1/_2$ cup dried apricots, finely chopped (about 3 ounces)

1 teaspoon grated peeled gingerroot

1 teaspoon grated lemon zest

2 tablespoons fresh lemon juice

In a medium bowl, toss together all the ingredients. Let stand for 10 minutes to let the flavors blend.

PER SERVING

calories 97
total fat 0.0 g
  saturated 0.0 g
  polyunsaturated 0.0 g
  monounsaturated 0.0 g
cholesterol 0 mg

sodium 33 mg
carbohydrates 23 g
  fiber 3 g
  sugar 16 g
protein 1 g

100 200 300 400

DIETARY EXCHANGES
1 fruit; 1$^1/_2$ vegetable

multicolored marinated slaw

Serves 8; ½ cup per serving

Marinated slaw provides a change of pace from the usual mixed green salad. Prepare at least 12 hours in advance to let the flavors blend.

dressing

⅓ cup white wine vinegar

¼ cup water

¼ cup sugar

1 tablespoon canola or corn oil

½ teaspoon garlic powder

½ teaspoon celery seeds

¼ teaspoon dry mustard

⅛ teaspoon salt

⅛ teaspoon pepper

slaw

1 small sweet onion, thinly sliced, cut into bite-size pieces

½ medium head green cabbage, coarsely shredded (about 4 cups)

1 medium red bell pepper, cut into strips

1 medium cucumber, peeled, seeded, and thinly sliced

1 large carrot, thinly sliced

1 medium rib of celery, thinly sliced

In a large bowl, whisk together the dressing ingredients.

Add all the slaw ingredients. Toss. Transfer to a large resealable plastic bag. Seal the bag and refrigerate the slaw for at least 12 hours, turning occasionally to distribute the dressing through the slaw. The slaw will keep for several days in the refrigerator.

PER SERVING

calories 82
total fat 2.0 g
 saturated 0.0 g
 polyunsaturated 0.5 g
 monounsaturated 1.0 g
cholesterol 0 mg

sodium 66 mg
carbohydrates 15 g
 fiber 3 g
 sugar 11 g
protein 2 g

100   200   300   400

DIETARY EXCHANGES
1½ vegetable; ½ other carbohydrate; ½ fat

mango-avocado salad

Serves 6; $^1/_2$ cup per serving

The addition of avocado gives this salad a creamy touch. It's the perfect match for any grilled or roasted entrée.

1	medium avocado, cut into $^1/_2$-inch cubes
1$^1/_2$	cups diced fresh or bottled mango or fresh or frozen unsweetened peaches, thawed if frozen (fresh preferred)
$^1/_4$	cup finely chopped red onion
$^1/_4$	cup snipped fresh cilantro
$^1/_4$	cup fresh lime juice
1	teaspoon sugar

In a medium bowl, gently toss all the ingredients.

Serve immediately or refrigerate for up to 2 hours to allow the flavors to blend.

COOK'S TIP: For fruit salsa, simply finely chop the avocado and mango.

PER SERVING

calories 89
total fat 5.0 g
  saturated 0.5 g
  polyunsaturated 0.5 g
  monounsaturated 3.5 g
cholesterol 0 mg

sodium 4 mg
carbohydrates 12 g
  fiber 3 g
  sugar 8 g
protein 1 g

100 200 300 400 **DIETARY EXCHANGES**
1 fruit; 1 fat

asian citrus salad

Serves 6; $^1/_2$ cup per serving

Experimenting with produce and seasonings can be interesting and fun. This salad uses a large pomelo—similar to a grapefruit but sweeter—and a honey infused with five-spice powder and fresh mint.

1 large pomelo

1 medium orange

1 small tangerine

3 tablespoons honey

1 tablespoon chopped fresh mint

$^1/_2$ teaspoon five-spice powder

Grate 1 teaspoon zest from the pomelo or from a combination of the pomelo, orange, and tangerine. Set the zest aside.

Cut both ends from the pomelo. Cut away all the remaining thick peel. Using a knife with a thin blade, cut each segment of fruit from the tough white membrane. Put the fruit in a medium bowl. Peel the orange and tangerine. Divide into segments and remove any seeds. Add the segments to the pomelo.

In a small saucepan, stir together the reserved zest, honey, mint, and five-spice powder. Cook over medium-low heat for 1 to 2 minutes, or until the mixture is warmed through, stirring occasionally.

Pour the mixture over the fruit, stirring gently to coat. Serve with the topping still warm, or cover and refrigerate to serve chilled.

COOK'S TIP ON POMELO: Choose a pomelo that is heavy for its size, smells sweet, and is bright yellow, pinkish, or light green.

COOK'S TIP ON FIVE-SPICE POWDER: Five-spice powder usually can be found in the spice section of your grocery and in Asian markets. It is a fragrant blend of star anise, cloves, fennel, cinnamon, and Szechwan peppercorns.

PER SERVING

calories 90	sodium 2 mg
total fat 0.0 g	carbohydrates 24 g
saturated 0.0 g	fiber 3 g
polyunsaturated 0.0 g	sugar 21 g
monounsaturated 0.0 g	protein 1 g
cholesterol 0 mg	

100   200   300   400   DIETARY EXCHANGES
1 1/2 fruit

black-eyed pea salad
Serves 10; $^1/_2$ cup per serving

An old southern tradition suggests that eating black-eyed peas on New Year's Day brings good luck for the coming year. This salad is so tasty that you won't want to wait for the holiday to prepare it.

salad

1 medium cucumber

15-ounce can no-salt-added black-eyed peas (cowpeas), rinsed and drained

1 medium red bell pepper, chopped

1 medium rib of celery, chopped

4 medium green onions (green and white parts), chopped

1 tablespoon chopped fresh basil leaves

2 ounces fat-free or low-fat feta cheese, crumbled

dressing

3 tablespoons fresh lemon juice

2 tablespoons coarsely chopped fresh oregano leaves

$1^1/_2$ tablespoons olive oil (extra-virgin preferred)

$^1/_2$ teaspoon red hot-pepper sauce

$^1/_8$ teaspoon pepper

Cut the cucumber in half lengthwise. Discard the seeds. Cut the cucumber crosswise into $^1/_4$-inch slices. Put in a large bowl.

Stir in the remaining salad ingredients.

In a small bowl, whisk together the dressing ingredients.

To serve, pour the dressing over the salad mixture. Toss to coat. Serve or cover and refrigerate until needed.

PER SERVING

calories 75

total fat 2.0 g

  saturated 0.5 g

  polyunsaturated 0.0 g

  monounsaturated 1.5 g

cholesterol 0 mg

sodium 97 mg

carbohydrates 10 g

  fiber 3 g

  sugar 3 g

protein 4 g

100　200　300　400

DIETARY EXCHANGES

$^1\!/_2$ starch; $^1\!/_2$ lean meat

greek potato and artichoke salad

Serves 4; ½ cup per serving

Steamed potatoes and green beans are tossed with marinated artichokes, red bell pepper, and capers to give a fresh twist to an old favorite.

8 ounces red potatoes, cut into ½-inch cubes

2 ounces fresh green beans, trimmed, cut into ½-inch pieces (optional)

6-ounce jar marinated artichoke hearts, drained and coarsely chopped

½ medium red bell pepper, finely chopped

¼ cup finely chopped red onion

¼ cup snipped fresh parsley

2 tablespoons capers, rinsed and drained

2 tablespoons cider vinegar

¾ teaspoon dried oregano, crumbled

½ medium garlic clove, minced

Steam the potatoes and beans for 7 to 8 minutes, or until just tender. Drain in a colander and run under cold water to cool. Drain well.

Meanwhile, in a medium bowl, stir together the remaining ingredients.

Add the potatoes and beans. Toss gently. Let stand for 30 minutes to allow the flavors to blend.

PER SERVING

calories 82
total fat 3.0 g
  saturated 0.0 g
  polyunsaturated 0.0 g
  monounsaturated 0.0 g
cholesterol 0 mg

sodium 242 mg
carbohydrates 16 g
  fiber 3 g
  sugar 2 g
protein 2 g

100 200 300 400

DIETARY EXCHANGES
$1/2$ starch; 1 vegetable; $1/2$ fat

lemony rice and bean salad with feta

Serves 4; $^{1}/_{2}$ cup per serving

Turn this salad into a meatless entrée for four by tripling the recipe.

$^{2}/_{3}$ cup water

$^{1}/_{2}$ cup uncooked quick-cooking brown rice

$^{1}/_{2}$ 16-ounce can no-salt-added navy beans, rinsed and drained

$^{1}/_{4}$ cup finely chopped red onion

$^{3}/_{4}$ ounce reduced-fat feta cheese with sun-dried tomatoes and basil, crumbled

2 teaspoons olive oil (extra-virgin preferred)

1 teaspoon dried dillweed

1 teaspoon grated lemon zest

2 to 3 teaspoons fresh lemon juice

$^{1}/_{2}$ teaspoon dried oregano, crumbled

$^{1}/_{2}$ medium garlic clove, minced (optional)

$^{1}/_{4}$ teaspoon salt

In a small saucepan, bring the water to a boil over high heat. Stir in the rice. Reduce the heat and simmer, covered, for about 10 minutes, or until the water is absorbed. Spoon the rice in a single layer onto a baking sheet. Let stand for 5 to 7 minutes to cool completely. Transfer the cooled rice to a medium mixing bowl.

Add the remaining ingredients. Toss gently. Serve or cover and refrigerate for up to 8 hours.

PER SERVING

calories 126
total fat 3.0 g
  saturated 0.5 g
  polyunsaturated 0.5 g
  monounsaturated 2.0 g
cholesterol 2 mg

sodium 221 mg
carbohydrates 19 g
  fiber 3 g
  sugar 2 g
  protein 5 g

100 200 300 400 **DIETARY EXCHANGES**
1½ starch; ½ fat

tuna pasta provençal

Serves 4; 1½ cups per serving

This dish almost transports you to the south of France with its blend of tuna, black olives, and red bell pepper, along with garlic, tarragon, and Dijon mustard.

4 ounces dried whole-wheat or spinach rotini or small pasta shells

2 teaspoons olive oil

1 large sweet onion, such as Vidalia or Walla Walla, chopped

1 large red bell pepper, chopped

1 medium garlic clove, minced

12-ounce can albacore tuna packed in spring or distilled water, rinsed, drained, and flaked

¼ cup chopped black olives, rinsed and drained

⅓ cup fat-free or low-fat plain yogurt

¼ cup fat-free or light mayonnaise dressing

1½ tablespoons snipped fresh tarragon or ½ tablespoon dried, crumbled

2 teaspoons Dijon mustard

½ teaspoon pepper

Prepare the pasta using the package directions, omitting the salt and oil. Drain in a colander. Rinse with cold water and drain well. Transfer the pasta to a large bowl.

Meanwhile, heat a large nonstick skillet over medium heat. Pour the oil into the skillet and swirl to coat the bottom. Cook the onion, bell pepper, and garlic for 5 to 6 minutes, or until the onion is soft, stirring frequently.

When the pasta is ready, stir in the onion mixture, tuna, and olives.

In a small bowl, whisk together the remaining ingredients. Spoon over the pasta mixture, tossing to coat. Cover and refrigerate for 1 to 24 hours before serving.

PER SERVING

calories 300

total fat 6.5 g
  saturated 1.0 g
  polyunsaturated 1.5 g
  monounsaturated 3.0 g
cholesterol 36 mg

sodium 344 mg
carbohydrates 33 g
  fiber 5 g
  sugar 8 g
  protein 27 g

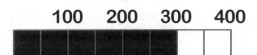

100 200 300 400

DIETARY EXCHANGES
2 starch; 1 vegetable;
3 lean meat

herbed chicken and roasted beet salad

Serves 4; 2 cups salad and 2$\frac{1}{4}$ ounces chicken per serving

This salad is a celebration of flavors, textures, and temperatures with the chilled, crisp, and slightly bitter frisée; the soft, sweet-tart orange sections; and warm, smooth beets.

4 medium beets

12 ounces boneless, skinless chicken breasts

1 tablespoon dried basil, crumbled

1 tablespoon dried parsley, crumbled

2 medium oranges

2 teaspoons sherry vinegar, raspberry vinegar, or balsamic vinegar

$\frac{1}{2}$ teaspoon salt

$\frac{1}{4}$ teaspoon pepper

1 medium head frisée

Preheat the oven to 350°F.

Discard all but 1 to 2 inches of the beet greens. Cut a thin piece from the root end of each beet, leaving on the skin. Put the beets in a single layer in a small baking dish. Add ¼ inch of water. Cover with aluminum foil. Bake for 10 minutes.

Meanwhile, line a rimmed baking sheet with cooking parchment. Place the chicken with the smooth side up on the parchment. Sprinkle with the basil and parsley. Add enough water to cover the bottom of the baking sheet to a depth of about ⅛ inch (about 4 cups).

When the beets have cooked for 10 minutes, put the chicken in the oven. Bake the chicken and the beets for 35 minutes, or until a sharp knife easily pierces the beets and the chicken reaches 165°F when tested with an instant-read thermometer. Let the beets and chicken rest for 10 minutes.

Using disposable plastic gloves so you don't stain your hands, peel the beets. Cut the beets and chicken into thin strips. Peel and section the oranges, reserving 2 tablespoons juice.

In a small bowl, stir together the orange juice, vinegar, salt, and pepper.

To assemble, remove 1½ inches from the base of the frisée and pull apart the leaves. Put in a medium bowl or on a platter. Pour the orange juice mixture over the frisée. Add the orange sections and lightly toss. Arrange the beets and chicken strips on top. Do not toss or stir. Serve immediately.

COOK'S TIP: Frisée, a member of the chicory family, is the ideal choice for this salad because the warm ingredients won't wilt it.

TIME-SAVER: Substitute 9 ounces of warmed boneless, skinless cooked chicken or turkey breast (cooked without added salt) for the baked chicken.

PER SERVING

calories 170
total fat 1.5 g
  saturated 0.5 g
  polyunsaturated 0.5 g
  monounsaturated 0.5 g
cholesterol 49 mg

sodium 412 mg
carbohydrates 20 g
  fiber 7 g
  sugar 13 g
protein 22 g

100 200 300 400

DIETARY EXCHANGES
$\frac{1}{2}$ fruit; 2 vegetable;
$2\frac{1}{2}$ very lean meat

chicken and toasted walnut salad

Serves 4; 1/2 cup per serving

Serve this sweet and crunchy chicken salad as is, on a bed of spring greens or slices of cantaloupe, in an open-face sandwich—even in hollowed-out apples for a fun presentation.

12 ounces chicken tenders
     Vegetable oil spray
1/4 cup fat-free or light sour cream
  2 tablespoons fat-free half-and-half or fat-free milk
  2 tablespoons fat-free or light mayonnaise dressing
1/2 teaspoon curry powder (optional)
1/4 teaspoon salt
1/4 teaspoon pepper
3/4 cup halved green or red seedless grapes
  1 medium rib of celery, thinly sliced
1/2 cup finely chopped red onion
1/4 cup finely chopped dried apricots
1/4 cup finely chopped walnut pieces, dry-roasted

Discard all visible fat from the chicken. Heat a large nonstick skillet over medium heat. Remove from the heat and lightly spray with vegetable oil spray (being careful not to spray near a gas flame). Cook the chicken for 5 minutes on each side, or until no longer pink in the center. Transfer to a cutting board to cool slightly.

Meanwhile, in a medium bowl, whisk together the sour cream, half-and-half, mayonnaise, curry powder, salt, and pepper until completely blended.

Stir in the remaining ingredients except the chicken.

Chop the cooled chicken into bite-size pieces. Stir into the salad. Serve or cover and refrigerate for up to 24 hours.

PER SERVING

calories 231

total fat 6.0 g

  saturated 1.0 g

  polyunsaturated 4.0 g

  monounsaturated 1.0 g

cholesterol 52 mg

sodium 297 mg

carbohydrates 21 g

  fiber 2 g

  sugar 12 g

protein 23 g

100 200 300 400

DIETARY EXCHANGES

1 fruit; 1 vegetable;
3 lean meat

mexican beef salad

Serves 4; 2 cups per serving

What a great way to use leftover beef!

6 ounces cooked lean beef, cooked without salt, all visible fat discarded

2 tablespoons fat-free or light Italian salad dressing

2 tablespoons fresh lime juice

1/3 cup snipped fresh cilantro

2 small Anaheim chile peppers or 1/2 medium green bell pepper

1 or 2 medium fresh jalapeños or 1/8 to 1/4 teaspoon crushed red pepper flakes (optional)

10 ounces mixed salad greens (spring greens preferred)

1/2 medium cucumber, peeled and sliced

1/2 cup thinly sliced red onion

1/4 cup plus 2 tablespoons fat-free or light Italian salad dressing

2 ounces crumbled blue cheese or fat-free or reduced-fat feta cheese or 2 ounces shredded part-skim mozzarella or fat-free or reduced-fat Cheddar cheese

Thinly slice the beef. Put in a medium bowl.

Stir in 2 tablespoons salad dressing and lime juice until the beef is coated.

Add the cilantro. Toss gently.

Wearing disposable plastic gloves, discard the seeds and ribs of the Anaheim and jalapeño peppers. Cut the Anaheim peppers into thin rounds and mince the jalapeños. If using bell pepper, thinly slice lengthwise. (Gloves are not needed.) Transfer the peppers to a large bowl.

Add the salad greens, cucumber, onion, and remaining salad dressing to the peppers. Toss together.

To serve, place the greens mixture on plates. Top with the beef mixture. Sprinkle with the blue cheese.

PER SERVING

calories 182
total fat 6.5 g
  saturated 3.5 g
  polyunsaturated 0.5 g
  monounsaturated 2.0 g
cholesterol 40 mg

sodium 524 mg
carbohydrates 14 g
  fiber 2 g
  sugar 6 g
protein 17 g

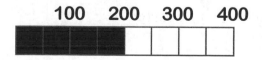

100 200 300 400

DIETARY EXCHANGES
1 vegetable;
$\frac{1}{2}$ other carbohydrate;
2 lean meat

flank steak salad
with sesame-lime dressing

Serves 4; 1¹/₂ cups salad, 2 ounces steak, and 2 tablespoons dressing per serving

The dressing in this recipe is a fine complement for the Honey-Lime Flank Steak (page 464) or other grilled steak saved from a previous meal.

salad

3 cups shredded napa cabbage (about ¹/₂ medium)

2 cups torn mixed salad greens (spring greens preferred)

8-ounce can sliced water chestnuts, rinsed and drained

7-ounce jar pickled baby corn, rinsed and drained

8 grape tomatoes or cherry tomatoes

4 medium green onions (green and white parts), sliced

dressing

¹/₄ teaspoon grated lime zest

¹/₃ cup fresh lime juice

2 tablespoons honey

1 tablespoon plain rice vinegar

2 teaspoons sesame seeds, dry-roasted

Dash of cayenne

8 ounces grilled flank steak (such as reserved from Honey-Lime Flank Steak), thinly sliced on the diagonal, warmed if desired

¼ cup slivered almonds, dry-roasted

In a large bowl, toss together the salad ingredients.

In a small bowl, whisk together the dressing ingredients. Pour over the salad. Toss gently.

To assemble, put the salad on plates. Arrange the steak slices over the salad. Sprinkle with the almonds.

PER SERVING ···

calories 271
total fat 9.5 g
 saturated 2.5 g
 polyunsaturated 1.5 g
 monounsaturated 4.5 g
cholesterol 33 mg

sodium 170 mg
carbohydrates 26 g
 fiber 6 g
 sugar 16 g
protein 22 g

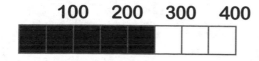

100 200 300 400

DIETARY EXCHANGES
3 vegetable;
½ other carbohydrate;
2½ lean meat; ½ fat

cannellini and black bean salad

Serves 6; 1 cup bean salad and $\frac{2}{3}$ cup spinach per serving

This colorful salad has it all—smooth and crunchy textures; tart, sweet, and hot flavors; and protein, fruit, and vegetables.

2 small fresh jalapeños

2 cups grape tomatoes or chopped tomatoes

1 cup no-salt-added cannellini beans, rinsed and drained

1 cup no-salt-added black beans, rinsed and drained

1 cup peeled jícama in 1-inch strips (about 10 ounces)

1 large mango, chopped

1 small onion, chopped

¼ cup snipped fresh cilantro

3 tablespoons fresh lime juice

1 tablespoon white wine vinegar

1 teaspoon salt

¼ teaspoon pepper

4 cups fresh baby spinach leaves

Wearing disposable plastic gloves, discard the seeds and ribs of the jalapeños. Dice the jalapeños. Transfer to a large bowl. Add the remaining ingredients except the spinach. (You can refrigerate the mixture, covered, for up to one day before serving.)

To serve, place the spinach on plates. Top with the bean mixture.

TIME-SAVER: For a shortcut, substitute 3 cups of prepared pico de gallo for the tomatoes, onions, jalapeño, cilantro, and 1 tablespoon of the lime juice. You can find pico de gallo in the produce section of your grocery store.

PER SERVING

calories 142
total fat 0.5 g
  saturated 0.0 g
  polyunsaturated 0.0 g
  monounsaturated 0.0 g
cholesterol 0 mg

sodium 415 mg
carbohydrates 30 g
  fiber 7 g
  sugar 12 g
protein 7 g

---

100 200 300 400

DIETARY EXCHANGES
1 starch; $\frac{1}{2}$ fruit;
1$\frac{1}{2}$ vegetable;
$\frac{1}{2}$ very lean meat

seafood

Fish Tacos with Tomato and
Avocado Salsa

Cornmeal-Crusted Catfish with
Lemon-Ginger Tartar Sauce

Parmesan-Topped Salmon

Salmon Florentine

Salmon with Creamy Caper Sauce

Skillet-Poached Salmon with Wasabi
and Soy Sauce

Pasta with Salmon, Roasted
Mushrooms, and Asparagus

Baked Almond-Crunch Sea Bass

Cajun-Creole Stuffed Sole

Lime-Cilantro Swordfish with Mixed
    Bean and Pineapple Salsa

Tilapia en Papillote

Tilapia Champignon

Tilapia and Spinach Roll-Ups
    with Shallot and
    White Wine Sauce

Hazelnut-Crusted Trout
    with Balsamic Glaze

Tuna Steaks with Tarragon Sour
    Cream

Gourmet Tuna-Noodle Casserole

Tropical Tuna Hero Sandwiches

Tuna and Broccoli with
    Lemon-Caper Brown Rice

Grilled Fish with Cucumber Salsa

Scallop and Spinach Sauté

Cumin Shrimp and Rice Toss

Shrimp and Lemon-Basil Pasta

Tomato-Caper Shrimp
    with Herbed Feta

fish tacos with tomato and avocado salsa

Serves 4; 1 taco per serving

Finely chopped fresh vegetables absorb the lime and cilantro flavors more evenly, producing a very tasty salsa.

tomato and avocado salsa

1 medium tomato, finely chopped (about 3/4 cup)
1/2 medium avocado, chopped
1/2 medium green bell pepper, finely chopped
1/3 cup snipped fresh cilantro
1/4 cup finely chopped red onion
1 to 2 tablespoons fresh lime juice
1/4 teaspoon salt

4 mild, thin fish fillets, such as tilapia (about 4 ounces each)
1/2 teaspoon ground cumin
1/8 teaspoon salt
Paprika to taste
Vegetable oil spray
4 8-inch fat-free or low-fat flour tortillas
2 cups shredded lettuce

In a medium bowl, stir together the salsa ingredients. Set aside.

Rinse the fish and pat dry with paper towels. Sprinkle the fish with the cumin, $\frac{1}{8}$ teaspoon salt, and paprika.

Heat a 12-inch nonstick skillet over medium-high heat. Remove from the heat and lightly spray with vegetable oil spray (being careful not to spray near a gas flame). With the skillet away from the heat, add the fish. Lightly spray the fish with vegetable oil spray. Cook for 3 minutes on each side, or until the fish flakes easily when tested with a fork.

Meanwhile, warm the tortillas using the package directions.

To serve, top each tortilla with lettuce, fish, and salsa. Serve open-face or as a wrap.

COOK'S TIP ON AVOCADOS: The buttery, slightly nutty-tasting avocado is actually a fruit, not a vegetable. Although it is high in fat, most of the fat is monounsaturated. When purchasing avocados, look for those that feel heavy for their size and have no blemishes. Because avocados don't start to ripen until they are taken off the tree, they probably will be hard when you purchase them. Let them ripen at room temperature for two to six days, until they yield to firm pressure but don't feel very soft. Drizzling or tossing avocados with citrus juice or combining them with tomatoes will help keep the avocados from darkening for an hour or so. The discoloration doesn't affect the flavor but does make the fruit look unappealing.

PER SERVING

calories 252	sodium 596 mg
total fat 5.0 g	carbohydrates 31 g
saturated 0.5 g	fiber 5 g
polyunsaturated 0.5 g	sugar 3 g
monounsaturated 2.5 g	protein 22 g
cholesterol 43 mg	

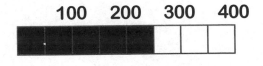

100   200   300   400

DIETARY EXCHANGES
1½ starch; 1½ vegetable; 3 lean meat

cornmeal-crusted catfish with lemon-ginger tartar sauce

Serves 4; 3 ounces fish and 1 tablespoon tartar sauce per serving

Catfish goes from common to chic with this classy dish. The fillets are dusted with a lemon-pepper cornmeal coating, pan-seared until crisp, and topped with a zesty tartar sauce. A carrot, cabbage, and broccoli slaw is a good choice for a side dish.

lemon-ginger tartar sauce

¼ cup fat-free or light mayonnaise dressing
1 tablespoon sweet pickle relish
1 teaspoon grated peeled gingerroot
1 teaspoon grated lemon zest
1 teaspoon fresh lemon juice

4 catfish fillets (about 4 ounces each)
¼ cup fat-free or low-fat buttermilk
½ teaspoon salt-free lemon pepper
¼ cup whole-wheat flour
¼ cup yellow cornmeal
Vegetable oil spray
1 teaspoon canola or corn oil

In a small bowl, stir together the tartar sauce ingredients. Cover and refrigerate until ready to serve. (The tartar sauce will keep for up to three days in the refrigerator.)

Rinse the fish and pat dry with paper towels.

In a large, shallow bowl, stir together the buttermilk and lemon pepper. Dip the fish in the buttermilk, turning to coat. Let the fillets soak for 10 minutes at room temperature or up to 4 hours covered in the refrigerator.

In a medium, shallow bowl, stir together the flour and cornmeal. Remove one fillet from the buttermilk. Coat on both sides with the cornmeal mixture, shaking off any excess. Place the fillet on a flat work surface. Repeat with the remaining fillets.

Heat a large nonstick skillet over medium-high heat. Remove from the heat and lightly spray with vegetable oil spray (being careful not to spray near a gas flame). Pour the oil into the skillet and swirl to coat the bottom. Cook the fillets for 4 to 5 minutes, or until browned on one side. Remove the pan from the heat and lightly spray the top of the fillets with vegetable oil spray. Turn the fillets. Cook for 4 to 5 minutes, or until the fish is golden brown and flakes easily when tested with a fork.

To serve, transfer the fillets to plates. Serve with the tartar sauce on the side or spoon a dollop of sauce onto each fillet.

PER SERVING

calories 201
total fat 5.0 g
  saturated 1.0 g
  polyunsaturated 1.5 g
  monounsaturated 2.0 g
cholesterol 66 mg

sodium 222 mg
carbohydrates 17 g
  fiber 2 g
  sugar 3 g
protein 21 g

100 200 300 400

DIETARY EXCHANGES
1 starch; 3 lean meat

parmesan-topped salmon
Serves 4; 3 ounces fish per serving

In less than half an hour, you can prepare this delicious salmon dish from start to finish—perfect for those busy days!

Vegetable oil spray
4 salmon fillets (about 4 ounces each)
1 tablespoon plus 1 teaspoon fat-free or light mayonnaise dressing
1 medium garlic clove, minced
Dash of white pepper (optional)
2 tablespoons shredded or grated Parmesan cheese
1/2 teaspoon paprika

Preheat the oven to 375°F.

Lightly spray a shallow roasting pan with vegetable oil spray. Rinse the fish and pat dry with paper towels. Place the fish in the pan.

In a small bowl, stir together the mayonnaise, garlic, and white pepper. Lightly spread on each fillet. Sprinkle with the Parmesan and paprika.

Bake for 15 to 20 minutes, or until the fish flakes easily when tested with a fork.

COOK'S TIP ON PAPRIKA: Paprika is often thought of as a garnish, simply imparting its vibrant color to food without adding much flavor. However, paprika is actually a spice made from ground red-pepper pods, so it does provide flavor. Many people prefer Hungarian paprika, one of the mildest types, yet one that gives a sweet, rich flavor and lovely color. You can use Hungarian paprika anytime paprika or sweet paprika is called for. Hungarians consume about 6,000 pounds of paprika each year, making it the single most important spice—and one of the most important ingredients overall—used in their cooking.

PER SERVING

calories 149
total fat 4.5 g
 saturated 1.0 g
 polyunsaturated 1.5 g
 monounsaturated 1.5 g
cholesterol 61 mg

sodium 161 mg
carbohydrates 1 g
 fiber 0 g
 sugar 1 g
protein 24 g

100   200   300   400

DIETARY EXCHANGES
3 lean meat

salmon florentine

Serves 4; 3 ounces fish and ½ cup spinach per serving

The large amount of spinach cooks down into a flavorful bed for the salmon in this one-dish entrée.

Vegetable oil spray
4 salmon fillets (about 4 ounces each)
1 tablespoon salt-free all-purpose seasoning blend
1 teaspoon olive oil
1 teaspoon pepper
1 teaspoon paprika
2 medium garlic cloves, minced
1 teaspoon water
¼ teaspoon salt
6 to 8 cups fresh baby spinach leaves
6-ounce jar marinated artichoke hearts, drained and chopped

Preheat the oven to 375°F. Lightly spray a 13 × 9 × 2-inch baking pan with vegetable oil spray.

Rinse the fish and pat dry with paper towels.

In a small bowl, combine the seasoning blend, oil, pepper, paprika, garlic, water, and salt. Brush the seasoning mixture over both sides of the fish.

To assemble, put the spinach in the baking pan, covering the bottom. Put the salmon and artichokes on the spinach. Lightly spray with vegetable oil spray.

Bake, uncovered, for 15 to 20 minutes, or until the fish flakes easily when tested with a fork.

salmon with creamy caper sauce

Serves 4; 3 ounces fish and 2 tablespoons sauce per serving

If you need immediate elegance, you can depend on this dish. While the salmon cooks, toss the sauce together. Then sit back and enjoy your guests.

Vegetable oil spray
4 salmon fillets with skin (about 5 ounces each)
1/4 teaspoon pepper

creamy caper sauce

1/3 cup fat-free or low-fat plain yogurt
2 tablespoons capers, rinsed and drained
2 teaspoons fat-free milk
1 teaspoon dried dillweed, crumbled
3/4 teaspoon stone-ground Dijon mustard
1/2 medium garlic clove, minced
1/4 teaspoon coarsely ground pepper

Preheat the oven to 350°F. Line a baking sheet with aluminum foil. Lightly spray with vegetable oil spray.

Rinse the fish and pat dry with paper towels. Place the fish with the skin side down on the baking sheet. Sprinkle with 1/4 teaspoon pepper.

Bake, uncovered, for 18 to 20 minutes, or until the fish flakes easily when tested with a fork and is opaque in the center.

Meanwhile, in a small bowl, stir together the sauce ingredients.

To serve, place the fish on plates. Spoon 2 tablespoons sauce over each fillet.

COOK'S TIP: Lining the baking sheet with aluminum foil will make cleanup easy.

PER SERVING

calories 160
total fat 4.5 g
  saturated 0.5 g
  polyunsaturated 1.5 g
  monounsaturated 1.0 g
cholesterol 65 mg

sodium 240 mg
carbohydrates 2 g
  fiber 0 g
  sugar 2 g
protein 26 g

100 200 300 400 **DIETARY EXCHANGES**

3 lean meat

skillet-poached salmon with wasabi and soy sauce

Serves 4; 3 ounces fish, $1/2$ cup sugar snap peas, and 2 tablespoons sauce per serving

A pungent blend of wasabi, soy sauce, and fresh ginger makes an unusual, delicious poaching liquid for salmon. With sugar snap peas added, the sauce is then reduced to a tempting glaze. Serve with soba noodles and fresh orange slices.

$1/2$ cup fat-free, low-sodium chicken broth
2 medium green onions (green and white parts), chopped
2 tablespoons light brown sugar
2 tablespoons low-salt soy sauce
1 teaspoon grated peeled gingerroot
1 teaspoon wasabi paste
1 teaspoon toasted sesame oil
1 medium garlic clove, minced
4 salmon fillets (about 4 ounces each)
2 cups sugar snap peas (about 8 ounces), trimmed

In a large skillet, bring the broth, green onions, brown sugar, soy sauce, gingerroot, wasabi paste, sesame oil, and garlic to a simmer over medium-high heat.

Add the salmon. Spoon the sauce mixture over the salmon to coat. Reduce the heat and simmer, covered, for 8 to 9 minutes, or until the fish is almost cooked through.

Stir in the sugar snap peas. Increase the heat to medium high. Occasionally spooning the sauce over the salmon, cook, uncovered, for 2 to 3 minutes, or until the fish flakes easily when tested with a fork, the peas are tender, and the sauce is slightly reduced and is the consistency of a glaze.

PER SERVING
calories 205
total fat 5.5 g
  saturated 1.0 g
  polyunsaturated 2.0 g
  monounsaturated 1.5 g
cholesterol 59 mg

sodium 311 mg
carbohydrates 13 g
  fiber 2 g
  sugar 9 g
protein 25 g

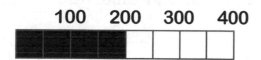

100 200 300 400

DIETARY EXCHANGES
1 vegetable; ½ other
carbohydrate;
3 lean meat

pasta with salmon, roasted mushrooms, and asparagus

Serves 4; 1½ cups per serving

While the vegetables are roasting, the pasta is cooking for this all-in-one meal, featuring salmon in a pouch. Fit in some extra veggies with a tossed salad.

Vegetable oil spray

3 tablespoons red wine vinegar or balsamic vinegar

1 tablespoon low-salt soy sauce or light teriyaki sauce

2 teaspoons sugar

2 medium garlic cloves, minced

1 teaspoon minced peeled gingerroot

¼ teaspoon pepper

8 ounces baby portobellos or other fresh mushrooms, thickly sliced

8 ounces fresh asparagus, trimmed and cut diagonally into 1-inch pieces

2 tablespoons sesame seeds

6 ounces whole-wheat or spinach elbow macaroni

7.1-ounce pouch skinless, boneless pink salmon

2 teaspoons toasted sesame oil

2 medium green onions (green and white parts), chopped

Preheat the oven to 425°F. Lightly spray a rimmed baking sheet with vegetable oil spray.

In a large bowl, stir together the vinegar, soy sauce, sugar, garlic, gingerroot, and pepper.

Add the mushrooms and asparagus, stirring to coat. Arrange in a single layer on the baking sheet. Spoon the vinegar mixture over the vegetables. Sprinkle with the sesame seeds.

Bake for 10 minutes. Stir. Bake for 5 minutes, or until the vegetables begin to caramelize, or brown richly.

Meanwhile, cook the pasta using the package directions, omitting the salt and oil. Drain well in a colander. Transfer to a large bowl.

To serve, stir the salmon, roasted vegetables with accumulated pan juices, and sesame oil into the pasta. Sprinkle with the green onions.

COOK'S TIP ON GINGERROOT:

When purchasing fresh gingerroot, look for firm, unwrinkled pieces with thin skin. Peel it with a small, sharp paring knife or a vegetable peeler and then grate, mince, chop, or slice as your recipe recommends.

PER SERVING

calories 299
total fat 7.5 g
  saturated 1.5 g
  polyunsaturated 2.5 g
  monounsaturated 2.0 g
cholesterol 18 mg

sodium 357 mg
carbohydrates 42 g
  fiber 9 g
  sugar 7 g
protein 19 g

100   200   300   400

DIETARY EXCHANGES
2 starch; 2 vegetable;
1½ lean meat

baked almond-crunch sea bass

Serves 4; 3 ounces fish, $^1/_2$ cup carrots, and $^1/_2$ baked potato per serving

Simplify dinnertime by baking everything in one pan. Add a green salad for a delicious meal with very little cleanup.

Vegetable oil spray

2 medium baking potatoes, such as russet

2 cups baby carrots

$^1/_2$ teaspoon salt

Pepper to taste

4 sea bass, salmon, or halibut steaks or fillets (about 4 ounces each)

Pepper to taste

2 tablespoons Dijon mustard

1 tablespoon stick margarine, melted

1 tablespoon plus 1 teaspoon honey

$^1/_4$ cup plain dry bread crumbs

$^1/_4$ cup sliced almonds

2 tablespoons fresh snipped parsley or 1 teaspoon dried, crumbled

2 tablespoons fresh snipped cilantro or 1 teaspoon dried, crumbled

$^1/_4$ teaspoon salt

Preheat the oven to 375°F. Lightly spray a large baking sheet with vegetable oil spray.

Leaving the peel on, cut the potatoes lengthwise into ½-inch-thick strips.

Place the potatoes and carrots in a single layer on the baking sheet. Lightly spray with vegetable oil spray. Sprinkle with the ½ teaspoon salt and pepper.

Bake for 15 minutes.

Meanwhile, rinse the fish and pat dry with paper towels. Sprinkle the fish with pepper.

In a small bowl, stir together the mustard, margarine, and honey. Brush on the fish.

In another small bowl, combine the bread crumbs, almonds, parsley, and cilantro. Pat the mixture on the fish.

Remove the vegetables from the oven. Increase the temperature to 450°F. Using a spatula, turn the potatoes and carrots, making room in the middle of the baking sheet for the fish. Without disturbing the crumb topping, gently place the fish on the baking sheet with the vegetables.

Bake for 10 minutes for each inch of thickness, or until the fish flakes easily when tested with a fork.

PER SERVING ....

calories 306
total fat 9.5 g
 saturated 1.5 g
 polyunsaturated 2.5 g
 monounsaturated 4.0 g
cholesterol 47 mg

sodium 776 mg
carbohydrates 32 g
 fiber 4 g
 sugar 12 g
 protein 26 g

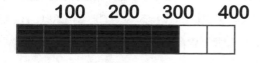

100 200 300 400   **DIETARY EXCHANGES**
                      1½ starch; 1½ vege-
                      table; 3 lean meat

cajun-creole stuffed sole

Serves 4; 3 ounces fish and $\frac{1}{2}$ cup rice stuffing per serving (plus 3 cups rice stuffing reserved)

Ideal for a Mardi Gras celebration, these sole fillets get a double dose of Louisiana tradition. They are stuffed with a jazzed-up jambalaya mix (with leftovers for another dish), then coated with Cajun or Creole seasoning.

Vegetable oil spray
1 medium onion, diced
1 medium red bell pepper, diced
2 medium ribs of celery, thinly sliced
$\frac{1}{4}$ cup snipped fresh parsley
2 medium garlic cloves, minced
$2\frac{1}{2}$ cups water
8-ounce box jambalaya mix with seasoning packet
2 sole fillets (about 8 ounces each)
1 teaspoon Cajun or Creole seasoning blend

Heat a medium saucepan over medium-high heat. Remove from the heat and lightly spray with vegetable oil spray (being careful not to spray near a gas flame). Cook the onion, bell pepper, celery, parsley, and garlic for 3 to 4 minutes, or until tender, stirring occasionally.

Stir in the water. Bring to a simmer, stirring occasionally. Stir in the jambalaya mix with seasoning. Reduce the heat and simmer, covered, for 20 to 25 minutes, or until the rice is tender (no stirring needed).

Measure 2 cups of the jambalaya mixture and set aside. Cover and refrigerate the remaining mixture for another use (see facing recipe for a suggestion).

Preheat the oven to 400°F. Lightly spray an 8-inch square baking dish with vegetable oil spray.

Rinse the fish and pat dry with paper towels. Cut each fillet in half lengthwise. Spoon 1/2 cup jambalaya mixture onto the middle of each fillet. Bring the ends to the center to enclose the filling. Place the fillets with the seam side down in the baking dish. Lightly spray the tops with vegetable oil spray. Sprinkle with the seasoning blend.

Bake, covered, for 15 minutes. Uncover and bake for 5 minutes, or until the fish flakes easily when tested with a fork and the filling is warmed through.

jambalaya

Serves 6; about 1½ cups per serving

3 cups cooked jambalaya mix (see above)

1 cup chopped, cooked lean meat, cooked without salt, such as chicken, turkey, beef, or pork tenderloin, or 1/2 cup chopped, cooked low-fat, lower-sodium ham

15-ounce can no-salt-added beans, such as navy, pinto, or red

In a 1½-quart microwaveable casserole, stir together all the ingredients. Microwave at 100 percent power (high) for 2 to 3 minutes, or until warm. Or stir the ingredients together in a nonstick casserole dish and warm in a preheated 350°F oven for 20 to 25 minutes.

CAJUN-CREOLE STUFFED SOLE

PER SERVING

calories 226
total fat 1.5 g
 saturated 0.5 g
 polyunsaturated 0.5 g
 monounsaturated 0.5 g
cholesterol 54 mg

sodium 595 mg
carbohydrates 26 g
 fiber 5 g
 sugar 3 g
 protein 26 g

100   200   300   400   DIETARY EXCHANGES
1 starch; 2 vegetable;
3 very lean meat

JAMBALAYA

PER SERVING

calories 282
total fat 1.0 g
 saturated 0.5 g
 polyunsaturated 0.5 g
 monounsaturated 0.5 g
cholesterol 30 mg

sodium 558 mg
carbohydrates 43 g
 fiber 9 g
 sugar 3 g
 protein 21 g

100   200   300   400   DIETARY EXCHANGES
3 starch;
2 very lean meat

lime-cilantro swordfish with mixed bean and pineapple salsa

Serves 4; 3 ounces fish and ¾ cup salsa per serving

This tropically inspired dish will transport you to summer. Prepare the salsa several hours in advance, if possible, to allow the flavors to blend.

4 swordfish steaks (about 4 ounces each)

marinade

Juice of 2 medium limes

1 tablespoon olive oil (extra-virgin preferred)

1 tablespoon honey

¼ teaspoon salt

Pepper to taste

salsa

1 cup drained canned no-salt-added black beans, rinsed

1 cup drained canned no-salt-added pink or pinto beans, rinsed

1 cup finely diced fresh pineapple

½ cup snipped fresh cilantro

1 tablespoon olive oil (extra-virgin preferred)

Juice of 2 medium limes

2 tablespoons minced red onion

½ teaspoon ground cumin

⅛ teaspoon salt

Dash of pepper

....

1 tablespoon snipped fresh cilantro (optional)

Rinse the fish and pat dry with paper towels.

In a glass baking dish, stir together the marinade ingredients. Put the fish in the marinade and turn to coat. Cover and refrigerate for 20 minutes to 2 hours, turning occasionally.

Meanwhile, stir together the salsa ingredients.

Preheat the grill or a large nonstick skillet over high heat.

Discard the marinade. Cook the fish for about 3 minutes on each side, or until it is seared, is the desired doneness, and flakes easily when tested with a fork.

To serve, place the fish on plates. Top with the salsa. Garnish with the cilantro.

COOK'S TIP ON SEA SALT: Sea salt is the least processed salt and therefore contains the most natural nutrients. Because it is very flavorful, if you want to substitute it in this and other recipes, use slightly less salt than is called for.

PER SERVING

calories 295
total fat 8.0 g
 saturated 1.5 g
 polyunsaturated 1.5 g
 monounsaturated 4.0 g
cholesterol 41 mg

sodium 315 mg
carbohydrates 27 g
 fiber 6 g
 sugar 8 g
protein 28 g

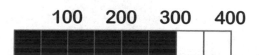

100 200 300 400

DIETARY EXCHANGES
1 1/2 starch; 1/2 fruit;
3 lean meat

tilapia en papillote
Serves 4; 3 ounces fish per serving

For tender, moist fish, steam it in parchment paper (**en papillote**). Serving each diner a puffed parchment pouch, with the top split open to release the aromatic steam, makes a dramatic presentation.

pico de gallo

$\frac{1}{2}$ medium fresh jalapeño

$\frac{1}{2}$ cup chopped tomato

$\frac{1}{2}$ cup chopped onion

$\frac{1}{4}$ cup snipped fresh cilantro

1 tablespoon fresh lime juice

Vegetable oil spray

4 tilapia fillets (about 4 ounces each)

Dash of salt

Dash of pepper

2 medium limes, each cut into 4 to 8 thin slices

Preheat the oven to 450°F.

Using plastic gloves, discard the seeds and ribs of the jalapeño. Dice the jalapeño. Transfer to a small bowl.

Stir the remaining pico de gallo ingredients into the jalapeño. Set aside.

Fold four pieces of cooking parchment, each about 14 × 12 inches, in half lengthwise. Cut each piece into a heart shape using the fold as the center of the heart and cutting half a heart. Open one paper heart and set it on a flat surface with the point of the heart toward you. Lightly spray the center of one half with vegetable oil spray. Place a fish fillet lengthwise on the sprayed area. Sprinkle with salt and pepper. Top with pico de gallo. Cover with slices of lime. Fold the other half over. Starting at the top of the heart, create a tight seam by folding about 1 inch of the paper toward you. Work your way down the side, toward the point, by folding over another 1 inch of paper, starting in the middle of the first 1-inch foldover. (It will look like a chain.) Continue down the side. When you reach the bottom of the heart, turn the last edge under the parchment pouch. Repeat for each fillet. Place the pouches on a baking sheet.

Bake for 8 minutes.

To serve, place the pouches on plates. Cut into the pouches at the top, being careful to avoid a steam burn.

VARIATION: Try different types of fish and vegetables to create your own signature dishes. Sole, cod, and catfish are just a few fish you can use for this dish. Instead of the pico de gallo, experiment with slices of mushrooms, zucchini, carrots, or shallots placed under the fillet, and top with dill, thyme, or basil and lemon slices. Prepare as directed above.

TIME-SAVER: Buy prepared pico de gallo and use 1 cup of it in place of the pico de gallo in this recipe.

PER SERVING

calories 89

total fat 1.0 g

  saturated 0.0 g

  polyunsaturated 0.0 g

  monounsaturated 0.0 g

cholesterol 43 mg

sodium 68 mg

carbohydrates 5 g

  fiber 1 g

  sugar 2 g

protein 17 g

DIETARY EXCHANGES

3 very lean meat;
1 vegetable

100   200   300   400

tilapia champignon
Serves 4; 3 ounces fish per serving

Mushrooms and wine combine magnificently with tilapia to create a delicate entrée. It's easy to prepare, yet elegant enough for guests.

Vegetable oil spray (olive oil spray preferred)
1/4 cup dry white wine (regular or nonalcoholic)
8 ounces sliced fresh button mushrooms
2 medium garlic cloves, minced
2 1/2 tablespoons plain dry bread crumbs
2 tablespoons shredded or grated Romano cheese
2 teaspoons salt-free all-purpose seasoning blend
1 teaspoon dried parsley, crumbled
1 teaspoon paprika
4 tilapia or sole fillets (about 4 ounces each)
1/4 cup dry white wine (regular or nonalcoholic)
1 medium lemon, quartered

Preheat the oven to 375°F. Lightly spray a 13 × 9 × 2-inch baking pan with vegetable oil spray. Set aside.

Heat a large nonstick skillet over medium-high heat. Pour in 1/4 cup wine. Add the mushrooms and cook for 7 to 10 minutes, or until tender, stirring occasionally. Stir in the garlic. Cook for 1 minute.

Meanwhile, in a small bowl, stir together the bread crumbs, Romano cheese, seasoning blend, parsley, and paprika.

Rinse the fish and pat dry with paper towels. Place the fillets side by side in the baking pan. Pour the mushroom mixture over the fish. Pour ¼ cup wine around, not over, the fish. Sprinkle the fish with the breadcrumb mixture.

Bake, uncovered, for 15 to 18 minutes, or until the fish flakes easily when tested with a fork.

Squeeze the lemon over the fish and serve.

PER SERVING

calories 136
total fat 2.0 g
  saturated 0.5 g
  polyunsaturated 0.0 g
  monounsaturated 0.5 g
cholesterol 44 mg

sodium 107 mg
carbohydrates 7 g
  fiber 1 g
  sugar 2 g
protein 20 g

100   200   300   400

DIETARY EXCHANGES
½ starch; 3 very lean meat

tilapia and spinach roll-ups with shallot and white wine sauce

Serves 4; 3 ounces fish per serving

Mild-flavored tilapia, which blends so nicely with other foods, is complemented here with baby spinach leaves and a topping of crushed walnuts.

4 tilapia fillets (about 4 ounces each)

1/4 teaspoon salt

Pepper to taste

5 ounces fresh baby spinach leaves

1/2 cup shredded or grated Parmesan cheese

1 cup dry white wine (regular or nonalcoholic), plus more as needed

1/2 cup fat-free, low-sodium chicken broth or low-sodium vegetable broth, plus more as needed

1 medium shallot, minced

2 tablespoons walnuts, crushed

Preheat the oven to 375°F.

Rinse the tilapia and pat dry with paper towels. Place the fish on a flat surface. Sprinkle the fish with the salt and pepper. Place the spinach on the fish. Sprinkle with the Parmesan. Starting at a short end, roll each fillet jelly-roll style. Secure each roll-up with a wooden toothpick. Place the fillets in a glass 13 × 9 × 2-inch baking dish.

Pour the wine and broth over the fish, using enough liquid to fill the dish to a depth of about ½ inch.

Sprinkle the shallot over the fish.

Bake, covered, for 30 minutes, or until the fish flakes easily when tested with a fork.

To serve, using a slotted pancake turner, transfer the roll-ups to plates. Sprinkle with the walnuts.

PER SERVING

calories 188
total fat 6.0 g
 saturated 2.0 g
 polyunsaturated 2.0 g
 monounsaturated 1.0 g
cholesterol 50 mg

sodium 383 mg
carbohydrates 3 g
 fiber 1 g
 sugar 0 g
protein 22 g

100 200 300 400 **DIETARY EXCHANGES**
1 vegetable; 3 lean meat

hazelnut-crusted trout with balsamic glaze

Serves 4; 3 ounces fish and 1 tablespoon glaze per serving

An almost effortless, intense balsamic glaze is the crowning touch to pan-seared trout fillets coated with crunchy hazelnut breading.

    3 tablespoons all-purpose flour
 1/4 cup fat-free or low-fat buttermilk
 1/4 cup plain dry bread crumbs
    2 tablespoons finely chopped hazelnuts
    4 rainbow, speckled, or brook trout fillets with skin
      (about 5 ounces each)
    1 teaspoon olive oil
      Vegetable oil spray (olive oil spray preferred)
 1/2 cup balsamic vinegar
    2 medium shallots, finely chopped
    1 tablespoon light brown sugar

Put the flour and buttermilk in separate shallow bowls. In a third bowl, stir together the bread crumbs and hazelnuts. Set the bowls in a row, assembly-line fashion.

Lightly coat both sides of a fillet with flour, shaking off the excess. Coat only the flesh side of the fillet with the buttermilk, then with the bread-crumb mixture. Place the fillet on a cutting board or plate. Repeat with the remaining fillets.

Heat a large nonstick skillet over medium-high heat. Pour the oil into the skillet and swirl to coat the bottom. Cook the fillets with the flesh side down for 3 to 4 minutes, or until the hazelnut crust is golden brown. Remove the pan from the heat. Lightly spray the skin side of the fish with vegetable oil spray. Cook with the skin side down for 3 to 4 minutes, or until the fish flakes easily when tested with a fork.

Meanwhile, in a small saucepan, stir together the vinegar and shallots. Bring to a simmer over medium-high heat. Adjusting the heat as needed, simmer without stirring for 5 minutes, or until the mixture is reduced by half (to about 1/4 cup).

Stir in the brown sugar. Simmer without stirring for 1 minute, or until the sugar is dissolved and the flavors have blended.

To serve, remove the fish skin with tongs if desired. Carefully place the fillets with the crust side up on plates. Drizzle the glaze over the fish.

PER SERVING

calories 267
total fat 8.0 g
 saturated 1.5 g
 polyunsaturated 2.0 g
 monounsaturated 4.0 g
cholesterol 68 mg

sodium 111 mg
carbohydrates 22 g
 fiber 1 g
 sugar 12 g
 protein 26 g

100 200 300 400 DIETARY EXCHANGES
1 1/2 starch; 3 lean meat

tuna steaks with tarragon sour cream

Serves 4; 3 ounces tuna and 2 tablespoons sour cream mixture per serving

The rich flavor of tuna blends perfectly with this bold yet creamy tarragon-lime sauce.

sauce

- 1/3 cup fat-free or light sour cream
- 2 tablespoons fat-free or light mayonnaise dressing
- 2 teaspoons fresh lime juice
- 3/4 teaspoon dried tarragon, crumbled
- 1/2 teaspoon pepper
- 1/4 teaspoon salt

- 1/4 teaspoon paprika
- 1/8 teaspoon garlic powder
- 1/8 teaspoon salt
- 4 tuna steaks (about 4 ounces each)
  Vegetable oil spray
- 1 medium lime, quartered

In a small bowl, stir together the sauce ingredients.

In another small bowl, combine the paprika, garlic powder, and 1/8 teaspoon salt. Sprinkle over both sides of the tuna.

Heat a large nonstick skillet over medium-high heat. Remove from the heat and lightly spray with vegetable oil spray (being careful not to spray near a gas flame). Cook the tuna for 2 minutes on each side, or until very pink in the center, for rare. Be careful not to overcook.

To serve, transfer the tuna to plates. Drizzle with the sauce. Place the lime wedges on the side.

PER SERVING

calories 157

total fat 1.0 g

  saturated 0.5 g

  polyunsaturated 0.5 g

  monounsaturated 0.0 g

cholesterol 54 mg

sodium 339 mg

carbohydrates 6 g

  fiber 0 g

  sugar 2 g

protein 28 g

100	200	300	400

DIETARY EXCHANGES
$1/2$ other carbohydrate;
3 very lean meat

gourmet tuna-noodle casserole

Serves 6; 1½ cups per serving

Flecks of spinach, crunchy water chestnuts, and a burst of lemon zest and fresh dill enhance this dish.

8 ounces dried whole-wheat pasta, such as rotini
  Vegetable oil spray
  12-ounce can albacore tuna in spring or distilled water, drained and flaked
  10.75-ounce can low-fat, reduced-sodium condensed cream of chicken soup
10 ounces frozen chopped spinach, thawed and squeezed dry
  8-ounce can sliced water chestnuts, rinsed and drained, coarsely chopped if desired
½ cup fat-free milk
½ cup fat-free or light sour cream
2 medium green onions (green and white parts), thinly sliced
1 tablespoon snipped fresh dillweed
2 teaspoons grated lemon zest
½ teaspoon salt
½ cup cornflake crumbs (about 1¼ cups flakes)

Prepare the pasta using the package directions, omitting the salt and oil. Drain well in a colander. Transfer to a large bowl.

Meanwhile, preheat the oven to 350°F. Lightly spray a 13 × 9 × 2-inch baking pan with vegetable oil spray.

Stir the remaining ingredients except the cornflake crumbs into the pasta. Spoon the mixture into the baking pan, smoothing the top. Sprinkle with the cornflake crumbs.

Bake for 30 minutes, or until the mixture is warmed through and the cornflake topping is crisp and golden brown.

PER SERVING

calories 321

total fat 3.0 g

  saturated 1.0 g

  polyunsaturated 1.0 g

  monounsaturated 0.5 g

cholesterol 30 mg

sodium 571 mg

carbohydrates 51 g

  fiber 8 g

  sugar 7 g

  protein 23 g

100   200   300   400

DIETARY EXCHANGES
3 starch; 1 vegetable;
2 very lean meat

tropical tuna hero sandwiches
Serves 4; 1 sandwich per serving

Macadamia nuts, basil, and orange zest are some of the ingredients that make this delightful filling unlike any other tuna salad you've ever eaten. Serve with slices of chilled honeydew melon.

4 hoagie-style rolls

tuna salad

9-ounce can albacore tuna in spring or distilled water, drained and flaked

8-ounce can pineapple tidbits in their own juice, drained

1/4 cup fat-free or light mayonnaise dressing

2 tablespoons chopped macadamia nuts

1 tablespoon imitation bacon bits

1 teaspoon grated orange zest

1/2 teaspoon dried basil, crumbled

1/8 teaspoon pepper

1/2 cup roasted red bell peppers, rinsed and drained if bottled

8 slices Bibb lettuce

Preheat the oven to 350°F.

Split the hoagie rolls and place them with the cut side up on a nonstick baking sheet.

Bake for 5 minutes, or until lightly toasted.

Meanwhile, in a medium bowl, stir together the tuna salad ingredients.

To assemble, spread the tuna salad on the bottom half of each hoagie roll. Place the bell peppers and lettuce on the tuna. Cover with the hoagie roll tops. Cut the sandwiches in half if desired.

PER SERVING

calories 358

total fat 10.0 g

  saturated 3.5 g

  polyunsaturated 2.0 g

  monounsaturated 4.0 g

cholesterol 27 mg

sodium 578 mg

carbohydrates 43 g

  fiber 3 g

  sugar 10 g

protein 23 g

100   200   300   400

DIETARY EXCHANGES

2$\frac{1}{2}$ starch; $\frac{1}{2}$ fruit;
2$\frac{1}{2}$ lean meat

tuna and broccoli with lemon-caper brown rice

Serves 4; 1 cup tuna mixture and ½ cup rice per serving

Although this dish tastes like a casserole, it's prepared on the stovetop.

1¼ cups fat-free, low-sodium chicken broth
1 tablespoon capers, rinsed and drained
1 teaspoon grated lemon zest
1 cup uncooked instant brown rice
1½ cups fat-free, low-sodium chicken broth
3 tablespoons all-purpose flour
½ teaspoon salt-free all-purpose seasoning
¼ teaspoon salt
½ cup fat-free half-and-half
2 cups frozen broccoli florets, thawed
9-ounce can albacore tuna in spring or distilled water, drained
¼ cup shredded or grated Parmesan cheese

In a medium saucepan, bring the 1¼ cups broth, capers, and lemon zest to a simmer over medium-high heat. Stir in the rice. Reduce the heat and simmer, covered, for 8 to 10 minutes, or until the rice is tender and has absorbed the liquid. Cover partially to keep warm.

Meanwhile, in a separate medium saucepan, whisk together the 1½ cups broth, flour, all-purpose seasoning, and salt until smooth. Bring to a simmer over medium-high heat. Simmer for 2 to 3 minutes, or until thickened, whisking occasionally. Whisk in the half-and-half. Cook on medium for 2 to 3 minutes, or until warmed through, whisking occasionally.

Stir in the broccoli, tuna, and Parmesan. Cook for 2 to 3 minutes, or until warmed through.

To serve, spoon the rice into bowls. Top with the tuna mixture.

PER SERVING

calories 257
total fat 4.5 g
 saturated 1.5 g
 polyunsaturated 1.0 g
 monounsaturated 1.5 g
cholesterol 30 mg

sodium 444 mg
carbohydrates 30 g
 fiber 4 g
 sugar 3 g
 protein 25 g

100   200   300   400

DIETARY EXCHANGES
1½ starch; 1 vegetable;
2½ very lean meat

grilled fish with cucumber salsa

Serves 4; 3 ounces fish and $\frac{1}{2}$ cup salsa per serving

Serve this on a summer night when you don't want to heat up the kitchen.

Vegetable oil spray

cucumber salsa

1 medium cucumber, finely chopped (about 1 cup)

$\frac{1}{2}$ medium green bell pepper, finely chopped

$\frac{1}{2}$ medium avocado, finely chopped

$\frac{1}{3}$ cup snipped fresh parsley

$\frac{1}{2}$ teaspoon grated lemon zest

1 to 2 tablespoons fresh lemon juice

$\frac{1}{2}$ teaspoon salt

$\frac{1}{4}$ teaspoon red hot-pepper sauce

4 fish fillets, such as halibut (about 4 ounces each)

$\frac{1}{2}$ teaspoon chili powder

$\frac{1}{4}$ teaspoon salt

1 medium lemon, quartered

Spray the grill rack with vegetable oil spray. Preheat the grill on medium high.

Meanwhile, in a medium bowl, gently stir together the salsa ingredients. Set aside.

Rinse the fish and pat dry with paper towels. Sprinkle the fish with the chili powder and ¼ teaspoon salt. Lightly spray both sides of the fish with vegetable oil spray. Grill for 3 minutes on each side, or until it flakes easily when tested with a fork.

To serve, transfer the fish to plates. Squeeze a lemon wedge over each serving. Spoon the salsa to the side.

PER SERVING

calories 167

total fat 5.0 g

  saturated 1.0 g

  polyunsaturated 1.0 g

  monounsaturated 3.0 g

cholesterol 40 mg

sodium 493 mg

carbohydrates 6 g

  fiber 3 g

  sugar 2 g

protein 24 g

100 200 300 400

DIETARY EXCHANGES

1 vegetable; 3 lean meat

scallop and spinach sauté

**Serves 4; 3 ounces scallops and
$^1\!/_2$ cup spinach per serving**

Seafood is ideal for busy days because it cooks so fast. Here, tender scallops are combined with leeks and baby spinach for a quick meal that is sure to impress. Brown rice is excellent with this dish.

1 teaspoon olive oil

2 medium leeks (white part only), thinly sliced

1 pound fresh bay scallops (about 2 cups), rinsed and patted dry with paper towels

1 tablespoon snipped fresh dillweed or 1 teaspoon dried, crumbled

1 teaspoon grated lemon zest

1 pound baby spinach leaves (about 10 cups)

2-ounce jar diced pimientos, rinsed and drained

1 tablespoon capers, rinsed and drained

Heat a large nonstick skillet over medium-high heat. Pour the oil into the skillet and swirl to coat the bottom. Cook the leeks for 1 to 2 minutes, or until tender-crisp, stirring occasionally.

Add the scallops, dillweed, and lemon zest. Cook for 30 seconds. Stir. Cook for 1 minute, stirring occasionally. (If the scallops have ever been frozen, they may need to cook for an additional 1 to 2 minutes to evaporate the extra liquid they may release.)

Stir in the spinach, pimientos, and capers. Cook for 1 to 2 minutes, or until the spinach is wilted, stirring occasionally.

PER SERVING

calories 167

total fat 2.5 g

  saturated 0.5 g

  polyunsaturated 0.5 g

  monounsaturated 1.0 g

cholesterol 37 mg

sodium 342 mg

carbohydrates 14 g

  fiber 4 g

  sugar 3 g

protein 23 g

100   200   300   400

DIETARY EXCHANGES

3 vegetable;

3 very lean meat

cumin shrimp and rice toss
Serves 4; 1½ cups per serving

Squeezing a generous amount of fresh lime over this dish raises it from good to great.

Vegetable oil spray

1 medium poblano or green bell pepper

1 medium yellow summer squash, cut into ¼-inch rounds

1 medium onion, cut into ½-inch wedges

12 cherry tomatoes

1 cup uncooked quick-cooking brown rice

1 pound peeled raw medium shrimp, rinsed and patted dry

½ tablespoon chili powder

1 teaspoon ground cumin

¼ teaspoon cayenne

⅛ teaspoon salt

1 tablespoon olive oil (extra-virgin preferred)

¼ teaspoon salt

⅓ cup snipped fresh cilantro

2 medium limes, quartered

Preheat the broiler. Line a broiler pan with aluminum foil. Lightly spray with vegetable oil spray.

Wearing disposable plastic gloves, discard the seeds and ribs of the poblano. Cut the poblano into 1-inch pieces. (Gloves are not needed if you are using bell pepper.)

Arrange the poblano, squash, onion, and tomatoes on the broiler pan in a single layer. Lightly spray the vegetables with vegetable oil spray.

Broil about 4 inches from the heat for 10 minutes. Stir gently. Broil for 2 minutes, or until tender-crisp and beginning to richly brown on the edges. Transfer the vegetables to a medium bowl. Cover with plastic wrap and let stand to allow the flavors to blend.

Meanwhile, prepare the rice using the package directions, omitting the salt and margarine.

Lightly spray any browned bits remaining in the skillet with vegetable oil spray. Heat over medium heat. Add the shrimp, chili powder, cumin, cayenne, and $1/8$ teaspoon salt. Stir. Cook for 5 minutes, or until the shrimp are opaque in the center, stirring frequently.

Stir the rice, oil, and $1/4$ teaspoon salt into the vegetable mixture.

To serve, transfer the rice and vegetable mixture to a platter. Top with the shrimp and any accumulated juices. Sprinkle with the cilantro. Serve with the lime wedges.

PER SERVING

calories 247

total fat 5.5 g
 saturated 1.0 g
 polyunsaturated 1.0 g
 monounsaturated 3.0 g
cholesterol 168 mg

sodium 434 mg
carbohydrates 27 g
 fiber 4 g
 sugar 6 g
protein 22 g

100   200   300   400   **DIETARY EXCHANGES**
1 starch; 2 vegetable;
3 lean meat

shrimp and lemon-basil pasta
Serves 4; 1$\frac{1}{2}$ cups per serving

Lots of lemon adds sparkle to this so-easy one-pot meal.

4 quarts water
8 ounces dried rotini
1 pound peeled raw medium shrimp
2 tablespoons olive oil (extra-virgin preferred)
1 tablespoon dried basil, crumbled
$\frac{1}{2}$ tablespoon dried oregano, crumbled
2 teaspoons Dijon mustard
2 medium garlic cloves, minced
$\frac{1}{2}$ teaspoon grated lemon zest
3 to 4 tablespoons fresh lemon juice
$\frac{1}{2}$ teaspoon salt
$\frac{1}{4}$ teaspoon pepper
$\frac{3}{4}$ cup grape tomatoes, halved (about 4 ounces)
$\frac{1}{2}$ cup finely snipped fresh parsley
1 medium lemon, quartered

In a large saucepan, bring the water to a boil over high heat. Stir in the pasta. Boil for 6 minutes. Stir in the shrimp. Boil for 5 minutes, or until the shrimp are opaque in the center and the pasta is tender. Drain well in a colander.

Meanwhile, in a large bowl, stir together the oil, basil, oregano, mustard, garlic, lemon zest, lemon juice, salt, and pepper.

Add the pasta mixture to the oil mixture. Toss gently to coat.

Add the tomatoes and parsley. Toss gently. Serve with the lemon wedges.

COOK'S TIP: The heat of the pasta and shrimp gently cooks the fresh garlic.

PER SERVING

calories 381	sodium 548 mg
total fat 9.0 g	carbohydrates 48 g
saturated 1.5 g	fiber 3 g
polyunsaturated 1.5 g	sugar 4 g
monounsaturated 5.5 g	protein 26 g
cholesterol 168 mg	

100 200 300 400 **DIETARY EXCHANGES**
3 starch; 3 lean meat

tomato-caper shrimp with herbed feta

Serves 4; 1½ cups per serving

Cooking the shrimp with the pasta is a definite step saver.

3 quarts water

6 ounces dried bow-tie pasta

1 pound peeled raw medium shrimp

3 medium tomatoes, diced

1 teaspoon dried basil, crumbled

½ teaspoon dried oregano, crumbled

1 medium garlic clove, minced

⅛ teaspoon crushed red pepper flakes

2 tablespoons capers, rinsed and drained

1 tablespoon olive oil (extra-virgin preferred)

¼ teaspoon salt

1 ounce feta cheese with sun-dried tomatoes and basil, crumbled

In a large saucepan, bring the water to a boil over high heat. Stir in the pasta. Boil for 6 minutes. Stir in the shrimp. Return to a boil. Boil for 3 to 5 minutes, or until the shrimp are opaque in the center and the pasta is tender. Drain well in a colander.

Meanwhile, heat a large nonstick skillet over medium-high heat. Cook the tomatoes, basil, oregano, garlic, and red pepper flakes for 5 minutes, or until the tomatoes are soft, stirring frequently. Remove from the heat. Stir in the capers, oil, and salt.

To serve, transfer the pasta and shrimp to a serving bowl. Top with the tomato mixture. Sprinkle with the feta.

PER SERVING
calories 294
total fat 4.5 g
  saturated 1.0 g
  polyunsaturated 1.0 g
  monounsaturated 1.5 g
cholesterol 171 mg

sodium 557 mg
carbohydrates 37 g
  fiber 3 g
  sugar 5 g
protein 26 g

100   200   300   400

DIETARY EXCHANGES
2 starch; 1½ vegetable;
3 very lean meat

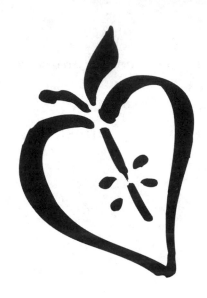

poultry

Sunday-Best Roast Chicken Breasts

Southwest Lime Chicken

Bistro Chicken with Fresh Asparagus

Salsa Chicken

Chicken with Herbed Mustard and
Green Onion Sauce

Chicken Breasts with Spinach,
Apricots, and Pine Nuts

Chicken with Zesty Apricot Sauce

Black-Pepper Chicken

Chicken Parmesan Supreme

Chicken Breasts Stuffed with Goat
Cheese, Dates, and Spinach

Stuffed Chicken Breasts
   in Lemon-Oregano Tomato Sauce

Chicken Fajitas

Slow-Cooker Chicken and Noodles

Chicken and Bow-Ties
   with Green Beans

Chicken with Penne Pasta
   and Mixed Greens

Risotto with Porcini Mushrooms
   and Chicken

Chicken and Veggies with Noodles

Chicken Enchiladas

Chicken Pot Pie

Barbecue Chicken Pizza

Slow-Roasted Sage Turkey Breast

Turkish Meatballs

Open-Face Broiled Turkey Sandwiches
   with Herb-Garlic Spread

Italian Turkey Sausage and Peppers
   with Whole-Wheat Fettuccine

Artichoke and Bell Pepper Lasagna

sunday-best roast chicken breasts

Serves 4; 3 ounces chicken per serving

Slide a layer of herbs, lemon, garlic, and pepper under the skin of chicken breasts to provide moist, tantalizing roast chicken for dinner on Sunday or any other day.

3 tablespoons snipped fresh parsley or 1 tablespoon dried, crumbled

1 tablespoon chopped fresh sage or 1 teaspoon dried

2 teaspoons grated lemon zest

1 tablespoon fresh lemon juice

2 medium garlic cloves, minced

1/8 teaspoon pepper

4 chicken breast halves with bone and skin (about 6 ounces each), all visible fat discarded

Preheat the oven to 350°F.

In a small bowl, stir together all the ingredients except the chicken.

With your hands or a spoon, carefully loosen the skin from the meat of one breast, leaving the skin attached at the sides. Spoon about 1 tablespoon parsley mixture between the meat and the skin. Put the breast with the skin side up in an ungreased 13 × 9 × 2-inch baking pan. Repeat with the remaining chicken.

Bake for 1 hour to 1 hour 15 minutes, or until the chicken is no longer pink in the center. Put the pan on a cooling rack and let cool for 5 minutes, or until you can easily remove the skin with a fork. Discard the skin and any remaining visible fat before serving the chicken.

PER SERVING

calories 127
total fat 1.5 g
  saturated 0.5 g
  polyunsaturated 0.5 g
  monounsaturated 0.5 g
cholesterol 64 mg

sodium 74 mg
carbohydrates 1 g
  fiber 0 g
  sugar 0 g
protein 26 g

100　200　300　400

DIETARY EXCHANGES
3 very lean meat

southwest lime chicken

Serves 4; 3 ounces chicken per serving

The combination of hot pepper and lime provides just the right balance of spiciness in this dish.

2 tablespoons all-purpose flour
1 tablespoon snipped fresh parsley
2 teaspoons grated lime zest
1 teaspoon salt-free all-purpose seasoning blend
1/2 teaspoon garlic powder
1/8 to 1/4 teaspoon cayenne
1/8 teaspoon paprika
4 boneless, skinless chicken breast halves or turkey cutlets (about 4 ounces each), all visible fat discarded
   Vegetable oil spray
1 tablespoon olive oil
   Juice of 1 medium lime

In a small bowl, stir together the flour, parsley, lime zest, seasoning blend, garlic powder, cayenne, and paprika.

Put the chicken with the smooth side up between two pieces of wax paper or plastic wrap. Using a tortilla press, the smooth side of a meat mallet, or a rolling pin, lightly flatten the breasts to a thickness of 1/4 inch, being careful not to tear the meat. (No flattening is needed for the turkey cutlets.) Coat with the flour mixture, shaking off the excess.

Heat a large nonstick skillet over medium-high heat. Remove from the heat and lightly spray with vegetable oil spray (being careful not to spray near a gas flame). Pour the oil into the skillet and swirl to coat the bottom. Once the oil is hot, cook the chicken for 4 minutes on each side, or until no longer pink in the center.

Sprinkle with the lime juice. Cook for 10 to 20 seconds, turning once.

PER SERVING

calories 174
total fat 5.0 g
  saturated 1.0 g
  polyunsaturated 0.5 g
  monounsaturated 3.0 g
cholesterol 66 mg

sodium 75 mg
carbohydrates 4 g
  fiber 0 g
  sugar 0 g
protein 27 g

100   200   300   400

DIETARY EXCHANGES
3 lean meat

bistro chicken with fresh asparagus

Serves 4; 3 ounces chicken, ⅓ cup mushroom mixture, and 2 asparagus spears per serving

The next time you have dinner guests, serve this easy-to-prepare chicken dish.

½ cup plain dry bread crumbs

1 tablespoon shredded or grated Parmesan cheese

½ teaspoon salt-free lemon pepper

½ teaspoon salt-free all-purpose seasoning blend

½ teaspoon garlic powder

½ teaspoon dried oregano, crumbled

2 tablespoons Dijon honey mustard

4 boneless, skinless chicken breast halves or turkey cutlets (about 4 ounces each), all visible fat discarded

Vegetable oil spray

½ cup dry white wine (regular or nonalcoholic), divided use

8 ounces sliced fresh button mushrooms

1 small onion, chopped

8 fresh asparagus spears, trimmed

1 medium tomato, seeded and chopped

1 tablespoon capers, rinsed and drained

In a small resealable plastic bag, combine the bread crumbs, Parmesan, lemon pepper, seasoning blend, garlic powder, and oregano.

Put the chicken with the smooth side up between two pieces of wax paper or plastic wrap. Using a tortilla press, the smooth side of a meat mallet, or a rolling pin, lightly flatten the breasts to a thickness of 1/4 inch, being careful not to tear the meat. (No flattening is needed for the turkey cutlets.)

Spread the mustard on both sides of the chicken. Add the chicken to the plastic bag, one piece at a time, and shake to coat. Shake to remove excess coating. Put the chicken on a plate. Repeat with the remaining chicken.

Heat a large nonstick skillet over medium-high heat. Remove from the heat and lightly spray with vegetable oil spray (being careful not to spray near a gas flame). Put the chicken in the skillet. Pour 2 tablespoons of the wine over the chicken. Cook for 2 minutes. Turn the chicken and pour in another 2 tablespoons of the wine. Cook for 1 to 2 minutes, or until the chicken is no longer pink in the center. Transfer the chicken to a platter. Cover with aluminum foil. Set aside.

Heat the skillet over medium-high heat. Remove from the heat and lightly spray with vegetable oil spray (being careful not to spray near a gas flame). Cook the mushrooms and onion for 2 to 3 minutes, or until lightly browned, stirring frequently.

Stir in the asparagus and remaining ¼ cup wine. Cook, covered, for 2 to 4 minutes, or until the asparagus is tender-crisp. Stir in the tomato.

To serve, spoon the mushroom mixture over the chicken and sprinkle with the capers.

PER SERVING

calories 261

total fat 3.0 g

  saturated 1.0 g

  polyunsaturated 0.5 g

  monounsaturated 0.5 g

cholesterol 67 mg

sodium 267 mg

carbohydrates 21 g

  fiber 3 g

  sugar 6 g

  protein 32 g

100 200 300 400

DIETARY EXCHANGES
1 starch; 1½ vegetable; 3 very lean meat

salsa chicken

**Serves 4; 3 ounces chicken
and 2 tablespoons salsa per serving**

Warm baked chicken and cool, spicy salsa provide an appealing contrast in flavor and texture. Crisp baked whole-wheat tortilla or pita wedges would pair nicely with this dish.

salsa

1 small fresh jalapeño or ½ teaspoon bottled pickled jalapeño juice

1 small tomato, chopped (about ½ cup)

⅓ cup snipped fresh cilantro or Italian, or flat-leaf, parsley

2 medium green onions (green and white parts), chopped

¼ cup low-sodium mixed vegetable juice or low-sodium tomato juice

2 medium garlic cloves, minced

1 teaspoon grated lemon or lime zest

1 tablespoon fresh lemon or lime juice

½ teaspoon ground cumin

4 boneless, skinless chicken breast halves (about 4 ounces each) or 1 pound boneless, skinless turkey breast

1 teaspoon grated lemon or lime zest

½ cup yellow cornmeal

2 tablespoons snipped fresh cilantro or Italian, or flat-leaf, parsley, loosely packed

1/4 teaspoon crushed red pepper flakes

2 tablespoons fresh lemon or lime juice

2 teaspoons canola or corn oil

Using disposable plastic gloves, discard the seeds and ribs of the jalapeño. Mince the jalapeño.

In a large bowl, stir together the salsa ingredients. Set aside.

Discard all visible fat from the chicken. Put the chicken with the smooth side up between two pieces of plastic wrap. Using a tortilla press, the smooth side of a meat mallet, or a rolling pin, lightly flatten the breasts to a thickness of 1/4 inch, being careful not to tear the meat.

In a shallow dish or pie pan, stir together the lemon zest, cornmeal, cilantro, and red pepper flakes. Sprinkle both sides of the chicken with 2 tablespoons lemon juice. Lightly coat the chicken with the cornmeal mixture, shaking off the excess.

Heat a large nonstick skillet over medium-high heat. Pour the oil into the skillet and swirl to coat the bottom. Cook the chicken for 3 to 4 minutes on each side, or until lightly browned and no longer pink in the center.

To serve, spoon the salsa over the chicken.

PER SERVING

calories 228
total fat 4.0 g
  saturated 0.5 g
  polyunsaturated 1.0 g
  monounsaturated 2.0 g
cholesterol 66 mg

sodium 89 mg
carbohydrates 19 g
  fiber 2 g
  sugar 2 g
protein 28 g

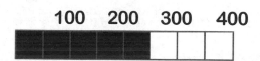

100 200 300 400

DIETARY EXCHANGES
1 starch; 1 vegetable;
3 very lean meat

chicken with herbed mustard and green onion sauce

Serves 4; 1 chicken breast and 2 tablespoons sauce per serving

Perfect for a warm-weather luncheon and sophisticated enough for candlelight, this dish features chicken breasts smothered in a delicate Dijon sauce seasoned with tarragon, rosemary, and mild green onions.

2 medium green onions

4 boneless, skinless chicken breast halves (about 4 ounces each)

1/4 teaspoon dried rosemary, crushed

1/4 teaspoon dried tarragon, crumbled

1/4 teaspoon salt

Vegetable oil spray

1/4 cup fat-free half-and-half

1/4 cup fat-free or light sour cream

1 tablespoon Dijon mustard

1/2 cup dry white wine (regular or nonalcoholic) or fat-free, low-sodium chicken broth

2 teaspoons olive oil (extra-virgin preferred)

1/4 teaspoon salt

Pepper to taste

1 medium lemon or lime, quartered (optional)

Chop the green part of the onions. Set aside. Fincly chop the white part, keeping separate from the green part.

Discard all visible fat from the chicken. Place the breasts with the smooth side up between two pieces of plastic wrap. Using a tortilla press, the smooth side of a meat mallet, or a rolling pin, lightly flatten the breasts to 1/4-inch thickness, being careful not to tear the meat. Sprinkle both sides of the chicken with the rosemary, tarragon, and 1/4 teaspoon salt.

Heat a 12-inch nonstick skillet over medium heat. Remove from the heat and lightly spray with vegetable oil spray (being careful not to spray near a gas flame). Cook the chicken for 5 minutes on each side, or until no longer pink in the center. Transfer to a plate. Cover with aluminum foil and set aside.

Meanwhile, in a small bowl, whisk together the half-and-half, sour cream, and mustard.

Increase the heat to high. Stir in the wine and white part of the green onions. Bring to a boil. Cook for 1 1/2 minutes, or until most of the liquid has evaporated, scraping the bottom and side frequently. Remove from the heat. Transfer to a separate plate.

Pour the half-and-half mixture into the skillet. Set over medium-low heat. Stir in the wine mixture, scraping the bottom and side of the skillet. (Be careful not to boil, or the sauce will break down.) Remove from the heat.

Stir in the oil and ¼ teaspoon salt. To assemble, place the chicken on plates. Pour the sauce over the chicken. Sprinkle with the pepper. Sprinkle with the green onion tops and lemon wedges.

PER SERVING

calories 201
total fat 4.0 g
 saturated 0.5 g
 polyunsaturated 0.5 g
 monounsaturated 2.0 g
cholesterol 68 mg

sodium 490 mg
carbohydrates 7 g
 fiber 0 g
 sugar 2 g
protein 29 g

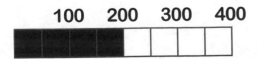

100 200 300 400

DIETARY EXCHANGES
½ other carbohydrate;
3 lean meat

chicken breasts with spinach, apricots, and pine nuts

Serves 4; 3 ounces chicken, scant ½ cup apricots, and ¼ cup spinach per serving

This elegant dish is a feast for your eyes as well as your taste buds.

 10-ounce can apricot halves in extra-light syrup
4 boneless, skinless chicken breast halves (about 4 ounces each)
 Whites of 3 large eggs
¾ cup plain dry bread crumbs
3 tablespoons pine nuts, crushed or finely chopped
¼ teaspoon salt
 Pepper to taste
2 teaspoons olive oil
5 ounces fresh baby spinach leaves

Drain the apricots well and reserve the syrup. Set aside.

Discard all the visible fat from the chicken. Put the chicken with the smooth side up between two pieces of plastic wrap. Using a tortilla press, the smooth side of a meat mallet, or a rolling pin, lightly flatten the breasts to a thickness of ¼ inch, being careful not to tear the meat.

In a pie pan or shallow bowl, lightly beat the egg whites. In another pie pan or shallow bowl, combine the bread crumbs, pine nuts, salt, and pepper. Set the containers side by side.

Dip the chicken in the egg whites. Coat with the bread-crumb mixture, shaking off any excess.

Heat a large skillet over medium-high heat. Pour the oil into the skillet and swirl to coat the bottom. Cook the chicken for 3 to 5 minutes, or until golden. Turn the chicken over.

Add the apricots to the skillet. Cook for 3 to 5 minutes, or until the chicken is browned on the outside and no longer pink in the center.

Pour in $1/4$ to $1/2$ cup reserved apricot syrup, depending on how much sauce you wish. Cook until the liquid has reduced by half and is the desired consistency.

Heat another large skillet over medium-high heat. Cook the spinach just until wilted, 2 to 3 minutes, stirring constantly.

To serve, arrange the spinach on plates. Top with the chicken and apricots.

PER SERVING

calories 310
total fat 8.0 g
 saturated 1.5 g
 polyunsaturated 2.0 g
 monounsaturated 3.5 g
cholesterol 66 mg

sodium 439 mg
carbohydrates 26 g
 fiber 3 g
 sugar 10 g
 protein 34 g

100 200 300 400

DIETARY EXCHANGES
1 starch; $1/2$ fruit;
$3^{1}/2$ lean meat

chicken with zesty apricot sauce

Serves 4; 3 ounces chicken and 2 tablespoons sauce per serving

Cooked rice tossed with green onions and slivers of sweet red bell pepper would make a colorful side for this sweet-tart entrée.

1 teaspoon chili powder

¼ teaspoon ground cumin

⅛ teaspoon salt

4 boneless, skinless chicken breast halves (about 4 ounces each)

Vegetable oil spray

½ cup all-fruit apricot spread

2 tablespoons cider vinegar

2 teaspoons sugar

⅛ teaspoon crushed red pepper flakes

⅛ teaspoon salt

1 medium lemon, quartered

In a small bowl, combine the chili powder, cumin, and ⅛ teaspoon salt.

Discard all visible fat from the chicken. Sprinkle the chili powder mixture over the smooth side of the chicken.

Heat a large skillet over medium-high heat. Remove from the heat and lightly spray with vegetable oil spray (being careful not to spray near a gas flame). Cook the chicken with the seasoned side down for 3 minutes. Turn over. Reduce the heat to medium and cook the chicken for 3 to 4 minutes, or until no longer pink in the center.

Meanwhile, in a small saucepan, stir together the apricot spread, vinegar, sugar, and red pepper flakes. Cook over medium heat for 2 minutes, or until the apricot spread has melted and the sugar is dissolved, stirring frequently. Spoon 2 tablespoons mixture onto each plate. With the back of the spoon, spread to a 6-inch diameter.

Sprinkle ⅛ teaspoon salt over the chicken. Place the chicken on the apricot mixture. Squeeze the lemon over the chicken.

PER SERVING

calories 219	sodium 226 mg
total fat 1.5 g	carbohydrates 24 g
saturated 0.5 g	fiber 0 g
polyunsaturated 0.5 g	sugar 19 g
monounsaturated 0.5 g	protein 26 g
cholesterol 66 mg	

100   200   300   400

DIETARY EXCHANGES
1½ fruit; 3 very lean meat

black-pepper chicken

Serves 4; 3 ounces chicken per serving

Sear chicken coated with black pepper over very high heat, then quickly reduce the sauce. That's all it takes to get these chicken tenders ready to serve. Make extra to use in soups, salads, sandwiches, casseroles—just about anything except dessert!

1 pound chicken tenders

1/2 teaspoon black pepper, or to taste

1 tablespoon olive oil, divided use

1/2 cup water

1/4 teaspoon salt

Discard all visible fat from the chicken. Sprinkle both sides of the chicken with the pepper.

Heat a 12-inch nonstick skillet over high heat. Pour 1/2 tablespoon of the oil into the skillet and swirl to coat the bottom. Cook the chicken for 2 minutes. Reduce the heat to medium. Pour in the remaining oil and swirl to coat the bottom of the skillet. Turn the chicken. Cook for 2 minutes, or until no longer pink in the center. Transfer the chicken to a platter.

Add the water and salt to the skillet. Increase the heat to high. Bring to a boil. Boil for 1 1/2 to 2 minutes, or until the liquid is reduced to 2 tablespoons, scraping to dislodge any browned bits from the bottom. Pour the sauce over the chicken. Turn the chicken to coat evenly.

COOK'S TIP: Be sure to use a 12-inch skillet for this dish. If you use a smaller size, it will crowd the chicken, causing it to simmer, not brown.

PER SERVING

calories 155
total fat 5.0 g
 saturated 1.0 g
 polyunsaturated 0.5 g
 monounsaturated 3.0 g
cholesterol 66 mg

sodium 220 mg
carbohydrates 0 g
 fiber 0 g
 sugar 0 g
protein 26 g

100	200	300	400	**DIETARY EXCHANGES**

3 lean meat

chicken parmesan supreme

Serves 4; 3 ounces chicken, $\frac{1}{2}$ cup sauce, and $\frac{1}{2}$ cup pasta per serving

If you enjoy chicken Parmesan, you'll love this calorie-trimmed version served in grand style. Breaded chicken is baked until moist, covered with a jazzed-up spaghetti sauce with shredded vegetables, and topped with just the right amount of melted cheese.

Vegetable oil spray

4 boneless, skinless chicken breast halves (about 4 ounces each)

$\frac{1}{3}$ cup fat-free or reduced-fat buttermilk

3 tablespoons whole-wheat flour or all-purpose flour

$\frac{1}{3}$ cup plain dry bread crumbs

3 tablespoons shredded or grated Parmesan cheese

1 teaspoon salt-free Italian seasoning

$\frac{1}{2}$ medium onion, thinly sliced

4 ounces sliced button mushrooms

1 cup shredded broccoli slaw

$1\frac{1}{2}$ cups fat-free, reduced-sodium spaghetti sauce

2 tablespoons chopped fresh basil leaves or 1 teaspoon dried, crumbled

4 ounces dried whole-wheat spaghetti

$\frac{1}{2}$ cup shredded part-skim mozzarella cheese

Preheat the oven to 350°F. Lightly spray a 13 × 9 × 2-inch baking pan with vegetable oil spray.

Discard all visible fat from the chicken. Put the chicken with the smooth side up between two pieces of plastic wrap. Using a tortilla press, the smooth side of a meat mallet, or a rolling pin, lightly flatten the breasts to a thickness of ½ inch, being careful not to tear the meat.

Put the buttermilk and flour in separate shallow bowls. In a third shallow bowl, stir together the bread crumbs, Parmesan, and Italian seasoning. Set the bowls and the baking pan in a row, assembly-line fashion.

Coat a chicken breast with the flour, shaking off the excess. Coat the chicken with the buttermilk, then the bread-crumb mixture. Place in the baking pan. Repeat with the remaining chicken.

Bake for 40 to 45 minutes, or until the chicken is no longer pink in the center.

Meanwhile, heat a medium saucepan over medium-high heat. Remove from the heat and lightly spray with vegetable oil spray (being careful not to spray near a gas flame). Cook the onion and mushrooms for 3 to 4 minutes, or until tender, stirring occasionally.

Stir in the broccoli slaw. Cook for 1 to 2 minutes, or until tender-crisp.

Stir in the spaghetti sauce and basil. Reduce the heat to medium and cook for 3 to 4 minutes, or until warmed through, stirring occasionally.

While the chicken bakes and the sauce cooks, prepare the pasta using the package directions, omitting the salt and oil. Drain well in a colander.

Spoon ½ cup sauce over each chicken breast. Sprinkle with the mozzarella.

Bake, uncovered, for 5 minutes, or until the cheese is melted.

To serve, spoon the pasta onto plates. Place the chicken with sauce on the pasta.

PER SERVING

calories 395
total fat 6.5 g
  saturated 3.0 g
  polyunsaturated 1.0 g
  monounsaturated 1.5 g
cholesterol 77 mg

sodium 601 mg
carbohydrates 44 g
  fiber 8 g
  sugar 10 g
protein 41 g

100   200   300   400

DIETARY EXCHANGES
2 starch; 2½ vegetable;
4 very lean meat

chicken breasts stuffed with goat cheese, dates, and spinach

Serves 4; 1 stuffed chicken breast half per serving

Stuffing chicken breasts is easier than you might think. Once you know how, the variations are limited only by your imagination or the ingredients in your kitchen.

4 boneless, skinless chicken breast halves (about 4 ounces each)

2 ounces soft goat cheese

1/8 teaspoon cayenne

4 dried dates, pitted and chopped

2 cups fresh baby spinach leaves

1/2 teaspoon paprika

Preheat the oven to 425°F. Line a rimmed baking sheet with cooking parchment.

Discard all visible fat from the chicken. Put the chicken with the smooth side up between two pieces of plastic wrap. Using a tortilla press, the smooth side of a meat mallet, or a rolling pin, lightly flatten the breasts to a thickness of 1/4 inch, being careful not to tear the meat.

Place the chicken breasts with the smooth side down on the baking sheet. Spread each breast with 1 tablespoon goat cheese, leaving a 1/2-inch border uncovered.

Sprinkle with the cayenne and dates. Top with the spinach, still leaving the border uncovered. Beginning at the narrowest end, roll each piece jelly-roll style. Place with the seam side down on the baking sheet. Sprinkle with the paprika.

Bake for 20 minutes. Remove from the oven and let stand on the baking sheet for 5 minutes.

To serve, cut crosswise into 1/2-inch slices. (The slices will look like pinwheels.) Arrange the slices in a fanlike pattern on a platter or plates.

chicken breasts stuffed with fresh basil and red bell pepper

Omit the goat cheese, cayenne, dates, and spinach. Stuff the chicken with 2 ounces fat-free or reduced-fat cream cheese, softened; 2 teaspoons minced garlic; 1/4 cup chopped red bell pepper; and 8 to 12 fresh basil leaves. Prepare as directed. If you prefer, you may omit the cream cheese.

COOK'S TIP ON COOKING PARCHMENT: Cooking parchment keeps food from sticking to baking sheets without the need for added oil. It also keeps the bottom of the meat, vegetables, or baked goods from browning too quickly. Remember, however, that it cannot be used for broiling because it could ignite and cause a fire.

WITH GOAT CHEESE, DATES, AND SPINACH

PER SERVING

calories 260

total fat 4.5 g

  saturated 2.5 g

  polyunsaturated 0.5 g

  monounsaturated 1.0 g

cholesterol 72 mg

sodium 139 mg

carbohydrates 26 g

  fiber 5 g

  sugar 20 g

protein 30 g

100 200 300 400

DIETARY EXCHANGES

$3\frac{1}{2}$ lean meat; $1\frac{1}{2}$ fruit

WITH FRESH BASIL AND RED BELL PEPPER

PER SERVING

calories 145

total fat 1.5 g

  saturated 0.5 g

  polyunsaturated 0.5 g

  monounsaturated 0.5 g

cholesterol 68 mg

sodium 144 mg

carbohydrates 2 g

  fiber 0 g

  sugar 1 g

protein 28 g

100 200 300 400

DIETARY EXCHANGES

$3\frac{1}{2}$ very lean meat

stuffed chicken breasts in lemon-oregano tomato sauce

Serves 4; 1 stuffed chicken breast and 2 tablespoons sauce per serving

A touch of lemon juice marinates the chicken, which is stuffed with a combination of fresh tomatoes, parsley, olives, and feta cheese. The tomato sauce, enhanced with lemon zest and oregano, helps keep the chicken moist.

1/2 cup no-salt-added tomato sauce

1 teaspoon grated lemon zest

1 teaspoon dried oregano, crumbled

1/2 teaspoon crushed red pepper flakes

1/4 teaspoon salt

4 boneless, skinless chicken breast halves (about 4 ounces each)

1 tablespoon fresh lemon juice

2 medium Italian plum tomatoes, diced

1/4 cup crumbled fat-free or low-fat feta cheese

2 tablespoons snipped fresh parsley or 1 teaspoon dried, crumbled

2 tablespoons chopped kalamata olives

1 medium green onion (green part only), chopped

In a small bowl, stir together the tomato sauce, lemon zest, oregano, red pepper flakes, and salt.

Discard all visible fat from the chicken. Put the chicken with the smooth side up between two pieces of plastic wrap. Using a tortilla press, the smooth side of a meat mallet, or a rolling pin, lightly flatten the breasts to a thickness of 1/2 inch, being careful not to tear the meat.

Put the chicken in a glass bowl with the lemon juice. Let stand at room temperature for 10 minutes, or cover and refrigerate for up to 4 hours.

Preheat the oven to 350°F.

In a small bowl, stir together the remaining ingredients.

To assemble, remove the chicken from the lemon juice, discarding any leftover liquid. Place the chicken on a flat work surface. Spoon the tomato-feta mixture down the center of each breast. Starting with the short end, roll up the breasts jelly-roll style. Place the breasts with the seam side down in a nonstick 8-inch square baking pan. Spoon the tomato sauce over the breasts.

Bake, covered, for 40 to 45 minutes, or until the chicken is no longer pink in the center.

PER SERVING

calories 168
total fat 2.5 g
  saturated 0.5 g
  polyunsaturated 0.5 g
  monounsaturated 1.0 g
cholesterol 66 mg

sodium 438 mg
carbohydrates 6 g
  fiber 1 g
  sugar 3 g
protein 29 g

100 200 300 400

DIETARY EXCHANGES
1 vegetable;
3 very lean meat

chicken fajitas

Serves 4; 2 fajitas per serving

Cilantro, jalapeño, and cumin spice up the sour cream and yogurt sauce that tops these fajitas.

8 ounces boneless, skinless chicken breasts

2 tablespoons fresh lime juice

1 small fresh jalapeño

3/4 cup fat-free or light sour cream

1/4 cup fat-free or low-fat plain yogurt

2 tablespoons finely snipped fresh cilantro

1/8 teaspoon ground cumin

8 6-inch fat-free flour tortillas

1 large green bell pepper, thinly sliced

1 small red bell pepper, thinly sliced

1 large onion, thinly sliced

1/2 cup fat-free, low-sodium chicken broth

2 cups shredded lettuce

2 medium tomatoes, seeded, chopped, and drained

Discard all visible fat from the chicken. Cut the chicken into thin slices. Sprinkle with the lime juice. Let stand at room temperature for 15 minutes.

Meanwhile, wearing disposable plastic gloves, discard the ribs and seeds of the jalapeño. Finely chop enough of the jalapeño to measure 1 teaspoon.

In a small bowl, stir together the sour cream, yogurt, cilantro, jalapeño, and cumin.

Preheat the oven to 350°F.

Wrap the tortillas in aluminum foil. Let warm in the oven for 10 minutes. Keep covered until ready to serve.

Meanwhile, heat a large nonstick skillet over medium heat. Cook the bell peppers, onion, and broth for 1 minute. Stir in the chicken strips. Cook for 2 to 4 minutes, or until the chicken is no longer pink in the center and the liquid has evaporated.

To assemble, spoon the chicken-vegetable mixture down the center of each tortilla. Top with the sour cream mixture, lettuce, and tomatoes. Roll up jelly-roll style. Serve immediately.

COOK'S TIP: For a different meal for another day, double the chicken-vegetable filling. Microwave at 100 percent power (high) in a microwaveable dish until hot and serve over cooked rice.

COOK'S TIP ON BELL PEPPERS:

To safely slice a bell pepper, cut it in half lengthwise first. Discard the ribs and seeds. Slice the pepper from the inside, not the skin side. This will help prevent the knife from sliding on the slippery curved outer surface.

PER SERVING

calories 323
total fat 1.5 g
  saturated 0.5 g
  polyunsaturated 0.5 g
  monounsaturated 0.0 g
cholesterol 41 mg

sodium 513 mg
carbohydrates 51 g
  fiber 6 g
  sugar 12 g
protein 24 g

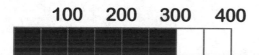

100 200 300 400

DIETARY EXCHANGES
3 starch; 1 vegetable;
2 very lean meat

slow-cooker chicken and noodles

Serves 6; 1½ cups per serving

Take advantage of the convenience of the slow cooker to prepare this heavenly comfort dish.

4 cups fat-free, low-sodium chicken broth
    10.75-ounce can low-fat, reduced-sodium condensed cream of chicken soup
1 pound chicken tenders or boneless, skinless chicken breasts, all visible fat discarded, cut into ½-inch-wide strips
1½ cups baby carrots
1 teaspoon poultry seasoning
½ teaspoon salt
¼ teaspoon pepper
2 cups yolk-free dumpling-style noodles (about 3 ounces)
1½ cups frozen green peas, thawed
1 teaspoon dried dillweed, crumbled

Put the broth, soup, chicken, carrots, poultry season-ing, salt, and pepper in a slow cooker. Stir well. Cook on low for 5 hours 15 minutes or on high for 3 hours 30 minutes.

Quickly stir in the noodles. Cook on low for 45 min-utes or on high for 30 minutes, or until the chicken and carrots are cooked through.

Quickly stir in the peas and dillweed. Cook on either heat setting for 10 minutes, or until the pasta is tender and the peas are warmed through.

PER SERVING

calories 214
total fat 2.0 g
 saturated 0.5 g
 polysaturated 0.5 g
 monosaturated 0.5 g
cholesterol 47 mg

sodium 524 mg
carbohydrates 23 g
 fiber 3 g
 sugar 5 g
protein 24 g

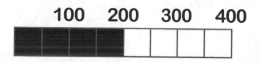

100   200   300   400

DIETARY EXCHANGES
1½ starch;
2½ very lean meat

chicken and bow-ties with green beans

Serves 4; 1½ cups per serving

Mild and creamy gorgonzola, added at the last minute, melts slightly to create a wonderfully aromatic dish.

3 quarts water
4 ounces dried bow-tie pasta
6 ounces whole fresh green beans, trimmed
Vegetable oil spray
12 ounces boneless, skinless chicken breasts, all visible fat discarded, cut into thin strips
½ cup finely chopped red onion
1 medium garlic clove, minced
2 ounces Gorgonzola cheese, crumbled
2 tablespoons chopped fresh basil leaves or 2 teaspoons dried, crumbled
2 teaspoons grated lemon zest
2 tablespoons lemon juice
2 teaspoons olive oil (extra-virgin preferred)

In a large saucepan, bring the water to a boil over high heat. Stir in the pasta. Boil for 6 minutes. Stir in the green beans. Boil for 5 minutes, or until the beans are tender-crisp. Drain well in a colander.

Meanwhile, heat a large nonstick skillet over medium-high heat. Remove from the heat and lightly spray with vegetable oil spray (being careful not to spray near a gas flame). Cook the chicken for 2 minutes, stirring constantly.

Stir in the onion and garlic. Cook for 1 to 2 minutes, or until the chicken is no longer pink in the center, stirring constantly. Remove from the heat. Cover to keep warm.

To serve, combine all the ingredients in a large bowl.

PER SERVING

calories 295
total fat 8.0 g
 saturated 3.5 g
 polyunsaturated 0.5 g
 monounsaturated 2.0 g
cholesterol 62 mg

sodium 253 mg
carbohydrates 28 g
 fiber 3 g
 sugar 3 g
protein 27 g

100 200 300 400

DIETARY EXCHANGES
$1\frac{1}{2}$ starch; 1 vegetable; 3 lean meat

chicken with penne pasta and mixed greens

Serves 5; 1½ cups per serving

A low-fat, three-cheese cream sauce takes center stage in this vitamin-rich entrée.

1 bunch or 5-ounce bag arugula

5 ounces fresh baby spinach leaves

1 bunch or 5-ounce bag Swiss chard

8 ounces dried penne pasta

cream sauce

1 cup fat-free or low-fat cottage cheese

3 ounces fat-free or light cream cheese, cut into 1-inch cubes

13 ounces fat-free evaporated milk

¼ cup plus 2 tablespoons shredded Parmesan or asiago cheese

12 ounces boneless, skinless chicken breasts

¼ teaspoon pepper

1 tablespoon olive oil

2 medium garlic cloves, minced

½ cup fat-free, low-sodium chicken broth or low-sodium vegetable broth

Coarsely chop the arugula, spinach, and Swiss chard. Set aside.

Prepare the pasta using the package directions, omitting the salt and oil. Drain well.

Meanwhile, in a food processor or blender, process the cottage cheese until smooth. Add the cream cheese. Process until smooth. Add the milk and Parmesan. Process until well blended. Set aside.

Discard all visible fat from the chicken. Cut the chicken into bite-size pieces. Season with the pepper.

Heat a large skillet over medium-high heat. Pour the oil into the skillet and swirl to coat the bottom. Cook the chicken and garlic for 2 to 3 minutes, or until the chicken is lightly browned on the outside and no longer pink in the center.

Pour in the broth, scraping to dislodge any browned bits from the bottom of the skillet.

Stir in the arugula, spinach, and Swiss chard. Cook, covered, for about 3 minutes, or until just wilted.

In a large bowl, stir together the pasta, chicken mixture, and cream sauce.

PER SERVING

calories 421
total fat 6.5 g
 saturated 2.0 g
 polyunsaturated 1.0 g
 monounsaturated 3.0 g
cholesterol 52 mg

sodium 567 mg
carbohydrates 49 g
 fiber 3 g
 sugar 13 g
protein 40 g

100 200 300 400

DIETARY EXCHANGES
$2\frac{1}{2}$ starch; 1 skim milk; $3\frac{1}{2}$ very lean meat

risotto with porcini mushrooms and chicken

Serves 4; 1 cup per serving

The key to a creamy risotto is the slow absorption of the liquid, which takes at least 20 minutes. If you take the time to make it right, you will be richly rewarded.

4 cups fat-free, low-sodium chicken broth or mushroom stock

1 1/2 cups dry white wine (regular or nonalcoholic)

1/2 cup dried porcini mushrooms

2 teaspoons olive oil

1 large onion, chopped

2 cups uncooked arborio rice

1/2 teaspoon salt

1/2 teaspoon pepper

8 ounces boneless, skinless chicken breasts, all visible fat discarded, cut into 1/2-inch pieces

1/2 cup shredded or grated Parmesan cheese

2 tablespoons finely snipped Italian, or flat-leaf, parsley

In a 4-quart saucepan, bring the broth and wine to a boil over high heat. Reduce the heat to a simmer. Stir in the dried mushrooms. Simmer, uncovered, for 5 minutes. Drain the mushrooms through a coffee filter to remove any dirt, reserving the broth. Chop the mushrooms into bite-size pieces. Return the broth to the saucepan. Bring to a simmer over low heat. Keep the broth at a simmer while preparing the risotto.

Meanwhile, heat a heavy 5-quart saucepan over medium-high heat. Pour the oil into the pan and swirl to coat the bottom. Cook the onion for 2 to 3 minutes, or until it starts to soften.

Stir in the rice, salt, and pepper, coating the rice grains with the oil mixture.

Pour in the simmering broth mixture 1 cup at a time, stirring until each addition of liquid is absorbed. (This takes time and patience.)

Meanwhile, heat a medium nonstick skillet over medium-high heat. Cook the chicken for 6 to 8 minutes, or until golden brown.

After the last addition of broth is absorbed by the rice mixture, stir in the chicken, Parmesan, and parsley.

COOK'S TIP: If you prefer a moister risotto, you can add a bit more broth or wine before serving. It is important to keep the liquid hot while adding it to risotto so the finished dish will be creamy.

PER SERVING

calories 388
total fat 6.0 g
  saturated 2.0 g
  polyunsaturated 0.5 g
  monounsaturated 3.0 g
cholesterol 40 mg

sodium 566 mg
carbohydrates 44 g
  fiber 2 g
  sugar 3 g
protein 24 g

100 200 300 400

DIETARY EXCHANGES
$2\frac{1}{2}$ starch; $1\frac{1}{2}$ vegetable; 2 lean meat

chicken and veggies with noodles

Serves 4; 1½ cups per serving

Chicken strips and vegetables in a creamy sauce, all served over noodles, is a family-pleasing combination.

Vegetable oil spray
1 pound boneless, skinless chicken breasts, all visible fat discarded, cut into thin strips
1 large onion, thinly sliced
1 large green bell pepper, thinly sliced
1 large rib of celery, thinly sliced
½ cup water
¾ teaspoon dried thyme, crumbled
⅛ teaspoon cayenne
4 ounces dried no-yolk egg noodles
10.75-ounce can low-fat, reduced-sodium condensed cream of chicken soup
¼ teaspoon salt

Heat a Dutch oven over medium-high heat. Remove from the heat and lightly spray with vegetable oil spray (being careful not to spray near a gas flame). Cook the chicken for 2 minutes, stirring constantly. Transfer to a plate.

Lightly spray the browned bits remaining in the Dutch oven with vegetable oil spray. Put the onion, bell pepper, and celery in the pot. Lightly spray the vegetables with vegetable oil spray. Cook for 4 minutes, or until the vegetables begin to brown, stirring frequently.

Stir in the chicken and any accumulated juices, water, thyme, and cayenne. Reduce the heat and simmer, covered, for 10 minutes, or until the celery is tender, stirring occasionally.

Meanwhile, prepare the noodles using the package directions, omitting the salt and oil.

When the celery is tender, stir in the soup and salt. Cook for 1 minute, or until heated through.

Spoon the pasta onto plates. Spoon the chicken mixture over the pasta.

COOK'S TIP: Adding the soup and the salt at the very end preserves the creaminess of the dish.

PER SERVING

calories 307

total fat 2.5 g
  saturated 1.0 g
  polysaturated 0.5 g
  monosaturated 0.5 g
cholesterol 70 mg

sodium 524 mg
carbohydrates 36 g
  fiber 4 g
  sugar 6 g
protein 32 g

100 200 300 400   **DIETARY EXCHANGES**
2 starch; 1 vegetable;
3 very lean meat

chicken enchiladas

Serves 6; 2 enchiladas per serving

If you want to challenge your heat barometer when eating this festive Mexican dish, increase the amount of jalapeño or leave in the seeds and ribs.

    Vegetable oil spray

filling

1 medium fresh jalapeño

1 large onion, diced

3/4 cup diced green bell pepper

3/4 cup diced carrots

3/4 cup diced zucchini

3 medium garlic cloves, minced

1/2 pound lean ground chicken breast, skin discarded before grinding

1 tablespoon chili powder

2 teaspoons dried oregano, crumbled

1 teaspoon ground cumin

19-ounce can no-salt-added black beans, rinsed and drained

1 cup fresh, frozen, or canned no-salt-added whole-kernel corn, cooked if fresh or frozen, rinsed and drained if canned

2 tablespoons fresh lime juice

2 tablespoons chopped fresh cilantro

....

12 6-inch corn tortillas

¼ cup low-fat Cheddar cheese

2½ cups fat-free, low-sodium salsa

½ cup low-fat Cheddar cheese

¾ cup fat-free or light sour cream

Preheat the oven to 350°F. Lightly spray a 15 × 11-inch glass baking dish with vegetable oil spray.

Wearing plastic gloves, discard the seeds and ribs of the jalapeño. Mince the jalapeño.

Heat a large skillet over medium heat. Remove from the heat and lightly spray with vegetable oil spray (being careful not to spray near a gas flame). Cook the onion, bell pepper, carrots, zucchini, and garlic for 5 minutes, or until the vegetables are softened.

Stir in the chicken. Cook for 1 minute, or until no longer pink, stirring constantly.

Stir in the jalapeño, chili powder, oregano, and cumin. Cook for 1 minute, stirring constantly. Remove from the heat.

Stir in the beans, corn, lime juice, and cilantro.

To assemble the enchiladas, spoon a heaping ¼ cup filling down the center of a tortilla. Sprinkle with 1 teaspoon Cheddar. Roll up jelly-roll style. Place with the seam down in the baking dish. Repeat with the remaining tortillas and filling.

Pour the salsa over the enchiladas, covering each one. Cover with aluminum foil.

Bake for 30 minutes. Sprinkle with ½ cup Cheddar. Bake, uncovered, for 5 minutes.

To serve, using a spatula, transfer the enchiladas to plates. Put a dollop of sour cream on each enchilada.

PER SERVING

calories 331

total fat 3.0 g

 saturated 1.0 g

 polyunsaturated 0.5 g

 monounsaturated 0.5 g

cholesterol 30 mg

sodium 584 mg

carbohydrates 53 g

 fiber 8 g

 sugar 13 g

protein 23 g

100 200 300 400

DIETARY EXCHANGES

2½ starch; 3 vegetable; 2 very lean meat

chicken pot pie

Serves 8; 1 wedge per serving

Turn leftovers into the epitome of comfort food with this recipe.

Vegetable oil spray

1 tablespoon olive oil

½ cup chopped onion

1 medium garlic clove, minced

2 medium ribs of celery, sliced

2 medium carrots, cut crosswise into ¼-inch slices

2 tablespoons olive oil

¼ cup all-purpose flour

1 cup fat-free, low-sodium chicken broth

3 cups chopped cooked chicken or turkey breast, cooked without salt, skin and all visible fat discarded

1 cup frozen baby green peas or leftover cooked or frozen vegetables

2 tablespoons chopped fresh Italian, or flat-leaf, parsley

1 cup fat-free, low-sodium chicken broth

¼ teaspoon salt

Pepper to taste

Mashed Potatoes (recipe follows) or about 4 cups leftover mashed potatoes, cooked without salt and margarine

Preheat the oven to 375°F. Lightly spray a 9-inch pie plate or baking dish with vegetable oil spray.

Pour 1 tablespoon oil into a 4-quart saucepan or Dutch oven and swirl to coat the bottom. Heat over medium-high heat. Cook the onion and garlic for 2 to 3 minutes, or until they begin to soften. Stir in the celery and carrots. Cook for 5 minutes, or until the celery begins to soften. Transfer the vegetables to a plate.

In the same saucepan, heat 2 tablespoons oil over medium heat. Whisk in the flour, thoroughly incorporating the oil. (The mixture will be dry.) Gradually pour in 1 cup broth, whisking constantly. Cook for 2 to 3 minutes, or until the mixture begins to thicken and turn golden and the flour loses its raw taste.

Stir in the chicken, peas, parsley, and enough of the remaining broth to achieve the desired consistency. Stir in the salt and pepper. Pour the mixture into the pie pan.

Spread the mashed potatoes over the chicken mixture.

Bake for 25 minutes, or until the potato crust is golden and the filling is bubbly.

mashed potatoes

- 1 pound Yukon gold potatoes, peeled and cut into 2-inch cubes
- 4 cups fat-free, low-sodium chicken broth
- 1 medium garlic clove

Put the potatoes in a 4-quart saucepan and add enough broth to cover. Add the garlic. Bring to a boil over high heat. Reduce the heat and cook at a low boil, uncovered, for 10 to 15 minutes, or until the potatoes are fork-tender. Drain the potatoes, reserving the cooking liquid.

In a large mixing bowl, beat the potatoes and garlic with an electric mixer until no large chunks remain. Gradually pour in the cooking liquid, beating after each addition, until the desired consistency is reached.

PER SERVING

calories 216
total fat 7.0 g
  saturated 1.0 g
  polyunsaturated 1.0 g
  monounsaturated 4.5 g
cholesterol 45 mg

sodium 177 mg
carbohydrates 19 g
  fiber 3 g
  sugar 3 g
protein 20 g

100 200 300 400

DIETARY EXCHANGES
1 starch; 1 vegetable;
2½ lean meat

barbecue chicken pizza

Serves 4; 2 slices per serving

Tangy barbecue sauce ties together the topping ingredients on this delicious pizza.

1 teaspoon olive oil

2 medium bell peppers (any color), thinly sliced

1 medium onion, thinly sliced

6 ounces sliced fresh mushrooms, such as button or baby portobellos

1 cup diced cooked skinless chicken breasts, cooked without salt (about 5 ounces)

1/4 cup barbecue sauce

1 teaspoon balsamic vinegar

12-inch prepared pizza crust

1/4 cup shredded part-skim mozzarella cheese

Preheat the oven to 425°F.

Heat a large skillet over medium-high heat. Pour the oil into the skillet and swirl to coat the bottom. Cook the bell peppers, onion, and mushrooms for 3 to 4 minutes, or until tender, stirring occasionally.

Stir in the chicken, barbecue sauce, and vinegar. Reduce the heat to medium and cook for 1 to 2 minutes, or until the mixture is slightly warmed through, stirring occasionally.

Put the pizza crust on an ungreased nonstick baking sheet. Spread the chicken mixture over the crust. Sprinkle with the mozzarella.

Bake for 10 to 12 minutes, or until the cheese is melted and the topping is warmed through. Cut into 8 wedges.

COOK'S TIP: Do some label comparisons when shopping for the ingredients for this pizza. Barbecue sauce can be high in sodium, and prepared pizza crust can be high in calories and fat as well as sodium.

PER SERVING

calories 346
total fat 8.0 g
  saturated 3.0 g
  polyunsaturated 0.5 g
  monounsaturated 2.0 g
cholesterol 34 mg

sodium 547 mg
carbohydrates 45 g
  fiber 4 g
  sugar 12 g
protein 23 g

100   200   300   400

DIETARY EXCHANGES
$2\frac{1}{2}$ starch; $1\frac{1}{2}$ vegetable; 2 lean meat

slow-roasted sage turkey breast

Serves 4; 3 ounces per serving (plus 1 pound reserved)

A thin coating of seasoning mixture and a squeeze of fresh lemon between the breast meat and the skin impart flavor that permeates the turkey as it slowly roasts. Try some of the leftover turkey in Open-Face Broiled Turkey Sandwiches with Herb Garlic Spread (page 448).

Vegetable oil spray
1/2 tablespoon dried sage
1 teaspoon paprika
3/4 teaspoon dried rosemary, crushed
1/4 teaspoon onion powder
1/4 teaspoon garlic powder
1/4 teaspoon pepper
3-pound boneless turkey breast with skin
1 medium lemon, halved crosswise

Preheat the oven to 325°F. Lightly spray a baking rack and pan with vegetable oil spray.

In a small bowl, combine the sage, paprika, rosemary, onion powder, garlic powder, and pepper.

Carefully pull back the skin from the turkey, leaving it attached at one end and trying not to tear the skin. Squeeze the lemon over the breast meat. Sprinkle with the sage mixture. Put the skin back in place. Put the turkey on the baking rack in the pan.

Roast, uncovered, for 1 hour 45 minutes, or until the internal temperature reaches 170°F when tested with a meat thermometer.

Transfer the turkey to a cutting board. Let stand for 10 minutes. Discard the skin before slicing the turkey.

PER SERVING

calories 122
total fat 1.0 g
 saturated 0.5 g
 polyunsaturated 0.5 g
 monounsaturated 0.0 g
cholesterol 73 mg

sodium 48 mg
carbohydrates 1 g
 fiber 0 g
 sugar 0 g
protein 26 g

100   200   300   400   DIETARY EXCHANGES
3 very lean meat

turkish meatballs

Serves 4; 4 meatballs and $\frac{1}{4}$ cup sauce per serving

These spicy but not hot meatballs and their tomato-wine sauce would partner well with whole-wheat couscous, brown rice, or orzo. Add a green salad, and dinner is served.

Vegetable oil spray
1 pound lean ground turkey breast, skin discarded before grinding
$\frac{1}{3}$ cup fat-free, low-sodium chicken broth
$\frac{1}{4}$ cup plain dry bread crumbs
$\frac{1}{4}$ cup finely chopped onion
$\frac{1}{2}$ medium rib of celery, finely chopped
$\frac{1}{4}$ cup snipped fresh Italian, or flat-leaf, parsley
$\frac{1}{2}$ teaspoon ground cinnamon
$\frac{1}{4}$ teaspoon ground allspice
$\frac{1}{4}$ teaspoon ground turmeric or curry powder
$\frac{1}{4}$ teaspoon pepper
1 small onion, thinly sliced
2 medium garlic cloves, minced

1 cup low-sodium mixed vegetable juice
or no-salt-added tomato sauce

1/3 cup dry red wine (regular or nonalcoholic)

1/4 teaspoon crushed red pepper flakes

Preheat the oven to 400°F. Lightly spray a 14 × 10-inch rack with vegetable oil spray. Place the rack on a 15 × 10 × 1/2-inch rimmed baking sheet.

In a large bowl, stir together the turkey, broth, bread crumbs, 1/4 cup onion, celery, parsley, cinnamon, all-spice, turmeric, and pepper. Shape the mixture into 16 balls. Place them on the rack on the baking sheet.

Bake for 12 to 15 minutes, or until light golden, turning the meatballs occasionally. Using tongs or a spatula, put the meatballs on paper towels to drain.

Heat a large nonstick skillet over medium heat. Remove from the heat and lightly spray with vegetable oil spray (being careful not to spray near a gas flame). Cook the sliced onion and garlic for 3 to 4 minutes, or until soft, stirring occasionally.

Stir in the remaining ingredients. Increase the heat to medium-high. Bring to a boil. Gently add the meatballs, spooning some of the sauce over them. Reduce the heat and simmer, covered, for 10 to 12 minutes, or until the meatballs are cooked through, turning them once in the sauce.

COOK'S TIP ON TURMERIC:

Turmeric is an herb often used in place of very expensive saffron—not for the flavor, which is quite different, but rather because of the similarity in their yellow-orange color. Turmeric also is a component in many prepared curry powder blends.

PER SERVING

calories 205
total fat 1.5 g
  saturated 0.5 g
  polyunsaturated 0.5 g
  monounsaturated 0.5 g
cholesterol 77 mg

sodium 151 mg
carbohydrates 13 g
  fiber 2 g
  sugar 5 g
protein 29 g

100 200 300 400

DIETARY EXCHANGES
1/2 starch; 1 1/2 vegetable;
3 very lean meat

open-face broiled turkey sandwiches with herb-garlic spread

Serves 4; 1 open-face sandwich per serving

What a wonderful way to take advantage of turkey leftovers! Pile a creamy herb-garlic spread, turkey slices, crunchy red onions, and mozzarella onto French bread and broil until the cheese melts.

2 tablespoons fat-free or light mayonnaise dressing

2 tablespoons fat-free or light sour cream

3/4 teaspoon dried basil, crumbled

1/2 medium garlic clove, minced

1/4 teaspoon dried oregano, crumbled

4 ounces French bread (not baguette), cut crosswise into 4 slices

4 ounces thinly sliced turkey breast, cooked without salt, skin and all visible fat discarded

1/4 cup very thinly sliced red onion

3 ounces grated part-skim mozzarella cheese

Preheat the broiler.

In a small bowl, stir together the mayonnaise, sour cream, basil, garlic, and oregano.

To assemble, spread the mayonnaise mixture on one side of each slice of bread. Place on a baking sheet. Top each slice with turkey, onion, and mozzarella.

Broil for 2 minutes, or until the mozzarella melts and begins to lightly brown.

PER SERVING

calories 172
total fat 1.0 g
  saturated 0.5 g
  polyunsaturated 0.5 g
  monounsaturated 0.5 g
cholesterol 29 mg

sodium 516 mg
carbohydrates 20 g
  fiber 2 g
  sugar 2 g
protein 19 g

100   200   300   400

DIETARY EXCHANGES
$1\frac{1}{2}$ starch;
2 very lean meat

italian turkey sausage and peppers with whole-wheat fettuccine

Serves 4; 3 ounces sausage and $\frac{3}{4}$ cup pasta per serving

Boldly flavored ingredients, such as the Italian turkey sausage used here, are desirable when you serve dishes featuring whole-wheat pasta. Add a splash of color with a variety of bell peppers.

6 ounces dried whole-wheat fettuccine

12 ounces hot Italian or sweet Italian turkey sausage, cut into $\frac{1}{2}$-inch slices

2 medium bell peppers, any color or combination, thinly sliced

1 medium onion, thinly sliced

1 medium garlic clove, minced

$\frac{1}{8}$ teaspoon salt

Pepper to taste

Prepare the pasta using the package directions, omitting the salt and oil. Drain well in a colander.

Meanwhile, heat a large nonstick skillet over medium-high heat. Cook the sausage, bell peppers, onion, and garlic for 8 to10 minutes, or until the sausage is no longer pink and the peppers and onion are soft, stirring occasionally.

In a large bowl, stir together all the ingredients.

PER SERVING

calories 311

total fat 8.5 g

  saturated 2.5 g

  polyunsaturated 2.0 g

  monounsaturated 3.5 g

cholesterol 72 mg

sodium 683 mg

carbohydrates 38 g

  fiber 7 g

  sugar 5 g

protein 19 g

100   200   300   400

DIETARY EXCHANGES
2 starch; 1 $\frac{1}{2}$ vegetable; 2 lean meat

artichoke and bell pepper lasagna

Serves 4; 5$\frac{1}{2}$ x 3$\frac{1}{2}$-inch piece per serving

Turkey pepperoni adds an unusual element to this vegetable-laden lasagna.

Vegetable oil spray
4 dried whole-wheat or regular lasagna noodles
3 medium green bell peppers, finely chopped
1 small zucchini, finely chopped
$\frac{1}{2}$ cup fat-free, reduced-sodium spaghetti sauce
$\frac{1}{2}$ tablespoon dried basil, crumbled
1 teaspoon dried oregano, crumbled
16 turkey pepperoni slices, quartered
14.5-ounce can artichokes, rinsed, drained, and finely chopped
2 ounces shredded part-skim mozzarella cheese
1 tablespoon shredded or grated Parmesan cheese

Preheat the oven to 350°F. Lightly spray an 11 × 7 × 2-inch baking dish with vegetable oil spray.

Prepare the noodles using the package directions, omitting the salt and oil. Drain well.

Meanwhile, heat a large skillet over medium-high heat. Remove from the heat and lightly spray with vegetable oil spray (being careful not to spray near a gas flame). Cook the bell peppers and zucchini for 5 minutes, or until beginning to brown, stirring frequently. Remove from the heat.

Place 2 noodles in the baking dish. Make sure the edges of the noodles are tucked under to keep them from drying out. Spoon 2 tablespoons spaghetti sauce over each noodle. Sprinkle with half of each of the following, in order: basil, oregano, pepperoni, artichokes, bell-pepper mixture, and mozzarella. Repeat the layers.

Lightly spray a sheet of aluminum foil with vegetable oil spray. Cover the baking dish with the foil with the sprayed side down.

Bake for 25 minutes, or until the mozzarella has melted.

Sprinkle with the Parmesan. Let stand for 10 minutes before cutting so the flavors can blend.

PER SERVING

calories 193	sodium 592 mg
total fat 2.0 g	carbohydrates 31 g
saturated 0.5 g	fiber 7 g
polyunsaturated 0.5 g	sugar 6 g
monounsaturated 0.5 g	protein 14 g
cholesterol 12 mg	

100 200 300 400 DIETARY EXCHANGES
1 starch; 3 vegetable;
1 very lean meat

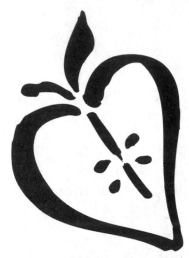

meats

Beef Tenderloin
with Horseradish Cream

Beef Tenderloin with Shallot and
Sweet-Onion Marmalade

Filet Mignon with Balsamic
Berry Sauce

Honey-Lime Flank Steak

Orange Beef Stir-Fry

Beef Stroganoff with Baby
Portobello Mushrooms

Slow-Cooker Shredded Beef on
Potato Mounds

Saucy Minute Steaks

Chicken-Fried Steak
with Creamy Gravy

Satay-Style Sirloin with Peanut
Dipping Sauce

Greek-Style Sirloin Cubes
and Olive-Feta Rice

Meat Loaf with a Twist

Baked Ziti with Beef
and Green Beans

Beefy Macaroni and Cheese

Tex-Mex Beef Casserole with
Cornbread Crust

Chopped Beef Hash

Ham and Broccoli with Rotini

Pork Tenderloin with Cranberry Salsa

Pork Tenderloin with Orange-Ginger
Sweet Potatoes

Thai Coconut Curry with Pork
and Vegetables

Pork Chops Parmesan

Sausage and White Beans
with Spinach

Veal Stew with Sweet Potatoes, Pearl
Onions, and Petit Pois Peas

Lamb Kebabs with Apricot-Rosemary
Dipping Sauce

beef tenderloin with horseradish cream

**Serves 4; 3 ounces meat
and 2 tablespoons sauce per serving**

Beef tenderloin with a heavenly horseradish cream adds a touch of elegance to that special celebration.

Vegetable oil spray

horseradish cream

3 tablespoons fat-free or low-fat plain yogurt

3 tablespoons fat-free or light sour cream

2 tablespoons chopped green onions (green and white parts)

2 teaspoons prepared white horseradish, or to taste

1/2 teaspoon low-sodium Worcestershire sauce

1-pound center-cut beef tenderloin, all visible fat and silver skin discarded

1 medium garlic clove, cut into 6 slices

1/2 tablespoon spicy brown mustard

1/2 teaspoon garlic powder

1/4 teaspoon pepper

Preheat the oven to 450°F. Lightly spray a shallow roasting pan with vegetable oil spray.

In a small bowl, stir together the horseradish cream ingredients. Cover and refrigerate for at least 30 minutes to allow the flavors to blend.

Meanwhile, cut 6 small, evenly spaced slits into the top of the meat. Insert a garlic slice into each slit. Thinly spread the mustard all over the meat. Sprinkle with the garlic powder and pepper. Put the meat in the roasting pan.

Roast, uncovered, for 20 minutes. Reduce the temperature to 350°F. Roast for 20 to 25 minutes, or until the meat registers 140°F on an instant-read meat thermometer for medium-rare doneness or 155°F for medium doneness. Remove from the oven. Cover the meat with aluminum foil. Let stand for at least 10 minutes before slicing; the temperature will rise about 5 degrees.

To serve, slice the meat. Serve with the horseradish cream on or to the side of the meat.

COOK'S TIP ON HORSERADISH:

Freshly opened bottled horseradish is much hotter than horseradish that was opened previously. Therefore, the amount of horseradish you use, such as in this recipe, may be governed by how long it has been since the horseradish was first opened.

PER SERVING

calories 200
total fat 7.5 g
  saturated 3.0 g
  polyunsaturated 0.5 g
  monounsaturated 3.0 g
cholesterol 78 mg

sodium 130 mg
carbohydrates 5 g
  fiber 0 g
  sugar 2 g
protein 27 g

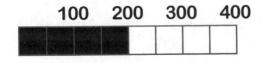

100 200 300 400   **DIETARY EXCHANGES**
½ other carbohydrate;
3 lean meat

beef tenderloin with shallot and sweet-onion marmalade

Serves 8; 3 ounces meat and $1/4$ cup marmalade per serving (plus 1 cup reserved)

When sweet onions are in season, reach for this recipe and invite friends over for dinner. The extra marmalade is a lovely condiment to serve with other lean roasted meats.

shallot and sweet-onion marmalade

1 tablespoon canola oil

8 large shallots, thinly sliced

8 medium sweet onions, such as Vidalia, halved crosswise and thinly sliced

3 cups fat-free, no-salt-added beef broth

2 cups sugar

2 tablespoons red wine vinegar

$1/2$ teaspoon fresh thyme leaves

1 teaspoon salt

$1/4$ teaspoon pepper

2-pound beef tenderloin, all visible fat and silver skin discarded

$1/2$ teaspoon salt

Pepper to taste

Heat a 6-quart saucepan or Dutch oven over high heat. Pour the oil into the pan and swirl to coat the bottom. Cook the shallots and onions for 8 to 10 minutes, or until they begin to soften, stirring occasionally.

Stir in the broth, sugar, vinegar, and thyme. Continue to stir until the sugar is dissolved.

Adjust the heat to keep the mixture just below the boil. Cook for about 45 minutes, or until most of the liquid has evaporated. Transfer to a serving bowl if serving warm, or put in an airtight container and chill for up to one week.

To roast the tenderloin, preheat the oven to 400°F.

Tuck the thin end of the meat under so the roast is an even thickness. Tie with kitchen twine to secure the tucked-under part. Sprinkle the salt and pepper on all sides of the meat. Put the meat in a roasting pan.

Roast, uncovered, in the center of the oven for 30 to 45 minutes, or until the desired doneness. Test for doneness by inserting an instant-read thermometer into the thickest section of the meat. Rare will read 120°F to 125°F, and medium 140°F to 145°F.

Remove from the oven and let stand for at least 10 minutes before slicing.

To serve, place the meat on a platter. Serve with the marmalade to spoon to the side.

COOK'S TIP: This is a good dish to cook early in the day, refrigerate, and serve later at room temperature. Let the roast cool completely before wrapping it tightly in aluminum foil. Refrigerate until 1 hour before serving time. You can adapt this recipe for almost any number of servings. The rule of thumb is four servings per pound of meat (raw weight) and ¼ teaspoon of salt for every pound.

COOK'S TIP ON SHALLOTS: Shallots are the small pinkish-skinned members of the onion family. They are formed like garlic, with multiple cloves, and have a very mild onion flavor.

PER SERVING

calories 364
total fat 8.5 g
  saturated 3.0 g
  polyunsaturated 0.5 g
  monounsaturated 3.5 g
cholesterol 76 mg

sodium 426 mg
carbohydrates 44 g
  fiber 2 g
  sugar 40 g
protein 28 g

100	200	300	400

DIETARY EXCHANGES
3 vegetable;
2 other carbohydrate;
3 lean meat

filet mignon with balsamic berry sauce

Serves 4; 3 ounces beef and 2 tablespoons sauce per serving

This beautiful cut of meat is served with a sweet, mellow, sophisticated sauce that is perfect for that intimate dinner party.

balsamic berry sauce

1/2 cup water

1/4 cup all-fruit blackberry spread

2 tablespoons balsamic vinegar

2 tablespoons low-salt soy sauce

2 tablespoons low-sodium Worcestershire sauce

Vegetable oil spray

4 filets mignons without bacon (about 4 ounces each), all visible fat discarded

1/4 teaspoon salt

1/4 teaspoon pepper

In a small bowl, whisk together the sauce ingredients.

Heat a large nonstick skillet over high heat. Remove from the heat and lightly spray with vegetable oil spray (being careful not to spray near a gas flame). Add the filets. Sprinkle with the salt and pepper. Cook for 2 minutes. Reduce the heat to medium. Turn the filets over and cook for 2 minutes. Turn again and cook for 2 minutes, or until desired doneness. Transfer to a plate. Cover to keep warm.

Increase the heat to high. Pour in the sauce. Bring to a boil, scraping any browned bits from the bottom of the skillet. Cook for 1 to 2 minutes, or until the liquid is reduced to ½ cup.

To serve, spoon the sauce over the filets.

PER SERVING

calories 238
total fat 9.0 g
  saturated 3.5 g
  polyunsaturated 0.5 g
  monounsaturated 3.5 g
cholesterol 70 mg

sodium 418 mg
carbohydrates 13 g
  fiber 0 g
  sugar 10 g
protein 24 g

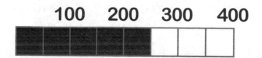

100 200 300 400

DIETARY EXCHANGES
1 other carbohydrate;
3 lean meat

honey-lime flank steak

Serves 4; 3 ounces steak per serving (plus 8 ounces reserved)

This one easy-to-prepare dish actually is the base for two meals. Serve part of the grilled flank steak for a delicious dinner with your choice of vegetables, and refrigerate the rest of the cooked steak to use in Flank Steak Salad with Sesame-Lime Dressing (page 334) later in the week.

marinade

Juice of 1 medium lime
3 tablespoons honey
2 tablespoons plain rice vinegar
1 tablespoon low-salt soy sauce
2 teaspoons toasted sesame oil
1 teaspoon grated peeled gingerroot
2 medium garlic cloves, minced

1 1/2 pounds flank steak, all visible fat and silver skin discarded
Vegetable oil spray (optional)

In a large resealable plastic bag or glass baking dish, stir together the marinade ingredients. Add the meat and turn to coat. Seal the bag or cover the dish and refrigerate for several hours or overnight, turning occasionally.

If using an outdoor grill, preheat on medium high. If using a ridged stovetop grill pan, lightly spray with vegetable oil spray.

Discard the marinade. Cook the meat over medium-high heat for 7 to 8 minutes on each side for medium rare, or until the desired doneness. Transfer to a cutting board. Let stand for 5 minutes. Cut diagonally across the grain into very thin slices. Reserve 8 ounces steak for another use.

COOK'S TIP ON MEASURING HONEY:
Lightly spray your measuring cup or spoon with vegetable oil spray before you measure honey. The honey will easily slide out of the measuring implement without sticking.

PER SERVING

calories 162
total fat 6.0 g
  saturated 2.5 g
  polyunsaturated 0.0 g
  monounsaturated 2.0 g
cholesterol 37 mg

sodium 127 mg
carbohydrates 0 g
  fiber 0 g
  sugar 0 g
protein 25 g

100 200 300 400

DIETARY EXCHANGES
1 vegetable;
$\frac{1}{2}$ other carbohydrate;
2 lean meat

orange beef stir-fry

**Serves 4; 3 ounces meat and
2 tablespoons sauce per serving**

You might want to make a double batch of this quick-cooking meal—it is every bit as tasty a day or two later. Use two woks or skillets if making extra so the meat isn't crowded and doesn't steam instead of stir-fry.

1 pound flank steak, partially frozen if possible
  Vegetable oil spray
1 teaspoon canola or corn oil
4 medium green onions (green and white parts), sliced
2 teaspoons grated peeled gingerroot
2 teaspoons grated orange zest
2 medium garlic cloves, minced
¼ cup fresh orange juice
2 tablespoons plain rice vinegar or white wine vinegar
1 tablespoon light teriyaki sauce or low-salt soy sauce
1½ tablespoons honey
1 teaspoon toasted sesame oil
2 teaspoons cornstarch
¼ cup cold water

Discard all the visible fat and the silver skin from the flank steak. Thinly slice the steak on the diagonal. Cut into bite-size pieces.

Heat a wok or large skillet over high heat. Remove from the heat and lightly spray with vegetable oil spray (being careful not to spray near a gas flame). Cook the steak for 2 minutes, or until browned, stirring frequently. Transfer to a medium bowl. Wipe the wok with paper towels.

Reduce the heat to medium. Pour the oil into the wok and swirl to coat the bottom. Cook the green onions, gingerroot, orange zest, and garlic for 3 minutes, or until the green onions are soft, stirring frequently. Stir in the steak with any accumulated juices.

Increase the heat to medium high. Stir in the orange juice, vinegar, teriyaki sauce, honey, and sesame oil. Cook for 1 to 2 minutes, or until the steak is the desired doneness and the mixture is hot, stirring occasionally.

Put the cornstarch in a cup. Add the water, stirring to dissolve. Stir the cornstarch mixture into the wok. Cook for 1 minute, or until thickened, stirring frequently.

COOK'S TIP ON SLICING
MEAT: Freezing meat for about 30 minutes before cutting it makes the task much easier.

PER SERVING ···

calories 235
total fat 8.5 g
  saturated 2.5 g
  polyunsaturated 1.0 g
  monounsaturated 3.5 g
cholesterol 37 mg

sodium 179 mg
carbohydrates 13 g
  fiber 1 g
  sugar 10 g
protein 25 g

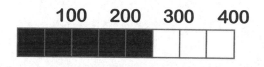

100   200   300   400

DIETARY EXCHANGES
1 vegetable; $\frac{1}{2}$ other carbohydrate; 3 lean meat

beef stroganoff with baby portobello mushrooms

Serves 4; 1 cup meat mixture and ½ cup noodles per serving

Delicate pearl onions and mini portobello mushrooms are cooked until they are so tender they seem to melt into the sauce of this stroganoff. Serve with a salad of crisp romaine lettuce, shredded carrots, and juicy red tomatoes.

3 ounces dried yolk-free noodles
1 pound boneless top round steak, all visible fat discarded, cut into thin slices
2 tablespoons all-purpose flour
½ teaspoon salt-free all-purpose seasoning
    Vegetable oil spray
1 teaspoon olive oil
1 pound sliced baby portobello mushrooms
1 cup frozen pearl onions
1 cup fat-free, no-salt-added beef broth
¼ cup dry white wine (regular or nonalcoholic) or fat-free, no-salt-added beef broth
2 tablespoons low-sodium steak sauce
¼ teaspoon salt
¼ teaspoon pepper
⅓ cup fat-free or light sour cream

Prepare the noodles using the package directions, omitting the salt and oil. Drain well in a colander. Cover to keep warm.

Meanwhile, put the steak, flour, and all-purpose seasoning in a medium resealable plastic bag. Seal the bag. Shake to coat the meat.

Heat a large nonstick skillet over medium-high heat. Remove from the heat and lightly spray with vegetable oil spray (being careful not to spray near a gas flame). Pour the oil into the skillet and swirl to coat the bottom. Add the meat mixture, including any flour remaining in the bag, and cook for 6 to 8 minutes, or until the meat is browned on the outside and slightly pink on the inside. Transfer the meat to a medium bowl or plate.

Add the mushrooms and pearl onions to the skillet. Cook for 3 to 4 minutes, or until the mushrooms are tender and the onions are almost thawed, stirring occasionally.

Stir in the remaining ingredients except the sour cream. Bring to a simmer over medium-high heat, stirring occasionally. Reduce the heat and simmer, covered, for 20 to 25 minutes, or until the beef is tender and the sauce is thickened (no stirring needed).

Stir a small amount of the beef mixture into the sour cream to prevent curdling. Stir the sour-cream mixture into the remaining beef mixture. Cook over low heat for 1 to 2 minutes, or until warmed through, stirring occasionally.

To serve, spoon the noodles onto each plate. Top each serving with the beef mixture.

PER SERVING

calories 350	sodium 278 mg
total fat 5.5 g	carbohydrates 37 g
saturated 1.5 g	fiber 3 g
polyunsaturated 0.5 g	sugar 7 g
monounsaturated 2.0 g	protein 34 g
cholesterol 67 mg	

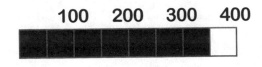

100 200 300 400 **DIETARY EXCHANGES**
1½ starch; 3 vegetable; 3 lean meat

slow-cooker shredded beef on potato mounds

Serves 4; 1 cup meat mixture and ¹/₂ cup potatoes per serving

When you know you won't have much time in the evening to prepare a hot meal, here's a go-to recipe the whole family will relish. The beef mixture (no potatoes) also makes a great filling for soft tortillas.

Vegetable oil spray

1 pound boneless round steak, all visible fat discarded

2 medium green bell peppers, thinly sliced

1 large onion, thinly sliced

8 ounce can no-salt-added tomato sauce

1 tablespoon low-sodium Worcestershire sauce

2 teaspoons sugar

¹/₄ teaspoon salt

¹/₄ teaspoon pepper

2 cups packaged refrigerated mashed potatoes

¹/₄ cup finely snipped fresh parsley

Lightly spray a slow cooker with vegetable oil spray. Put the steak in the pot. Top with the bell peppers and onion.

In a small bowl, stir together the tomato sauce, Worcestershire sauce, and sugar. Pour over the vegetables. Cook, covered, on low for 3½ hours, or until the steak is tender.

Transfer the steak to a cutting board. Shred the steak with a fork. Return to the slow cooker. Stir in the salt and pepper. Put the cover back on, but don't turn on the slow cooker.

Prepare the potatoes using the package directions.

To serve, spoon the potatoes in the center of shallow bowls. Top with the steak and its liquid. Sprinkle with the parsley.

PER SERVING ···

calories 277	sodium 505 mg
total fat 5.0 g	carbohydrates 29 g
saturated 1.5 g	fiber 4 g
polyunsaturated 0.0 g	sugar 11 g
monounsaturated 1.5 g	protein 27 g
cholesterol 58 mg	

100 200 300 400

DIETARY EXCHANGES
1 starch; 3 vegetable;
3 lean meat

saucy minute steaks

Serves 4; 1 patty and 2 to 3 tablespoons sauce per serving

Pop baking potatoes in the microwave while you prepare this easy dish.

sauce

3/4 cup water

2 tablespoons dry sherry

2 teaspoons cornstarch

2 teaspoons very low sodium beef bouillon granules

1 teaspoon low-sodium Worcestershire sauce

1/2 teaspoon dried oregano, crumbled

1/4 teaspoon sugar

1/8 teaspoon garlic powder

4 cube steaks (about 4 ounces each)
Vegetable oil spray

1/2 teaspoon dried oregano, crumbled

1/8 teaspoon pepper

2 teaspoons light tub margarine

2 tablespoons finely snipped fresh parsley

In a small bowl, whisk together the sauce ingredients until the cornstarch is completely dissolved. Set aside.

Sprinkle the steaks with the remaining oregano and the pepper. Heat a large nonstick skillet over high heat. Remove from the heat and lightly spray with vegetable oil spray (being careful not to spray near a gas flame). Cook the steaks for 3 minutes. Turn the steaks over. Cook for 2 minutes, or until slightly pink in the center. Transfer to a plate.

Reduce the heat to medium high. Stir the sauce into the skillet. Bring to a boil, scraping any browned bits from the bottom. Cook for 1 minute, or until thickened slightly, stirring constantly. Remove from the heat. Stir in the margarine and parsley. Spoon over the steaks.

PER SERVING

calories 169
total fat 4.5 g
 saturated 1.5 g
 polyunsaturated 0.5 g
 monounsaturated 2.0 g
cholesterol 65 mg

sodium 81 mg
carbohydrates 3 g
 fiber 0 g
 sugar 1 g
protein 26 g

100   200   300   400   DIETARY EXCHANGES
3 lean meat

chicken-fried steak
with creamy gravy

**Serves 4; 3 ounces meat and
2 tablespoons gravy per serving**

Whole-wheat cracker crumbs provide the crunchy crust you expect with chicken-fried steak, and chicken broth and fat-free half-and-half combine in a wonderful creamy gravy. All you *don't* get of this southern classic are the calories, saturated fats, and cholesterol.

1/4 cup all-purpose flour

1 teaspoon salt-free all-purpose seasoning

1/2 cup fat-free or low-fat buttermilk

3/4 cup finely crushed whole-wheat crackers (about 30 crackers)

4 cube steaks (about 4 ounces each), all visible fat discarded

2 teaspoons olive oil

Vegetable oil spray

1/4 cup fat-free, low-sodium chicken broth

1/4 cup fat-free half-and-half

1/4 teaspoon salt

In a shallow bowl, stir together the flour and all-purpose seasoning. Set aside 2 teaspoons of this mixture. Put the buttermilk and cracker crumbs in two separate shallow bowls. Set the bowls with the flour mixture, the buttermilk, and the cracker crumbs in a row, assembly-line fashion.

Coat a steak with the flour, shaking off the excess. Coat with the buttermilk, then with the cracker crumbs. Cover and refrigerate the steaks for 30 minutes to 4 hours. (This will help the coating adhere to the steak during cooking.)

Heat a large nonstick skillet over medium-high heat. Pour the oil into the skillet and swirl to coat the bottom. Cook the steaks on one side for 4 to 5 minutes, or until golden brown. Remove the skillet from the heat. Lightly spray the uncooked side of the steaks twice with vegetable oil spray (being careful not to spray near a gas flame). Turn the steaks. Cook for 4 to 5 minutes, or until golden brown on the outside and no longer pink in the center. Transfer the steaks to a platter. Cover with aluminum foil to keep warm. Remove the skillet from the heat to cool slightly. (A pan that is too hot at this point will evaporate the gravy liquid.)

In a small bowl, whisk together the broth, half-and-half, salt, and reserved flour mixture. Pour into the skillet. Cook over medium heat for 2 to 3 minutes, or until the mixture comes to a simmer and thickens, stirring occasionally.

To serve, place the steaks on plates. Spoon the sauce over the steaks or serve it on the side.

COOK'S TIP: Cube steaks are usually easy to find, but you can always ask the butcher to tenderize or "cube" eye-of-round, top round, or bottom round steaks if you don't spot them in the counter. You may also tenderize your own steaks at home with a meat-tenderizing mallet. Just pound both sides firmly with the mallet without tearing the meat.

PER SERVING

calories 290

total fat 9.0 g

  saturated 2.5 g

  polyunsaturated 1.5 g

  monounsaturated 4.0 g

cholesterol 65 mg

sodium 345 mg

carbohydrates 22 g

  fiber 2 g

  sugar 3 g

protein 30 g

100   200   300   400

DIETARY EXCHANGES

$1\frac{1}{2}$ starch; 3 lean meat

satay-style sirloin with peanut dipping sauce

Serves 4; 3 ounces steak and 2 tablespoons sauce per serving

Grilling individual marinated steaks saves you the time it takes to assemble traditional satay meat skewers.

1 pound boneless top sirloin steak

marinade

4 medium green onions (green and white parts), thinly sliced

2 tablespoons fresh lime juice

2 teaspoons low-salt soy sauce

1 teaspoon light brown sugar

1 teaspoon grated peeled gingerroot

1 teaspoon toasted sesame oil

2 medium garlic cloves, minced

peanut dipping sauce

1/3 cup fat-free half-and-half

2 tablespoons reduced-fat creamy peanut butter

2 teaspoons low-salt soy sauce

1/2 teaspoon coconut extract

1/2 teaspoon chili paste (optional)

Vegetable oil spray (optional)

Discard all the visible fat from the steak. Cut the steak into 4 equal pieces. In a medium resealable plastic bag or glass baking dish, stir together the marinade ingredients. Add the steaks and turn to coat. Seal the bag or cover the dish and refrigerate for 15 minutes to 8 hours, turning occasionally.

Meanwhile, in a small bowl, whisk together the dipping sauce ingredients. Cover and refrigerate until ready to use. (The sauce will keep for two days.)

Preheat the grill on medium high or preheat the broiler. If using a broiler, lightly spray the pan and rack with vegetable oil spray.

Remove the meat from the marinade. Discard the marinade.

Grill the steaks or broil about 6 inches from the heat for 8 to 10 minutes on each side for medium rare to medium, or until the desired doneness.

To serve, put the steaks on plates. Serve with the dipping sauce.

PER SERVING

calories 217
total fat 8.5 g
  saturated 2.5 g
  polyunsaturated 0.0 g
  monounsaturated 2.5 g
cholesterol 71 mg

sodium 265 mg
carbohydrates 7 g
  fiber 1 g
  sugar 2 g
protein 28 g

100   200   300   400

DIETARY EXCHANGES
1/2 other carbohydrate;
3 lean meat

greek-style sirloin cubes and olive-feta rice

Serves 4; 1½ cups per serving

This dish of tender beef offers just the right combination of flavor, texture, and color. Serve with a salad of mixed salad greens, red and yellow tomatoes, and red onions.

Vegetable oil spray
1 cup frozen pearl onions
14.5-ounce can no-salt-added diced tomatoes, undrained
¼ cup water
1 teaspoon grated lemon zest
1 teaspoon fresh lemon juice
1 teaspoon dried oregano, crumbled
¼ teaspoon salt
⅛ teaspoon pepper
1¼ cups fat-free, low-sodium chicken broth
2 tablespoons chopped kalamata olives
2 tablespoons slivered almonds, dry-roasted
1 cup uncooked instant brown rice
2 tablespoons crumbled fat-free or low-fat feta cheese
1 pound boneless top sirloin steak, all visible fat discarded, cut into ¾-inch cubes

Heat a medium saucepan over medium-high heat. Remove from the heat and lightly spray with vegetable oil spray (being careful not to spray near a gas flame). Cook the pearl onions for 4 to 5 minutes, or until almost thawed and slightly golden brown on the outside, stirring occasionally.

Stir in the undrained tomatoes, water, lemon zest, lemon juice, oregano, salt, and pepper. Bring to a simmer, stirring occasionally. Reduce the heat and simmer, covered, for 15 to 20 minutes, or until the flavors have blended, stirring occasionally. Set aside.

Meanwhile, stir together the broth, olives, and almonds. Bring to a simmer over medium-high heat. Stir in the rice. Reduce the heat and simmer, covered, for 10 minutes, or until the rice is tender. Stir in the feta. Remove from the heat and cover to keep warm.

Heat a large nonstick skillet over medium-high heat. Remove from the heat and lightly spray with vegetable oil spray (being careful not to spray near a gas flame). Cook the steak cubes for 5 to 6 minutes, or until browned on the outside and slightly pink in the center, stirring occasionally.

Add the steak to the tomato mixture. Cook over low heat for 1 minute, or until the mixture is warmed through, stirring occasionally.

To serve, spoon the rice onto plates. Spoon the steak and tomato mixture over the rice.

PER SERVING

calories 330	sodium 404 mg
total fat 9.0 g	carbohydrates 31 g
saturated 2.5 g	fiber 4 g
polyunsaturated 1.0 g	sugar 6 g
monounsaturated 4.5 g	protein 30 g
cholesterol 71 mg	

100   200   300   400

DIETARY EXCHANGES
1 starch; 1 vegetable;
3 lean meat

meat loaf with a twist

Serves 6; 1 slice per serving

Grated zucchini adds moisture and flavor to this traditional meat loaf. If you have leftovers, you can make delicious sandwiches.

Vegetable oil spray

meat loaf

1 medium zucchini
1 pound lean ground beef
1/2 cup uncooked rolled oats
1 small onion, chopped
Whites of 2 large eggs, lightly beaten
2 tablespoons shredded or grated Parmesan cheese
2 tablespoons fat-free milk
1 tablespoon snipped fresh parsley
2 medium garlic cloves, minced
1/2 teaspoon dried basil, crumbled
1/2 teaspoon dried oregano, crumbled
1/4 teaspoon salt

glaze

1/4 cup no-salt-added ketchup

1 tablespoon light brown sugar

1 teaspoon Dijon honey mustard

1 teaspoon prepared white horseradish

1/8 teaspoon salt

....

1/2 teaspoon paprika (optional)

Preheat the oven to 350°F.

Lightly spray a broiler pan and rack with vegetable oil spray. (You can also use a cooling rack. Cover it with aluminum foil and place it in a roasting pan. Lightly spray the foil with vegetable oil spray. Using a fork, poke holes in the foil to allow the fat to drain.)

Shred enough zucchini to measure 1 cup. Squeeze dry between paper towels. Pat dry with more paper towels. Cut the remaining zucchini crosswise into thin slices. Set the slices aside.

In a large bowl, combine the shredded zucchini with the remaining meat loaf ingredients. Place the mixture on the broiler pan. Shape into an 8 × 3½ × 2-inch loaf.

Bake for 1 hour.

Meanwhile, in a small bowl, stir together the glaze ingredients.

Remove the meat loaf from the oven. Spoon the glaze over the top and sides of the loaf. Garnish with the reserved zucchini slices. Sprinkle the paprika over the zucchini slices.

Bake for 10 to 15 minutes, or until the loaf reaches an internal temperature of 160°F and is no longer pink in the center. Let stand for 5 minutes before slicing.

PER SERVING

calories 209
total fat 9.0 g
  saturated 3.0 g
  polyunsaturated 0.5 g
  monounsaturated 3.5 g
cholesterol 45 mg

sodium 277 mg
carbohydrates 14 g
  fiber 2 g
  sugar 7 g
protein 19 g

100 200 300 400

DIETARY EXCHANGES
1 starch; 2½ lean meat

baked ziti with beef and green beans

Serves 4; 1½ cups per serving

This hearty casserole features tubes of pasta, lean ground beef, green beans, and a rich-tasting tomato sauce, all layered and baked. Serve with fruit salad.

4 ounces dried ziti (about 1 cup)

1 pound lean ground beef

½ medium onion, chopped

   14.5-ounce can no-salt-added diced tomatoes, undrained

1 cup fat-free, no-salt-added beef broth

2 tablespoons no-salt-added tomato paste

1 tablespoon imitation bacon bits

1 teaspoon dried oregano, crumbled

2 medium garlic cloves, minced

2 cups frozen green beans (about 8 ounces), thawed

1 cup shredded fat-free or part-skim mozzarella cheese

¼ cup shredded or grated Parmesan cheese

Prepare the pasta using the package directions, omitting the salt and oil. Drain well in a colander.

   Heat a large nonstick skillet over medium-high heat. Cook the beef for 8 to 10 minutes, or until browned, stirring occasionally to turn and break up the beef. Pour into a colander and rinse under hot water to remove excess fat. Drain well. Wipe the skillet with paper towels. Return the beef to the skillet.

Add the onion to the beef. Cook for 3 to 4 minutes, or until the onion is soft, stirring occasionally.

Stir in the undrained tomatoes, broth, tomato paste, bacon bits, oregano, and garlic. Bring to a simmer. Reduce the heat and simmer, covered, for 10 minutes, or until the flavors have blended.

Preheat the oven to 350°F.

To assemble the casserole, pour 1 cup pasta in a 9-inch square nonstick baking pan. Pour half the meat sauce over the pasta. Top with half the green beans. Sprinkle with half the mozzarella and half the Parmesan. Repeat the layers.

Bake, uncovered, for 20 to 25 minutes, or until the cheeses are melted and the mixture is warmed through.

PER SERVING

calories 362
total fat 6.0 g
  saturated 2.5 g
  polyunsaturated 0.5 g
  monounsaturated 2.5 g
cholesterol 60 mg

sodium 632 mg
carbohydrates 36 g
  fiber 6 g
  sugar 8 g
protein 39 g

100 200 300 400

DIETARY EXCHANGES
1½ starch; 3 vegetable;
4 very lean meat

beefy macaroni and cheese
Serves 6; 1¹/₂ cups per serving

No baking is required for this updated American classic, which cooks quickly on the stovetop.

1¹/₂ cups dried whole-wheat macaroni
  1 teaspoon salt-free all-purpose seasoning
  1 pound lean ground beef
10 ounces frozen broccoli florets
  1 medium green bell pepper, chopped
¹/₂ medium onion, chopped
  2 medium garlic cloves, chopped
³/₄ to 1 teaspoon chili powder
¹/₄ to ¹/₂ teaspoon crushed red pepper flakes (optional)
  1 cup fat-free milk
1¹/₂ tablespoons all-purpose flour
¹/₂ teaspoon salt
¹/₄ teaspoon pepper
  1 cup shredded fat-free or low-fat Cheddar cheese

Prepare the pasta using the package directions, omitting the salt and oil and adding the all-purpose seasoning. Drain well in a colander. Transfer to a bowl and set aside.

Meanwhile, heat a large nonstick skillet over medium-high heat. Cook the beef for 8 to 10 minutes, or until browned, stirring occasionally to turn and break up the beef. Pour into the colander and rinse under hot water to remove excess fat. Drain well. Wipe the skillet with paper towels. Return the beef to the skillet.

Add the broccoli, bell pepper, onion, garlic, chili powder, and red pepper flakes. Cook over medium-high heat for 4 to 5 minutes, or until the vegetables are tender and the broccoli is warmed through, stirring occasionally. Reduce the heat to low and keep warm, uncovered, stirring occasionally.

In a medium saucepan, whisk together the milk, flour, salt, and pepper. Bring to a simmer over medium-high heat. Adjusting the heat as necessary, simmer for 2 to 3 minutes, or until thickened, whisking occasionally. Turn off the heat, leaving the pan on the stove. Add the pasta and Cheddar, whisking until the cheeses are melted. Pour over the beef mixture.

Cook over low heat for 2 to 3 minutes, or until the mixture is warmed through, stirring occasionally.

PER SERVING

calories 251
total fat 3.5 g
  saturated 1.0 g
  polyunsaturated 0.5 g
  monounsaturated 1.0 g
cholesterol 38 mg

sodium 398 mg
carbohydrates 30 g
  fiber 4 g
  sugar 4 g
protein 27 g

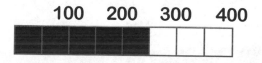

100 200 300 400

DIETARY EXCHANGES
1 1/2 starch; 1 1/2 vegetable; 3 very lean meat

tex-mex beef casserole with cornbread crust

Serves 4; 1½ cups per serving

Cornbread spiked with jalapeño (or milder green chiles) tops this satisfying casserole.

Vegetable oil spray

1 pound lean ground beef

2 teaspoons chili powder

1 teaspoon ground cumin

15-ounce can no-salt-added black beans, rinsed and drained

1 cup frozen whole-kernel corn, thawed

½ cup salsa

¼ teaspoon salt

1 medium fresh jalapeño or 2 tablespoons canned chopped green chiles, undrained

¾ cup yellow cornmeal

¼ cup whole-wheat flour or all-purpose flour

½ teaspoon baking powder

½ teaspoon baking soda

½ cup fat-free or low-fat buttermilk

Egg substitute equivalent to 1 egg, or 1 large egg

Preheat the oven to 425°F. Lightly spray an 8-inch square baking dish with vegetable oil spray.

In a large skillet, cook the beef over medium-high heat for 8 to 10 minutes, or until browned, stirring occasionally to turn and break up the beef. Pour into a colander and rinse under hot water to remove excess fat. Drain well. Wipe the skillet with paper towels. Return the beef to the skillet.

Stir in the chili powder and cumin. Reduce the heat to medium and cook for 1 to 2 minutes, or until the flavors have blended.

Stir in the beans, corn, salsa, and salt. Cook for 2 to 3 minutes, or until the mixture is warmed through. Transfer to the baking dish.

Meanwhile, wearing disposable plastic gloves, discard the seeds and ribs of the jalapeño. Finely chop the jalapeño. Put in a medium bowl.

Add the cornmeal, flour, baking powder, and baking soda to the jalapeño. Pour in the buttermilk and egg substitute, whisking just until the mixture is moistened (a few lumps may remain). Do not overmix or the topping will be tough. Pour over the meat mixture, smoothing the top with a spatula.

Bake for 24 to 26 minutes, or until a cake tester or wooden toothpick inserted into the topping comes out dry and the filling is warmed through.

PER SERVING

calories 405

total fat 5.5 g

  saturated 2.0 g

  polyunsaturated 0.5 g

  monounsaturated 2.0 g

cholesterol 52 mg

sodium 593 mg

carbohydrates 57 g

  fiber 8 g

  sugar 8 g

protein 33 g

100 200 300 400

DIETARY EXCHANGES

$3\frac{1}{2}$ starch; 1 vegetable; 3 very lean meat

chopped beef hash
Serves 4; 1½ cups per serving

Using frozen hash browns and leftover roast beef, you can have a home-style dinner on the table in just minutes.

1 teaspoon olive oil
1 medium red bell pepper, diced
1 medium green bell pepper, diced
1 medium onion, diced
  2-ounce jar diced pimientos, rinsed and drained
3 cups frozen diced hash browns, thawed
2 cups chopped cooked lean roast beef, cooked without salt (about 8 ounces), all visible fat discarded
1 teaspoon low-sodium Worcestershire sauce
1 teaspoon dried marjoram, crumbled
½ teaspoon dried thyme, crumbled
¼ teaspoon pepper

Heat a large nonstick skillet over medium-high heat. Pour the oil into the skillet and swirl to coat the bottom. Cook the bell peppers, onion, and pimientos for 3 to 4 minutes, or until tender, stirring occasionally.

Stir in the hash browns. Cook for 4 to 5 minutes, or until the potatoes are golden brown and warmed through, stirring occasionally.

Stir in the remaining ingredients. Cook for 3 to 4 minutes, or until the mixture is warmed through and the flavors have blended.

COOK'S TIP ON EASY ROAST BEEF: You can slow-cook a roast during the day or even overnight so you'll have it handy for use in recipes such as this one. Put a 2-pound eye-of-round roast (all visible fat discarded) in a slow cooker. Add 2 cups fat-free, no-salt-added beef broth and 1 tablespoon salt-free all-purpose seasoning. Cook on high for 5 to 6 hours or on low for 8 to 10 hours. Remove the roast from the slow cooker and let it set for at least 10 minutes before cutting. Serves 8; 3 ounces cooked meat per serving.

PER SERVING

calories 259

total fat 4.0 g

  saturated 1.0 g

  polyunsaturated 0.5 g

  monounsaturated 2.0 g

cholesterol 39 mg

sodium 76 mg

carbohydrates 36 g

  fiber 4 g

  sugar 4 g

protein 21 g

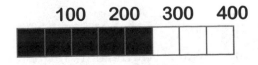

100 200 300 400

DIETARY EXCHANGES

2 starch; 1 1/2 vegetable;
2 very lean meat

ham and broccoli with rotini
Serves 4; 1¹⁄₂ cups per serving

Perfect for a rainy night, this one-dish meal is really quick and easy to prepare.

    4 quarts water
    6 ounces dried whole-wheat or regular rotini
1¹⁄₂ cups small broccoli florets
    1 large red bell pepper, cut into thin strips
    1 cup frozen whole-kernel corn, thawed
    4 slices reduced-fat American cheese
    3 ounces low-fat, lower-sodium ham, thinly sliced and chopped
    2 tablespoons fat-free milk
  ¹⁄₄ to ¹⁄₂ teaspoon dried thyme, crumbled
  ¹⁄₈ teaspoon salt
  ¹⁄₈ teaspoon cayenne

In a stockpot, bring the water to a boil over high heat. Boil the pasta for 7 minutes.

Stir in the broccoli and bell pepper. Cook for 2 to 3 minutes, or until the broccoli is tender-crisp. Drain well in a colander. Return to the pot.

Stir in the remaining ingredients. Spoon the mixture onto plates.

PER SERVING

calories 292
total fat 5.0 g
  saturated 2.5 g
  polyunsaturated 0.5 g
  monounsaturated 0.5 g
cholesterol 19 mg

sodium 587 mg
carbohydrates 48 g
  fiber 3 g
  sugar 7 g
protein 17 g

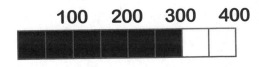

100 200 300 400 **DIETARY EXCHANGES**
3 starch; 1 vegetable; 1 lean meat

pork tenderloin with cranberry salsa

Serves 4; 3 ounces pork and ^{1}/2 cup salsa per serving

Pineapple, cranberries, and cinnamon combine in a tangy salsa that is great for the winter holidays and refreshing enough for a hot summer's day.

cranberry salsa

1 medium poblano pepper, seeds and ribs discarded, finely chopped

1 cup chopped fresh pineapple or canned pineapple chunks packed in their own juice, drained

1/2 cup dried sweetened cranberries

1/4 cup finely chopped red onion

1 teaspoon grated peeled gingerroot

1/2 teaspoon ground cinnamon

1-pound pork tenderloin, all visible fat and silver skin discarded

1/4 teaspoon paprika

1/4 teaspoon salt

1/4 teaspoon pepper

1/8 teaspoon garlic powder

Preheat the oven to 425°F.

Wearing disposable plastic gloves, discard the seeds and ribs of the poblano. Finely chop the poblano. Put in a medium bowl. Add the remaining salsa ingredients and toss gently. Set aside.

Place the pork on a baking sheet, tucking the narrow end under to allow the pork to cook evenly.

In a small bowl, stir together the remaining ingredients. Sprinkle over the pork.

Bake for 23 minutes, or until the pork is barely pink in the center and registers 150°F on an instant-read thermometer. Transfer to a cutting board. Let stand for about 5 minutes before slicing. (The pork will continue to cook during the standing time, reaching about 160°F.)

Serve the pork slices with the salsa on the side.

COOK'S TIP: For a milder dish or if poblanos are not available, use a medium green bell pepper instead. If you'd still like a little heat, toss in 1/8 teaspoon dried red pepper flakes.

PER SERVING

calories 222	sodium 205 mg
total fat 4.5 g	carbohydrates 21 g
saturated 1.5 g	fiber 3 g
polyunsaturated 0.5 g	sugar 16 g
monounsaturated 2.0 g	protein 25 g
cholesterol 74 mg	

---

100   200   300   400   **DIETARY EXCHANGES**
1 1/2 fruit; 3 lean meat

pork tenderloin with orange-ginger sweet potatoes

Serves 6; 3 ounces pork and about ³/4 cup sweet potato mixture per serving

You've probably eaten applesauce and pork together, but you may not have tried them quite like they're prepared in the following recipe. The applesauce makes a terrific coating that adds flavor and moistness to the pork.

1 teaspoon ground coriander

¹/2 teaspoon ground cumin

¹/2 teaspoon ground cinnamon

¹/2 teaspoon salt

Pepper to taste

1-pound pork tenderloin, all visible fat and silver skin discarded

¹/2 cup unsweetened applesauce

orange-ginger sweet potatoes

2 medium sweet potatoes

1 teaspoon olive oil

10-ounce can mandarin oranges, packed in water or light syrup, drained

¹/4 cup snipped fresh parsley

¹/4 teaspoon ground ginger

Preheat the oven to 450°F.

Line a baking sheet with cooking parchment. On the baking sheet, combine the coriander, cumin, cinnamon, salt, and pepper.

Tuck the narrow end of the tenderloin under so the pork is an even thickness. Tie with kitchen twine about every 2 inches so the pork will cook more evenly. Spread the applesauce over the pork. Roll the pork in the seasoning to coat.

Bake for 20 minutes, or until the pork reaches an internal temperature of 150°F and is no longer pink in the center. Transfer the pork to a cutting board and let it rest for about 5 minutes before slicing.

Meanwhile, pierce the potatoes in several places with a fork. Put the potatoes on a microwaveable plate or on the microwave turntable. Microwave at 100 percent power (high) for 3 to 4 minutes, or until pierced easily with a fork. Cut the potatoes into large chunks, about 2 inches.

Heat a large skillet over medium-high heat. Pour the oil into the skillet and swirl to coat the bottom. Cook the sweet potatoes, mandarin oranges, parsley, and ginger for 3 to 5 minutes, or until the potatoes are soft and the mixture is well blended, stirring frequently.

To serve, place the pork on plates. Spoon the sweet potato mixture on the side.

PER SERVING

calories 167

total fat 3.5 g

  saturated 1.0 g

  polyunsaturated 0.5 g

  monounsaturated 2.0 g

cholesterol 49 mg

sodium 251 mg

carbohydrates 18 g

  fiber 2 g

  sugar 8 g

protein 17 g

100 200 300 400

DIETARY EXCHANGES

$\frac{1}{2}$ starch; $\frac{1}{2}$ fruit; $2\frac{1}{2}$ very lean meat

thai coconut curry with pork and vegetables

Serves 4; 1½ cups per serving

Tempt your palate with the exciting flavors of Thai cuisine, including light coconut milk, lemongrass, and red curry paste. Serve with chilled slices of cantaloupe and honeydew melon.

1 cup uncooked instant brown rice

4 medium green onions (green and white parts), chopped

Vegetable oil spray

4 boneless center-cut pork chops (about 4 ounces each), all visible fat discarded, cut into ½-inch cubes

1 cup baby carrots

½ medium onion, cut into 1-inch pieces

1 stalk lemongrass or 1 teaspoon grated lemon zest

1½ cups fat-free, low-sodium chicken broth

1 teaspoon Thai red curry paste

½ cup light coconut milk

2 tablespoons cornstarch

4 ounces fresh broccoli florets (about 1 cup)

Prepare the rice using the package directions, omitting the salt and oil and adding the green onions. Set aside and keep warm.

Meanwhile, heat a large skillet over medium-high heat. Remove from the heat and lightly spray with vegetable oil spray (being careful not to spray near a gas flame). Cook the pork for 3 to 4 minutes, or until browned, stirring occasionally.

Stir in the carrots and onion. Cook for 3 to 4 minutes, or until the carrots are tender-crisp and the onion is soft.

Meanwhile, trim and discard about 6 inches from the slender tip of the lemongrass stalk. Remove the outer layer of leaves from the bottom part of the stalk. Cut the stalk in half lengthwise.

Stir the lemongrass, broth, and red curry paste into the pork mixture. Bring to a simmer. Reduce the heat and simmer, covered, for 15 to 20 minutes, or until the pork is no longer pink in the center and the vegetables are tender, stirring occasionally.

In a small bowl, whisk together the coconut milk and cornstarch until smooth. Stir into the pork mixture.

Add the broccoli. Simmer, covered, for 3 to 4 minutes, or until the mixture is thickened and the broccoli is tender, stirring occasionally. Remove the lemongrass.

To serve, spoon the rice into bowls. Ladle the pork mixture on top.

PER SERVING ···

calories 322

total fat 9.0 g

  saturated 3.5 g

  polyunsaturated 1.0 g

  monounsaturated 3.0 g

cholesterol 67 mg

sodium 137 mg

carbohydrates 30 g

  fiber 4 g

  sugar 5 g

protein 27 g

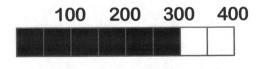

| 100 | 200 | 300 | 400 |

DIETARY EXCHANGES
1½ starch; 1½ vegetable; 3 lean meat

pork chops parmesan

Serves 4; 1 pork chop per serving

A coating of homemade soft bread crumbs and chopped fresh herbs keeps these pork chops moist while baking.

Vegetable oil spray

2 tablespoons all-purpose flour

Egg substitute equivalent to 1 egg, or 1 large egg, lightly beaten

2 slices whole-wheat bread

1/4 cup snipped fresh parsley or 1 tablespoon dried, crumbled

1/4 cup shredded or grated Parmesan cheese

10 medium to large fresh basil leaves or 1 teaspoon dried, crumbled

2 teaspoons fresh thyme leaves or 1/2 teaspoon dried, crumbled

2 teaspoons fresh oregano leaves or 1/2 teaspoon dried, crumbled

1 teaspoon garlic powder

1 teaspoon olive oil

1/4 teaspoon pepper

4 boneless center-cut pork chops (about 4 ounces each), all visible fat discarded

Preheat the oven to 375°F. Lightly spray an 8-inch square baking pan with vegetable oil spray.

Put the flour and egg substitute in two separate shallow bowls.

In a food processor, process the remaining ingredients except the pork chops until the bread is chopped into crumbs and the herbs are coarsely chopped. Put the mixture into a third shallow bowl. Set the bowls with the flour, egg substitute, and bread-crumb mixture and the baking pan in a row, assembly-line fashion.

Coat a pork chop with the flour, shaking off the excess. Coat it with the egg substitute, then with the bread-crumb mixture. Place in the baking pan. Repeat with the remaining pork chops.

Bake for 45 minutes, or until the pork is no longer pink in the center.

PER SERVING

calories 251

total fat 9.0 g
 saturated 3.0 g
 polyunsaturated 1.0 g
 monounsaturated 4.0 g
cholesterol 75 mg

sodium 267 mg
carbohydrates 11 g
 fiber 1 g
 sugar 3 g
protein 31 g

100 200 300 400   **DIETARY EXCHANGES**
½ starch; 3½ lean meat

sausage and white beans with spinach

Serves 4; 1$\frac{1}{2}$ cups per serving

The flavors of sausage and basil explode in this warm comfort dish—Mediterranean style.

Vegetable oil spray
6 ounces low-fat bulk breakfast sausage
1 tablespoon dried basil, crumbled
2 medium garlic cloves, minced
16-ounce can no-salt-added navy or cannellini beans, rinsed and drained
2 cups water, divided use
1$\frac{1}{2}$ cups uncooked quick-cooking brown rice
2 cups coarsely chopped spinach leaves (about 2 ounces)
$\frac{1}{2}$ teaspoon salt

Heat a 12-inch nonstick skillet over medium-high heat. Remove from the heat and lightly spray with vegetable oil spray (being careful not to spray near a gas flame). Cook the sausage for 3 to 4 minutes, or until no longer pink in the center, stirring constantly and breaking up any large pieces.

Stir in the basil and garlic. Cook for 15 seconds, stirring constantly.

Stir in the beans and $\frac{1}{4}$ cup water. Bring to a boil. Remove from the heat. Cover and set aside.

Meanwhile, in a medium saucepan, bring the remaining 1¾ cups water to a boil. Stir in the rice. Cook using the package directions, omitting the salt and margarine.

To serve, gently stir the rice into the bean mixture. Gently stir in the spinach and salt.

COOK'S TIP: The heat of the other ingredients gently warms and wilts the spinach without leaching out its brilliant color and rich vitamins.

PER SERVING

calories 286
total fat 2.5 g
 saturated 0.5 g
 polyunsaturated 0.5 g
 monounsaturated 0.5 g
cholesterol 21 mg

sodium 563 mg
carbohydrates 45 g
 fiber 6 g
 sugar 4 g
 protein 16 g

100 200 300 400 **DIETARY EXCHANGES**
3 starch;
1½ very lean meat

veal stew with sweet potatoes, pearl onions, and petit pois peas

Serves 8; 1$\frac{1}{2}$ cups per serving

Bite-size pieces of veal, small onions, and baby green peas add up to big flavor in this appealing stew.

1 cup all-purpose flour

$\frac{1}{4}$ teaspoon salt

Pepper to taste

1 pound lean veal stew meat, all visible fat discarded, cut into bite-size pieces

1 tablespoon olive oil

3 medium parsnips, peeled, cut into $\frac{1}{4}$-inch slices

1 large sweet potato, peeled, cut into $\frac{1}{2}$- to 1-inch cubes

2 medium garlic cloves, minced

4 cups fat-free, low-sodium chicken broth or mushroom stock

1 cup dry red wine (regular or nonalcoholic), such as burgundy

8 ounces frozen pearl onions

2 medium bay leaves

1 teaspoon dried basil, crumbled

8 ounces frozen petit pois (baby green peas)

1 cup fat-free, low-sodium chicken broth
or mushroom stock (optional)
½ cup all-purpose flour (optional)

In a shallow bowl, stir together the flour, salt, and pepper. Add the veal, turning to coat. Shake off any excess.

Heat a large stockpot over medium-high heat. Pour the oil into the pot and swirl to coat the bottom. Put in enough veal to make a single layer, not crowding the veal. Cook for 4 to 5 minutes, or until well browned on all sides, stirring occasionally. As it browns, transfer the veal to a plate. Repeat with the remaining veal.

Put the parsnips, potato, and garlic in the stockpot. Cook for 3 to 5 minutes, or until browned, stirring occasionally.

Return the veal to the pot. Stir in the broth, wine, onions, bay leaves, and basil. Increase the heat to high and bring to a boil. Reduce the heat and cook at a slow simmer, uncovered, stirring occasionally, for at least 1 hour 30 minutes, or until the meat and vegetables are tender and the flavors have blended. If preferred, transfer the stew to a slow cooker. Cook on low for 6 to 8 hours or on high for 3 to 4 hours.

Stir in the peas about 5 minutes before serving time.

For a thicker stew, in a small bowl, whisk together the 1 cup broth and ½ cup flour until smooth. Spoon a small amount of stew liquid into the flour mixture; whisk together. Whisk that mixture into the hot stew. Cook for 10 minutes to thicken the stew and cook the flour.

To serve, remove the bay leaves. Ladle the stew into bowls.

PER SERVING ···

calories 256
total fat 4.0 g
  saturated 1.0 g
  polyunsaturated 0.5 g
  monounsaturated 2.0 g
cholesterol 47 mg

sodium 199 mg
carbohydrates 34 g
  fiber 5 g
  sugar 6 g
protein 17 g

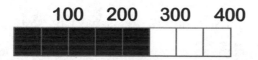

100   200   300   400

DIETARY EXCHANGES
2 starch; 1 vegetable;
2 very lean meat

lamb kebabs with apricot-rosemary dipping sauce

Serves 4; 2 kebabs and 2 tablespoons sauce per serving

Slowly warming this dipping sauce is the key to its excellent rosemary flavor.

1 pound boneless leg of lamb

marinade

2 tablespoons balsamic vinegar

2 medium garlic cloves, minced

1 medium bay leaf

1 teaspoon olive oil

1/4 teaspoon pepper

dipping sauce

1 teaspoon grated orange zest

1/4 cup fresh orange juice

1/4 cup all-fruit apricot spread

2 teaspoons chopped fresh rosemary or 1/2 teaspoon dried, crushed

Vegetable oil spray

Discard all visible fat from the lamb. Cut the lamb into 3/4-inch cubes.

In a medium resealable plastic bag or glass baking dish, stir together the marinade ingredients. Add the lamb and turn to coat. Seal the bag or cover the dish and refrigerate for 15 minutes to 8 hours, turning occasionally.

About 10 minutes before cooking the lamb, soak eight 8-inch wooden skewers in cold water.

Meanwhile, in a small saucepan, whisk together the sauce ingredients. Cook over low heat for 5 minutes, or until the mixture is warmed through, stirring occasionally. Turn the heat off, leaving the pan on the stove. Let stand until ready to serve.

Meanwhile, preheat the grill on medium high or preheat the broiler. If using the broiler, lightly spray the pan and rack with vegetable oil spray.

Remove the meat from the marinade. Discard the marinade. Thread the meat cubes onto the prepared skewers.

Grill the kebabs or broil about 6 inches from the heat for 8 to 10 minutes for medium, or until desired doneness, turning the kebabs four times.

To serve, put the kebabs on plates. Serve with the dipping sauce.

PER SERVING

calories 190
total fat 5.0 g
　saturated 1.5 g
　polyunsaturated 0.5 g
　monounsaturated 2.0 g
cholesterol 73 mg

sodium 69 mg
carbohydrates 12 g
　fiber 0 g
　sugar 9 g
　protein 23 g

100 200 300 400

DIETARY EXCHANGES
1 fruit; 3 lean meat

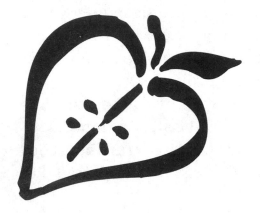

vegetarian entrées

Fresh Veggie Marinara with Feta

Penne with Matchstick Zucchini
and Mozzarella Cubes

Stuffed Shells with Arugula
and Four Cheeses

Make-Ahead Manicotti

Pesto Florentine Pasta

Soba Noodles in Peanut Sauce

Spinach and Bean Quesadillas
with Homemade Salsa

Braised Edamame with Bok Choy

Garden Veggie Tostadas

Mediterranean Wraps

Miami Wraps

Easy Two-Bean Chili

Mediterranean Vegetable Stew

Spinach and Ricotta Frittata

Cajun Red Beans and Brown Rice

Fried Rice with Snow Peas, Bell
    Pepper, and Water Chestnuts

Colossal Spring Rolls with Tofu
    and Vegetables

Creole Ratatouille

Mushroom and Artichoke Gnocchi
    with Capers

One-Pot Vegetable and Grain Medley

Couscous with Bell Pepper
    and Pine Nuts

Veggie Burgers with Gorgonzola

fresh veggie marinara with feta

Serves 4; 1 cup vegetable mixture and ½ cup pasta per serving

Here's a great opportunity to experience the joys of soy.

6 ounces dried whole-wheat penne pasta
   Vegetable oil spray
1 large zucchini, chopped
1 large green bell pepper, chopped
1 medium onion, chopped
1 tablespoon dried basil, crumbled
2 medium garlic cloves, minced
⅛ teaspoon crushed red pepper flakes
½ medium eggplant (about 8 ounces), diced, or 8 ounces sliced button mushrooms
1½ cups fat-free, reduced-sodium spaghetti sauce
6 ounces frozen soy protein crumbles (meatless crumbles), thawed
2 ounces feta cheese with sun-dried tomatoes and basil, crumbled

Prepare the pasta using the package directions, omitting the salt and oil. Drain well in a colander.

Meanwhile, heat a Dutch oven over medium-high heat. Remove from the heat and lightly spray with vegetable oil spray (being careful not to spray near a gas flame). Cook the zucchini, bell pepper, onion, basil, garlic, and red pepper flakes for 4 minutes, or until the onion is soft, stirring frequently.

Stir in the eggplant. Reduce the heat to medium low. Cook, covered, for 4 minutes, or until the eggplant is soft, stirring occasionally.

Stir in the spaghetti sauce. Cook, covered, for 5 minutes.

Stir in the crumbles. Cook, covered, for 2 minutes, or until heated thoroughly.

To serve, transfer the pasta to a platter. Top with the vegetable mixture. Sprinkle with the feta.

PER SERVING

calories 327

total fat 4.0 g

  saturated 2.0 g

  polyunsaturated 0.5 g

  monounsaturated 0.0 g

cholesterol 10 mg

sodium 569 mg

carbohydrates 55 g

  fiber 12 g

  sugar 12 g

protein 22 g

100 200 300 400

DIETARY EXCHANGES

2½ starch; 3 vegetable; 1½ lean meat

penne with matchstick zucchini and mozzarella cubes

Serves 4; 1$\frac{1}{2}$ cups per serving

Tube-shaped pasta, zucchini strips, and cheese cubes, along with sliced red bell pepper and chopped purplish-black olives, provide eye appeal in this intriguing dish.

4 ounces dried penne pasta
  Vegetable oil spray
1 large red bell pepper, thinly sliced
1 medium zucchini, cut into eighths lengthwise, then into 2-inch pieces
$\frac{1}{2}$ tablespoon dried oregano, crumbled
2 medium garlic cloves, minced
$\frac{1}{2}$ teaspoon dried basil, crumbled
12 kalamata olives, coarsely chopped
$\frac{1}{4}$ teaspoon salt
4 ounces part-skim mozzarella cheese, cut into $\frac{1}{2}$-inch cubes

Cook the pasta using the package directions, omitting any salt or oil. Drain well, reserving $\frac{1}{2}$ cup pasta water.

Meanwhile, heat a large nonstick skillet over medium-high heat. Remove from the heat and lightly spray with vegetable oil spray (being careful not to spray near a gas flame). Put the bell pepper, zucchini, oregano, garlic, and basil in the skillet and lightly spray with vegetable oil spray. Cook for 5 minutes, or until the bell pepper is tender-crisp and the zucchini is beginning to lightly brown.

Gently stir in the pasta, reserved pasta water, olives, and salt. Gently stir in the mozzarella.

PER SERVING

calories 247
total fat 9.5 g
  saturated 4.0 g
  polyunsaturated 1.0 g
  monounsaturated 4.0 g
cholesterol 15 mg

sodium 487 mg
carbohydrates 29 g
  fiber 2 g
  sugar 3 g
protein 12 g

100 200 300 400

DIETARY EXCHANGES
1½ starch;
1½ vegetable; 1 lean meat; 1 fat

stuffed shells with arugula and four cheeses

Serves 12; 3 shells per serving

These delicious stuffed shells are excellent to serve to a crowd, or use part for dinner and freeze individual portions for quick meals at a later time.

16 ounces dried jumbo pasta shells (about 36 shells)

marinara sauce

  1 tablespoon olive oil

  2 large garlic cloves, minced

¼ cup chopped fresh basil leaves

  2 tablespoons chopped fresh marjoram

  3 pints cherry tomatoes, halved (about 6 cups)

½ teaspoon pepper

   Dash of salt

  2 tablespoons snipped fresh Italian, or flat-leaf, parsley

filling

16 ounces fat-free or low-fat cottage cheese

15 ounces fat-free or low-fat ricotta cheese

2 cups fat-free or part-skim mozzarella cheese

1/4 cup shredded or grated Parmesan cheese

1/4 teaspoon salt

1/4 teaspoon pepper

4 ounces fresh arugula, chopped

1/2 cup chopped dry-packed sun-dried tomatoes

2 tablespoons snipped fresh Italian, or flat-leaf, parsley

Prepare the pasta shells using the package directions, omitting the salt and oil. Boil for 10 minutes. Do not overcook the shells; they should remain very firm so they hold up during baking. Drain the shells well and lay them on a dish towel to cool.

Preheat the oven to 375°F.

Heat a large skillet over high heat. Pour the oil into the skillet and swirl to coat the bottom. Cook the garlic for 1 to 2 minutes, or until fragrant.

Stir in the basil and marjoram. Cook for 1 minute.

Stir in the tomatoes, pepper, and salt. Reduce the heat and simmer, uncovered, for 10 minutes.

Stir in the parsley.

Meanwhile, in a food processor or blender, process the cottage cheese and ricotta until smooth. Transfer to a large bowl. Stir in the mozzarella, Parmesan, salt, and pepper. Stir in the arugula and sun-dried tomatoes.

Fill the shells with the cheese mixture. (A small ice cream scoop with a releasing handle works well for this.)

Ladle enough marinara sauce into a 13 × 9 × 2-inch casserole dish to cover the bottom (1½ to 2 cups). Place the shells with the seam side down on the sauce. Ladle the remaining sauce over the shells.

Bake, covered, for 30 minutes.

PER SERVING ···

calories 273	sodium 519 mg
total fat 2.5 g	carbohydrates 39 g
saturated 0.5 g	fiber 3 g
polyunsaturated 0.5 g	sugar 7 g
monounsaturated 1.0 g	protein 22 g
cholesterol 9 mg	

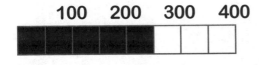

100 200 300 400   **DIETARY EXCHANGES**
2 starch; 2 vegetable;
2 very lean meat

make-ahead manicotti

Serves 7; 2 stuffed manicotti shells per serving

This dish is convenient because you don't pre-cook the pasta. Best of all, you can assemble the casserole the night before you need it.

Vegetable oil spray

tomato sauce

2 8-ounce cans no-salt-added tomato sauce

   14.5-ounce can no-salt-added stewed tomatoes, undrained

1 cup fat-free, reduced-sodium spaghetti sauce (tomato-basil preferred)

1 cup water

filling

15 ounces fat-free or low-fat ricotta cheese

10 ounces frozen chopped spinach, thawed and squeezed dry

   Whites of 2 large eggs

¼ cup shredded or grated Romano cheese

2 tablespoons chopped fresh basil leaves

1½ tablespoons sugar

2 medium garlic cloves, minced

⅛ teaspoon pepper

14 dried manicotti shells (about 8 ounces)

2 tablespoons shredded or grated Romano cheese

Lightly spray a 13 × 9 × 2-inch baking pan with vegetable oil spray.

In a medium bowl, stir together the tomato sauce ingredients, breaking up the large tomato pieces with a spoon. Spread 1 cup sauce in the baking pan.

In a large bowl, stir together the filling ingredients.

Stuff the uncooked manicotti shells with the filling. Arrange the shells in a single layer on the tomato sauce. Pour the remaining tomato sauce over the manicotti. Cover and refrigerate for 8 to 12 hours.

About 30 minutes before baking, remove the casserole from the refrigerator.

Preheat the oven to 350°F. Sprinkle the manicotti with 2 tablespoons Romano.

Bake, uncovered, for 40 to 45 minutes, or until heated through.

COOK'S TIP ON STUFFING MANICOTTI: You can use a small spoon, iced tea spoon, or butter knife to stuff manicotti. Another way is to turn a resealable plastic bag into a disposable pastry bag. Spoon the ricotta mixture into the bag, push the mixture toward a bottom corner, and twist the bag closed, pushing out any air. Make a ¾-inch diagonal cut in the corner of the bag with the filling. Squeeze it through the hole into the shells.

PER SERVING

calories 274
total fat 2.0 g
 saturated 1.0 g
 polyunsaturated 0.5 g
 monounsaturated 0.5 g
cholesterol 8 mg

sodium 365 mg
carbohydrates 44 g
 fiber 5 g
 sugar 13 g
protein 19 g

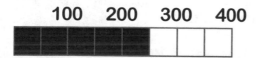

100 200 300 400

DIETARY EXCHANGES
2 starch; 3 vegetable;
1 very lean meat

pesto florentine pasta

Serves 6; 1 cup linguine and 2 tablespoons pesto per serving

Fresh baby spinach sneaks a nutrition boost into traditional pesto in this quick-to-prepare entrée.

12 ounces dried linguine or other flat pasta

pesto florentine

 3 cups fresh baby spinach leaves
 3 tablespoons shredded or grated Parmesan cheese
 2 tablespoons chopped fresh basil leaves
 1 tablespoon plus 1 teaspoon fresh lemon juice
 1 large garlic clove
 1/2 teaspoon salt
 1/4 teaspoon pepper
 1 1/2 tablespoons olive oil (extra-virgin preferred)

Prepare the pasta using the package directions, omitting the salt and oil. Drain well in a colander.

Meanwhile, in a food processor or blender, process the pesto ingredients except the oil for 25 seconds, or until smooth, scraping the side of the work bowl once with a rubber scraper. With the processor running, slowly pour the oil through the food chute. Process for 10 seconds, or until blended.

To serve, transfer the pasta to a large serving bowl. Stir in the pesto to coat thoroughly.

COOK'S TIP: You can easily double the amount of pesto in this recipe. The extra pesto makes a wonderful topping for chicken, fish, and roasted vegetables.

PER SERVING

calories 256
total fat 5.0 g
 saturated 1.0 g
 polyunsaturated 1.0 g
 monounsaturated 3.0 g
cholesterol 2 mg

sodium 252 mg
carbohydrates 44 g
 fiber 2 g
 sugar 2 g
protein 9 g

100   200   300   400

DIETARY EXCHANGES
3 starch; $\frac{1}{2}$ fat

soba noodles in peanut sauce

Serves 4; 1½ cups per serving

This is a dead ringer for the dish you'll find on the menu of almost every Chinese restaurant.

10 ounces soba (buckwheat) or whole-wheat noodles

peanut sauce

¼ cup plus 2 tablespoons hot water

2 tablespoons low-salt soy sauce or light teriyaki sauce

2½ tablespoons plain rice vinegar

2 tablespoons reduced-fat creamy peanut butter

1 tablespoon honey

2 teaspoons minced peeled gingerroot

2 medium garlic cloves, minced

¼ teaspoon pepper

¼ teaspoon crushed red pepper flakes

½ tablespoon toasted sesame oil

2 small ribs of celery, chopped

½ large green bell pepper, chopped

½ medium carrot, grated

4 medium green onions (green and white parts), thinly sliced

2 tablespoons sesame seeds

Prepare the noodles using the package directions, omitting the salt and oil. Drain well in a colander. Return the noodles to the pot.

Meanwhile, in a medium bowl, whisk together the peanut sauce ingredients.

Stir the remaining ingredients except the sesame seeds into the noodles. Pour the peanut sauce into the noodle mixture.

Sprinkle with the sesame seeds. Stir to coat.

PER SERVING

calories 377
total fat 8.0 g
  saturated 1.5 g
  polyunsaturated 2.0 g
  monounsaturated 2.0 g
cholesterol 0 mg

sodium 377 mg
carbohydrates 68 g
  fiber 6 g
  sugar 12 g
protein 14 g

100 200 300 400

DIETARY EXCHANGES
4 starch; 1$\frac{1}{2}$ vegetable;
1 fat

spinach and bean quesadillas with homemade salsa

Serves 4; 2 quesadillas and 2 tablespoons salsa per serving (plus 1 cup salsa reserved)

A healthful alternative to most restaurant varieties, these quesadillas get pizzazz from the cilantro-flavored salsa. As a bonus, there's salsa left over—perfect to use with baked chips or raw vegetables later in the week.

salsa

3 medium garlic cloves

1/2 cup snipped fresh cilantro

14.5-ounce can no-salt-added stewed tomatoes, undrained

Juice of 1/2 medium lime

1/4 teaspoon dried ground chipotle pepper (optional)

1/8 teaspoon salt

quesadillas

15-ounce can no-salt-added pinto beans, rinsed and drained

2 tablespoons snipped fresh cilantro

4 medium garlic cloves, minced

1 teaspoon salt-free onion-and-herb seasoning blend

1/8 teaspoon salt

4 8-inch fat-free or low-fat flour tortillas

10 ounces frozen leaf spinach, thawed and squeezed dry

1 medium red bell pepper, chopped

1½ ounces crumbled soft goat cheese

½ cup fat-free or light sour cream (optional)

Turn on a food processor or blender. With the motor running, drop in the garlic cloves. Process for 5 seconds, or until finely minced. Add the ½ cup cilantro and pulse until finely chopped. Add the remaining salsa ingredients. Pulse several times, until the tomatoes are the desired size. Pour the salsa into a small bowl. Set aside.

In the food processor or blender (no need to clean it first), process the beans for 15 to 20 seconds, or until almost smooth. Transfer to a separate small bowl. Stir in the 2 tablespoons cilantro, garlic, onion-and-herb seasoning, and salt.

Spread the bean mixture on half of each tortilla. Top the bean mixture with the spinach, bell pepper, and goat cheese. Fold the tortillas over to enclose the filling.

Heat a large nonstick skillet over medium-high heat. Cook 2 folded tortillas, covered, for 2 minutes on each side, or until golden brown and heated through.

Repeat with the remaining tortillas.

To serve, slice each tortilla in half. Top with the salsa and sour cream.

COOK'S TIP ON BEANS: Beans are an excellent source of fiber, with about 6 grams of fiber per ½ cup serving. Look for canned beans with no added salt because regular canned beans are typically extremely high in sodium. You can remove some of the sodium by rinsing the beans.

PER SERVING

calories 284

total fat 3.5 g

saturated 2.0 g

polyunsaturated 0.0 g

monounsaturated 0.5 g

cholesterol 5 mg

sodium 533 mg

carbohydrates 49 g

fiber 9 g

sugar 7 g

protein 15 g

100 200 300 400

DIETARY EXCHANGES
2½ starch; 2 vegetable; 1 very lean meat

WITH SOUR CREAM

PER SERVING

calories 319

total fat 3.5 g

saturated 2.0 g

polyunsaturated 0.0 g

monounsaturated 0.5 g

cholesterol 10 mg

sodium 558 mg

carbohydrates 54 g

fiber 9 g

sugar 7 g

protein 15 g

100 200 300 400

DIETARY EXCHANGES
2½ starch; 2 vegetable; 1 very lean meat

braised edamame with bok choy

Serves 4; 1½ cups per serving

Convenient frozen soy beans (edamame) cook so quickly that you'll make this Asian-style dish in no time. It is braised in toasted sesame oil and hoisin sauce and served over fluffy brown rice.

1 cup uncooked instant brown rice

1 teaspoon canola or corn oil

1 medium red bell pepper, diced

1 medium onion, diced

2 cups frozen shelled edamame

1 cup low-sodium vegetable broth

½ cup canned baby corn, rinsed and drained

3 tablespoons hoisin sauce

1 tablespoon light brown sugar

1 tablespoon plain rice vinegar

1 teaspoon toasted sesame oil

2 large stalks bok choy (green and white parts), cut into ½-inch pieces (about 2 cups)

Prepare the rice using the package directions, omitting the salt and oil. Cover to keep warm and set aside.

Meanwhile, heat a large saucepan over medium-high heat. Pour the oil into the saucepan and swirl to coat the bottom. Cook the bell pepper and onion for 2 to 3 minutes, or until tender, stirring occasionally.

Stir in the remaining ingredients except the bok choy. Bring to a simmer. Reduce the heat and simmer, covered, for 6 to 8 minutes, or until the edamame is tender.

Stir in the bok choy. Simmer, covered, for 2 to 3 minutes, or until the bok choy is tender-crisp, stirring occasionally.

To serve, spoon the rice into bowls. Ladle the edamame mixture on top.

PER SERVING

calories 293	sodium 173 mg
total fat 8.0 g	carbohydrates 40 g
saturated 1.5 g	fiber 9 g
polyunsaturated 3.5 g	sugar 10 g
monounsaturated 2.5 g	protein 14 g
cholesterol 0 mg	

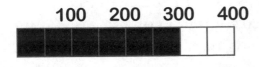

100   200   300   400   **DIETARY EXCHANGES**
2 starch; 2 vegetable;
1 very lean meat; 1 fat

garden veggie tostadas
Serves 4; 1 tostada per serving

These tostadas are made by layering tortillas with black beans, veggies, and cheese. A little taste of the Yucatán!

Vegetable oil spray

15-ounce can no-salt-added black beans, rinsed and drained

1/4 cup chopped red onion

1/4 cup fresh lime juice

2 tablespoons water

1 teaspoon ground cumin

1/8 teaspoon salt

4 6-inch corn tortillas

4-ounce can chopped green chiles, rinsed and drained

1 small yellow summer squash, thinly sliced

2 ounces sliced black olives, drained

1/4 cup snipped fresh cilantro

3 ounces grated fat-free mozzarella cheese

Preheat the oven to 425°F. Lightly spray a nonstick baking sheet with vegetable oil spray.

In a food processor or blender, process the beans, onion, lime juice, water, cumin, and salt until smooth, frequently scraping the side of the work bowl with a rubber scraper.

Put the tortillas on the baking sheet. Spoon the bean mixture over each tortilla, leaving a ½-inch border uncovered. In the order listed, top with the green chiles, squash, olives, cilantro, and mozzarella.

Bake for 7 minutes, or until the mozzarella has melted and the edges are beginning to lightly brown.

PER SERVING

calories 191

total fat 2.0 g

  saturated 0.5 g

  polyunsaturated 0.5 g

  monounsaturated 1.0 g

cholesterol 4 mg

sodium 575 mg

carbohydrates 30 g

  fiber 8 g

  sugar 5 g

  protein 14 g

100 200 300 400

DIETARY EXCHANGES

1½ starch; 1 vegetable; 1½ very lean meat

mediterranean wraps
Serves 4; 1 wrap per serving

With its many layers of color, this wrap is almost too pretty to eat.

1 cup no-salt-added chick-peas, rinsed and drained

1 medium cucumber, peeled, seeded, and chopped

1 small tomato, chopped

1/4 cup snipped fresh parsley

1/4 cup chopped red onion

2 tablespoons unsweetened dried cranberries

2 tablespoons soft goat cheese, crumbled

2 tablespoons fresh lemon juice

1 tablespoon capers, rinsed and drained

  Dash of pepper

4 10-inch fat-free flour tortillas

4 cups fresh spinach leaves

4 medium carrots, shredded

In a medium bowl, stir together the chick-peas, cucumber, tomato, parsley, onion, cranberries, goat cheese, lemon juice, capers, and pepper.

To assemble, on a griddle or in a large skillet, lightly heat 1 tortilla on medium-high heat for about 30 seconds on each side. This will make the tortilla supple and easier to wrap. Transfer the tortilla to a plate. Place 1 cup spinach on the tortilla, leaving a 1-inch border uncovered. Spread 1/2 cup carrots over the spinach. Spoon

½ cup chick-pea mixture 1 inch from the bottom. Roll up that edge. Fold over 1 inch from both sides. Starting at the bottom, roll up the tortilla jelly-roll style, pushing in any filling before reaching the top. Turn over the wrap. Place a toothpick about one-third from each end, securing the loose end. Slice the wrap in half on the diagonal. Set the wrap with the cut sides up on the plate. Repeat with the remaining ingredients.

PER SERVING

calories 371

total fat 4.5 g

  saturated 1.0 g

  polyunsaturated 1.0 g

  monounsaturated 1.5 g

cholesterol 3 mg

sodium 603 mg

carbohydrates 69 g

  fiber 13 g

  sugar 12 g

protein 16 g

100   200   300   400

DIETARY EXCHANGES

3½ starch; 3 vegetable; ½ very lean meat

miami wraps
Serves 4; 1 wrap per serving

If you could taste a cool breeze at the beach, it just might be like this refreshing wrap.

2 cups frozen whole-kernel corn, thawed

1 cup no-salt-added black beans, rinsed and drained

1 medium papaya, seeded and diced, or $1/2$ cup diced honeydew or Crenshaw melon or cantaloupe

$1/2$ cup snipped fresh cilantro

1 small red onion, or to taste, cut into rings

$1/4$ medium red bell pepper, diced

1 tablespoon fresh lime juice

1 tablespoon balsamic vinegar

$1/8$ teaspoon cayenne

Dash of salt

Dash of pepper

4 10-inch fat-free flour tortillas or 6-inch pita pockets

4 cups chopped romaine

In a medium bowl, stir together the corn, beans, papaya, cilantro, onion, bell pepper, lime juice, vinegar, cayenne, salt, and pepper.

To assemble, on a griddle or in a large skillet, lightly heat 1 tortilla on medium-high heat for about 30 seconds on each side. This will make the tortilla supple and easier to wrap. Transfer the tortilla to a plate. Place 1 cup romaine on the tortilla, leaving a 1-inch border uncovered. Spoon 1/2 cup corn mixture over the romaine. Roll up that edge. Fold over 1 inch from both sides. Starting at the bottom, roll up the tortilla jelly-roll style, pushing in any filling before reaching the top. Turn over the wrap. Place a toothpick about one-third from each end, securing the loose end. Slice the wrap in half on the diagonal. Set the wrap with the cut sides up on the plate. Repeat with the remaining ingredients.

PER SERVING

calories 341	sodium 508 mg
total fat 1.5 g	carbohydrates 73 g
saturated 0.0 g	fiber 10 g
polyunsaturated 0.5 g	sugar 12 g
monounsaturated 0.0 g	protein 13 g
cholesterol 0 mg	

100   200   300   400

DIETARY EXCHANGES
4 starch; 1/2 fruit; 1 vegetable

easy two-bean chili

Serves 4; 1½ cups per serving

This is a great meal to prepare when you don't have a lot of time to spend in the kitchen. The crunchiness of the celery contrasts nicely with the texture of the beans.

Vegetable oil spray

chili

1 teaspoon canola or corn oil

1 large onion, chopped

15-ounce can no-salt-added navy beans, undrained

15-ounce can no-salt-added dark red kidney beans, undrained

14.5-ounce can no-salt-added diced tomatoes, undrained

4-ounce can chopped green chiles

1 tablespoon snipped fresh cilantro

2 teaspoons chili powder, or to taste

1 teaspoon dry mustard

½ tablespoon cumin

½ teaspoon salt-free all-purpose seasoning blend

¼ teaspoon salt

½ teaspoon red hot-pepper sauce, or to taste

3 medium ribs of celery, cut into ¼-inch slices

garnishes (optional)

- 1/4 cup fat-free or light sour cream
- 1/4 cup plus 2 tablespoons shredded fat-free or reduced-fat sharp Cheddar cheese
- 1/4 cup chopped green onions (green and white parts)
- 1 1/2 tablespoons snipped fresh cilantro

Heat a Dutch oven over medium-high heat. Remove from the heat and lightly spray with vegetable oil spray (being careful not to spray near a gas flame). Pour the oil into the pan and swirl to coat the bottom. Cook the onion for about 5 minutes, or until golden.

Stir in the remaining chili ingredients except the celery. Increase the heat to high and bring to a boil. Reduce the heat and simmer, partially covered, for 15 minutes. Stir in the celery. Simmer for 5 minutes. (The celery should remain crisp.)

To serve, ladle the chili into bowls. Top each serving with sour cream, Cheddar, green onions, and cilantro.

PER SERVING

calories 247
total fat 2.0 g
  saturated 0.0 g
  polyunsaturated 0.5 g
  monounsaturated 0.5 g
cholesterol 0 mg

sodium 355 mg
carbohydrates 46 g
  fiber 13 g
  sugar 11 g
  protein 14 g

100   200   300   400

DIETARY EXCHANGES
$2\frac{1}{2}$ starch;
$1\frac{1}{2}$ vegetable;
$\frac{1}{2}$ very lean meat

WITH GARNISHES

PER SERVING

calories 284
total fat 2.0 g
  saturated 0.0 g
  polyunsaturated 0.5 g
  monounsaturated 0.5 g
cholesterol 4 mg

sodium 444 mg
carbohydrates 50 g
  fiber 13 g
  sugar 12 g
  protein 19 g

100   200   300   400

DIETARY EXCHANGES
3 starch; $1\frac{1}{2}$ vegetable;
1 very lean meat

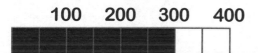

vegetarian entrées 543

mediterranean vegetable stew
Serves 6; 1²/₃ cups per serving

Eggplant, zucchini, and chick-peas team up for a hearty vegetarian stew with Mediterranean overtones.

1 medium to large zucchini
1 medium eggplant
½ teaspoon salt
1½ tablespoons olive oil
3 medium garlic cloves, minced
2 teaspoons Italian seasoning
28-ounce can no-salt-added diced tomatoes, undrained
2 10-ounce cans no-salt-added chick-peas, rinsed and drained
3 medium bay leaves
Pepper to taste
½ teaspoon salt

Thinly slice the zucchini into rounds and set aside.

Cut the eggplant into bite-size cubes. Place the pieces in a bowl and sprinkle with salt. (This will help keep the eggplant from absorbing too much oil.) After about 10 minutes, use paper towels to pat the moisture droplets from the eggplant.

Heat a large skillet over medium-high heat. Pour the oil into the skillet and swirl to coat the bottom. Cook the garlic and eggplant for 3 to 5 minutes, or until they begin to soften, stirring occasionally. Push to the side.

Put the Italian seasoning in the center of the skillet. Cook for 1 minute, or until the seasoning becomes fragrant.

Stir in the remaining ingredients, including the zucchini. Cook for 10 minutes, stirring occasionally.

Discard the bay leaves before serving the stew.

PER SERVING

calories 267
total fat 6.5 g
  saturated 0.5 g
  polyunsaturated 1.5 g
  monounsaturated 4.0 g
cholesterol 0 mg

sodium 460 mg
carbohydrates 43 g
  fiber 11 g
  sugar 10 g
protein 12 g

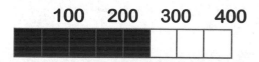

DIETARY EXCHANGES
2 starch; 2½ vegetable;
1 very lean meat; 1 fat

spinach and ricotta frittata
Serves 4; 1 wedge per serving

This dish is great for breakfast, lunch, or dinner. Serve it with fresh fruit or a tossed salad.

Vegetable oil spray
1/2 medium onion, sliced
Egg substitute equivalent to 4 eggs
1 cup fat-free or low-fat ricotta cheese
4 cups fresh baby spinach leaves (about 4 ounces)

Preheat the oven to 400°F.

Heat an 8-inch ovenproof skillet over medium-low heat. Remove from the heat and lightly spray with vegetable oil spray (being careful not to spray near a gas flame). Cook the onion for about 12 minutes, or until it begins to caramelize and turn brown on the edges, stirring occasionally.

Meanwhile, in a medium bowl, whisk together the egg substitute and ricotta.

Stir the spinach into the cooked onion. Cook for about 1 minute, or until lightly wilted, stirring constantly. Spread the mixture over the bottom of the skillet.

Pour in the egg substitute mixture, covering the vegetables.

Bake for 20 minutes, or until a knife inserted in the center comes out clean. Cut into 4 wedges and serve warm.

COOK'S TIP: Don't like spinach? You can make this frittata using leftover green beans, carrots, corn, chicken, turkey, black beans, or whatever else sounds good, is healthful, and is on hand. If you aren't fond of onions, try some roasted garlic instead. The ricotta adds body, so keep it to maintain the volume of this dish.

PER SERVING

calories 89
total fat 0.0 g
 saturated 0.0 g
 polyunsaturated 0.0 g
 monounsaturated 0.0 g
cholesterol 5 mg

sodium 269 mg
carbohydrates 6 g
 fiber 1 g
 sugar 4 g
protein 15 g

100 200 300 400

DIETARY EXCHANGES
1 vegetable;
2 very lean meat

cajun red beans and brown rice

Serves 6; 1 cup beans and $\frac{1}{2}$ cup rice per serving

In times past, cooks would simmer dried red beans all day while attending to the family's laundry. "Monday's Beans" provided a nutritious meal that required little attention while the cook labored at the washboard. Our updated version combines canned beans with a variety of seasonings. Dinner is ready in just about an hour—hardly enough time to do the wash!

Vegetable oil spray

red beans

2 15-ounce cans no-salt-added red beans, such as kidney beans, undrained

3 large ribs of celery, chopped

1 large onion, chopped

1 medium green bell pepper, chopped

8-ounce can no-salt-added tomato sauce

2 tablespoons snipped fresh parsley

2 tablespoons no-salt-added ketchup

6 medium garlic cloves, minced

2 teaspoons salt-free all-purpose seasoning blend

2 teaspoons low-sodium Worcestershire sauce

2 bay leaves

1 teaspoon chili powder or cayenne

¼ teaspoon salt

....

1 cup uncooked brown rice

Ground dried chipotle chiles to taste (optional)

Lightly spray a Dutch oven with vegetable oil spray. Put all the red beans ingredients in the Dutch oven. Bring to a boil over medium-high heat. Reduce the heat and simmer, covered, for 1 hour. Thin the mixture with water if needed.

Meanwhile, prepare the rice using the package directions, omitting the salt and margarine.

To serve, spoon the rice into bowls. Discard the bay leaves in the bean mixture. Ladle the bean mixture over the rice. Sprinkle with the ground chipotles.

COOK'S TIP ON CHIPOTLE CHILES: Chipotle chiles, which are dried smoked jalapeños, are available in several forms at the supermarket. The whole dried chiles are usually in the produce area, jars of ground dried chiles are in the international or spice section, and cans of chipotles in adobo sauce also are in the international area. Add your choice when you want a bit of heat and smoky flavor.

COOK'S TIP ON RICE COOKERS:

A rice cooker is the perfect appliance for cooking rice—it's quick and simple to use, and it's foolproof. As soon as the rice absorbs all the water and gets to the right temperature, the cooker changes from cooking mode to warming mode. It will keep the rice warm for hours. If your rice cooker has a brown rice setting, by all means, use that. If it has no such setting, try using two parts brown rice to three parts water.

PER SERVING

calories 284	sodium 150 mg
total fat 1.0 g	carbohydrates 58 g
saturated 0.0 g	fiber 9 g
polyunsaturated 0.5 g	sugar 8 g
monounsaturated 0.5 g	protein 13 g
cholesterol 0 mg	

100 200 300 400   **DIETARY EXCHANGES**
3 starch; $2\frac{1}{2}$ vegetable

fried rice with snow peas, bell pepper, and water chestnuts

Serves 4; 1½ cups per serving

Fresh gingerroot imparts its distinctive flavor to a delicious vegetable mixture.

½ cup uncooked brown rice

    Vegetable oil spray

    Egg substitute equivalent to 2 eggs, or 3 egg whites

1 tablespoon canola or corn oil

1 medium red bell pepper, coarsely chopped

4 medium green onions (green and white parts), sliced

2 medium ribs of celery, sliced on the diagonal

2 to 3 teaspoons minced peeled gingerroot

2 medium garlic cloves, minced

6 ounces (about 1½ cups) fresh or frozen snow peas or sugar snap peas, trimmed if fresh or thawed if frozen, halved if large

    8-ounce can sliced water chestnuts, rinsed and drained

¾ cup low-sodium vegetable broth or fat-free, low-sodium chicken broth

1½ tablespoons low-salt soy sauce or light teriyaki sauce

¼ teaspoon red hot-pepper sauce

Prepare the rice using the package directions, omitting the salt and margarine.

About 10 minutes before the rice is ready, heat a large nonstick skillet or wok over medium-high heat. Remove from the heat and lightly spray with vegetable oil spray (being careful not to spray near a gas flame). Pour in the egg substitute, swirling to distribute evenly over the bottom. Cook for about 1 minute, or until set. Using a spoon or whisk, break the egg "pancake" into small pieces. Transfer the pieces to a plate. Wipe the skillet with paper towels.

Reheat the skillet. Pour the oil into the skillet and swirl to coat the bottom. Cook the bell pepper, green onions, celery, gingerroot, and garlic for 3 to 4 minutes, or until tender-crisp, stirring frequently.

Stir in the snow peas. Cook for 2 to 3 minutes, or until tender-crisp, stirring occasionally.

Stir in the water chestnuts, rice, and egg pieces. Cook for 2 minutes, or until warmed through, stirring occasionally.

Stir in the remaining ingredients. Cook for 2 to 3 minutes, or until the mixture is hot, stirring occasionally.

PER SERVING

calories 201	sodium 257 mg
total fat 4.5 g	carbohydrates 33 g
saturated 0.5 g	fiber 6 g
polyunsaturated 1.5 g	sugar 5 g
monounsaturated 2.5 g	protein 8 g
cholesterol 0 mg	

100 200 300 400

DIETARY EXCHANGES
1½ starch; 2 vegetable; ½ fat

colossal spring rolls with tofu and vegetables

Serves 4; 1 spring roll and 2 teaspoons sauce per serving

One of the most widely enjoyed appetizers in Asian cuisine takes center stage as a dinner entrée. It features crispy baked phyllo dough instead of egg roll wrappers on the outside, tender shredded vegetables and tofu on the inside, and sweet chili sauce on top.

Vegetable oil spray

2 tablespoons low-salt soy sauce

1 tablespoon hoisin sauce

1 teaspoon cornstarch

1 teaspoon grated peeled gingerroot

1 teaspoon toasted sesame oil

1 medium garlic clove, minced

1 teaspoon canola or corn oil

2 cups shredded broccoli slaw

4 medium carrots, shredded

1 cup snow peas, trimmed and cut into thin strips

4 medium green onions (green and white parts), chopped

4 cups baby spinach leaves (about 4 ounces)

10.5-ounce package light tofu (firm or extra firm), diced

12 sheets (about 12 × 16½ inches) frozen phyllo
   dough, thawed

3 tablespoons sweet chili sauce, or 3 tablespoons
   sweet-and-sour sauce plus 2 to 3 drops red
   hot-pepper sauce

Preheat the oven to 400°F. Lightly spray a rimmed baking sheet with vegetable oil spray.

In a small bowl, whisk together the soy sauce, hoisin
sauce, cornstarch, gingerroot, sesame oil, and garlic until
the cornstarch is dissolved. Set aside.

For the filling, heat a large nonstick skillet over
medium-high heat. Pour the oil into the skillet and swirl
to coat the bottom. Cook the broccoli slaw, carrots,
snow peas, and green onions for 1 to 2 minutes, or until
the vegetables are tender-crisp, stirring constantly.

Stir in the spinach and tofu. Cook for 1 to 2 minutes,
or until the spinach is wilted, stirring occasionally.

Stir in the soy-sauce mixture. Cook for 1 minute, or
until the mixture has thickened, stirring occasionally.
Remove from the heat and let cool for 10 minutes.

Meanwhile, keeping the unused phyllo dough covered with a damp dish towel or damp paper towels to
prevent drying, place a short end of a piece of phyllo
dough toward you on a flat surface. Lightly spray one
side of the dough with vegetable oil spray. Stack another
sheet on the first. Lightly spray with vegetable oil spray.
Stack a third sheet and lightly spray with vegetable oil
spray. Spoon about ½ cup filling onto the dough about
2 inches from the short end nearest you. Fold about 2
inches of each long side toward the center of the dough.
Starting at the short end with the filling, roll the dough

jelly-roll style to enclose the filling (you'll have a cylinder shaped like a spring roll). Lightly spray with vegetable oil spray. Place the roll with the seam side down on the baking sheet. Repeat with the remaining phyllo dough and filling.

Bake for 18 to 20 minutes, or until the rolls are golden brown.

To serve, slice the spring rolls in half on the diagonal. Arrange two halves on each plate. Spoon 1/2 tablespoon chili sauce on each piece.

COOK'S TIP ON SWEET CHILI SAUCE: A popular condiment in Asian cooking, sweet chili sauce tastes like sweet-and-sour sauce, but with a kick. Find it in the Asian section of the grocery store.

PER SERVING

calories 371
total fat 5.0 g
  saturated 0.5 g
  polyunsaturated 2.0 g
  monounsaturated 2.0 g
cholesterol 0 mg

sodium 794 mg
carbohydrates 68 g
  fiber 7 g
  sugar 14 g
protein 13 g

100   200   300   400

DIETARY EXCHANGES
4 starch; 2 vegetable

creole ratatouille

Serves 4; 1 cup vegetable mixture and ½ cup rice per serving

French ratatouille (**ra-tuh-TOO-ee**) gets a Creole twist with celery, okra, thyme, parsley, and—of course—a dash of red hot-pepper sauce!

Vegetable oil spray

1 medium green bell pepper, cut into 1-inch pieces

1 medium onion, cut into ½-inch wedges

2 medium ribs of celery, chopped

2 cups fresh or frozen cut okra

14.5-ounce can no-salt-added tomatoes, undrained, or 1 pound fresh tomatoes, chopped

¾ cup water

2 teaspoons low-sodium Worcestershire sauce

½ teaspoon dried thyme, crumbled

½ teaspoon sugar

1 cup uncooked quick-cooking brown rice

½ cup snipped fresh parsley

1 teaspoon olive oil (extra-virgin preferred)

½ teaspoon salt

⅛ teaspoon red hot-pepper sauce, or to taste (optional)

2 ounces shredded part-skim mozzarella cheese

Heat a Dutch oven over medium heat. Remove from the heat and lightly spray with vegetable oil spray (being careful not to spray near a gas flame). Cook the bell pepper, onion, and celery for 6 minutes, or until beginning to brown on the edges, stirring frequently.

Stir in the okra, undrained tomatoes, water, Worcestershire sauce, thyme, and sugar. Increase the heat to high and bring to a boil. Reduce the heat and simmer, covered, for 20 minutes, or until the bell pepper is tender, stirring occasionally. Remove from the heat.

Meanwhile, prepare the rice using the package directions, omitting the salt and margarine.

Stir the parsley, oil, salt, and hot-pepper sauce into the okra mixture. Let stand, covered, for 10 minutes to allow the flavors to blend.

To serve, spoon the rice into bowls. Spoon the okra mixture over the rice. Top with the mozzarella.

COOK'S TIP: The flavors of this dish will improve if it is refrigerated overnight and reheated over medium heat. If you prefer a thinner consistency, pour in ¼ cup water before reheating.

PER SERVING

calories 203
total fat 5.0 g
  saturated 2.0 g
  polyunsaturated 0.5 g
  monounsaturated 2.0 g
cholesterol 8 mg

sodium 488 mg
carbohydrates 32 g
  fiber 6 g
  sugar 7 g
  protein 10 g

100   200   300   400

DIETARY EXCHANGES
1 starch; 3 vegetable;
½ lean meat; ½ fat

mushroom and artichoke gnocchi with capers

Serves 4; 1$\frac{1}{2}$ cups per serving

The combination of exotic and domestic mushrooms adds flavor depth to this hearty, rich-tasting vegetarian dish.

6 ounces frozen artichoke hearts
8 ounces fresh portobello mushrooms
4 ounces fresh shiitake mushrooms
4 ounces fresh button mushrooms
  cup fat-free, low-sodium chicken broth
$\frac{1}{2}$ cup fat-free half-and-half
2 tablespoons shredded or grated Parmesan cheese
2 tablespoons chopped fresh basil leaves or
  1 teaspoon dried, crumbled
2 tablespoons snipped fresh parsley or 1 teaspoon
  dried, crumbled
$\frac{1}{2}$ teaspoon garlic powder
  17.5-ounce package refrigerated potato gnocchi
2 tablespoons capers, rinsed and drained
$\frac{1}{4}$ teaspoon salt
  Pepper to taste
2 tablespoons shredded or grated Parmesan cheese

Prepare the artichokes using the package directions, omitting the salt. Cover and set aside.

Meanwhile, trim all the mushrooms. Chop into bite-size pieces. Transfer to a large saucepan.

Pour the broth into the saucepan. Bring to a simmer over medium heat. Simmer for 10 minutes, or until the broth has almost evaporated and the mushrooms are tender, stirring occasionally. Remove from the heat.

Stir in the half-and-half, 2 tablespoons Parmesan, basil, parsley, and garlic powder. Cover and set aside.

While the mushrooms cook, prepare the gnocchi using the package directions, omitting the salt and oil. Drain well.

Just before the gnocchi is ready, heat the sauce mixture over medium heat for 1 minute, stirring constantly. Do not boil.

To serve, stir the gnocchi into the sauce mixture. Gently stir in the artichokes, capers, salt, and pepper. Sprinkle with the 2 tablespoons Parmesan. Serve warm.

PER SERVING

calories 297
total fat 2.5 g
 saturated 1.0 g
 polyunsaturated 0.0 g
 monounsaturated 0.5 g
cholesterol 4 mg

sodium 666 mg
carbohydrates 55 g
 fiber 5 g
 sugar 4 g
protein 17 g

100 200 300 400 **DIETARY EXCHANGES**
3 starch; 2 vegetable;
1/2 very lean meat

one-pot vegetable and grain medley

Serves 4; 1½ cups per serving

As delicious as it is colorful, this recipe requires almost no effort to prepare. If there are any leftovers, you'll find they taste even better the next day. Serve with a bowl of fresh berries or sliced peaches.

1 teaspoon olive oil

2 medium bell peppers (orange and green preferred)

2 medium shallots, coarsely chopped

2 cups frozen whole-kernel corn

2 cups low-sodium vegetable broth

14.5-ounce can no-salt-added diced tomatoes, undrained

½ cup uncooked pearl barley

1 teaspoon dried oregano, crumbled

1 teaspoon dried rosemary, crushed

¼ teaspoon salt

¼ teaspoon pepper

¼ cup shredded or grated Parmesan cheese

Heat a Dutch oven or large saucepan over medium-high heat. Pour the oil into the pan and swirl to coat the bottom. Cook the bell peppers and shallots for 2 to 3 minutes, or until tender-crisp, stirring occasionally.

Stir in the remaining ingredients except the Parmesan. Bring to a simmer. Reduce the heat and simmer, covered, for 40 to 45 minutes, or until the barley is tender.

To serve, stir in the Parmesan. Ladle the mixture into bowls.

PER SERVING

calories 239

total fat 3.5 g

  saturated 1.0 g

  polyunsaturated 0.5 g

  monounsaturated 1.5 g

cholesterol 4 mg

sodium 302 mg

carbohydrates 47 g

  fiber 9 g

  sugar 8 g

protein 10 g

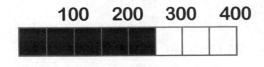

100 200 300 400

DIETARY EXCHANGES

$2\frac{1}{2}$ starch; 2 vegetable; $\frac{1}{2}$ fat

couscous with bell pepper and pine nuts

Serves 4; 1½ cups per serving

This colorful meatless entrée also makes a great side dish for entertaining when served in smaller portions.

1 cup water
5 ounces dried couscous
   Vegetable oil spray
1 large red bell pepper, thinly sliced
1 large onion, thinly sliced
¼ cup pine nuts, dry-roasted
1 tablespoon olive oil (extra-virgin preferred)
1 teaspoon ground cumin
½ teaspoon salt
¼ teaspoon ground cinnamon
⅛ teaspoon cayenne
1 cup frozen green peas, thawed
1½ ounces fat-free or low-fat feta cheese, crumbled

In a medium saucepan, bring the water to a boil over high heat. Stir in the couscous. Remove from the heat. Let stand, covered, for 5 minutes, or until all the water is absorbed. Fluff with a fork.

Meanwhile, heat a large nonstick skillet over medium-high heat. Remove the skillet from the heat and lightly spray with vegetable oil spray (being careful not to spray near a gas flame). Cook the bell pepper and onion for 4 minutes, or until tender-crisp, stirring frequently. Remove from the heat.

Stir in the pine nuts, oil, cumin, salt, cinnamon, and cayenne. Stir in the peas and feta.

To serve, spoon the couscous onto the center of a platter. Arrange the bell pepper and onion around the edge.

PER SERVING ···

calories 295
total fat 9.5 g
  saturated 1.0 g
  polyunsaturated 3.5 g
  monounsaturated 4.0 g
cholesterol 0 mg

sodium 501 mg
carbohydrates 42 g
  fiber 5 g
  sugar 8 g
  protein 11 g

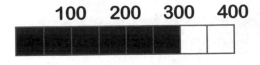

100   200   300   400   DIETARY EXCHANGES
2½ starch; 1½ vegetable; 1½ fat

veggie burgers with gorgonzola

Serves 4; 1 patty and $1/2$ cup vegetables per serving

Give classic cheeseburgers a healthful makeover with veggie patties topped with creamy Gorgonzola and hot cooked vegetables.

4 frozen reduced-fat vegetarian burgers, such as grilled soy protein burgers
1 large yellow summer squash, thinly sliced
1 medium onion, thinly sliced
1 medium green bell pepper, thinly sliced
$1/2$ teaspoon dried oregano, crumbled
$1/8$ teaspoon crushed red pepper flakes
Vegetable oil spray
$1/8$ teaspoon salt
2 ounces crumbled Gorgonzola or blue cheese

Cook the burgers using the package directions for the stovetop. Transfer to a platter. Do not cover.

Increase the heat to medium high. Add the squash, onion, bell pepper, oregano, and red pepper flakes to the pan. Lightly spray with vegetable oil spray. Cook for 5 minutes, or until the edges of the onion begin to lightly brown, stirring frequently. Remove from the heat.

Stir in the salt.

To serve, sprinkle the burgers with the Gorgonzola. Top with the vegetable mixture.

italian veggie burgers

Substitute 1 large zucchini, thinly sliced, for the yellow summer squash; 1 tablespoon fresh chopped basil or 1 teaspoon dried, crumbled, for the oregano; and part-skim mozzarella cheese for the Gorgonzola.

COOK'S TIP: Covering the cooked burgers to keep them warm might change the texture of the product. The heat from the cooked vegetables will reheat the patties while melting the cheese.

COOK'S TIP ON GORGONZOLA: Creamy, salty, soft, crumbly, pungent, rich tasting— all these adjectives describe Gorgonzola, an Italian blue cheese that is ivory-colored with bluish-green veins. Like other blue cheeses, Gorgonzola is high in fat and sodium; fortunately, the flavor is pronounced, so you won't need to use a lot. Gorgonzola and its British and French counterparts (Stilton and Roquefort, respectively) are sometimes called the "Kings of Cheeses."

VEGGIE BURGERS WITH GORGONZOLA

PER SERVING

calories 175
total fat 4.5 g
  saturated 3.0 g
  polyunsaturated 0.0 g
  monounsaturated 0.0 g
cholesterol 13 mg

sodium 549 mg
carbohydrates 26 g
  fiber 6 g
  sugar 7 g
protein 10 g

100   200   300   400

DIETARY EXCHANGES
1 ½ starch; 1 vegetable;
1 lean meat

ITALIAN VEGGIE BURGERS

PER SERVING

calories 160
total fat 2.5 g
  saturated 1.5 g
  polyunsaturated 0.0 g
  monounsaturated 0.5 g
cholesterol 9 mg

sodium 451 mg
carbohydrates 26 g
  fiber 5 g
  sugar 7 g
protein 10 g

100   200   300   400

DIETARY EXCHANGES
1 ½ starch; 1 vegetable;
1 very lean meat

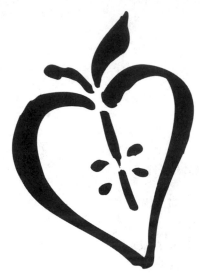

vegetables

Asparagus with Gremolata

Asparagus and Two Red Peppers
  with Orzo

Italian Barley and Mushrooms

Broccoli Bake with Three Cheeses

French Brussels Sprouts

Red Cabbage Braised with
  Balsamic Vinegar

Orange-Glazed Carrots

Cauliflower Mash

Oven-Fried Eggplant

Roasted Green Beans and Walnuts

Braised Mustard Greens with
  Pearl Onions

and
side dishes

Creole Lentils

Orzo with Tomato and Capers

Stir-Fried Sugar Snap Peas with
   Shallots and Walnuts

Smashed Potatoes with
   Aromatic Herbs

Lemon-Herb Brown Rice

Pesto and Pecan Rice

Spinach with Almonds and
   Lemon Zest

Stewed Zucchini and
   Cherry Tomatoes

Mixed Vegetable Grill

asparagus with gremolata
Serves 4; about 6 spears per serving

One of the best ways to cook fresh asparagus is to lightly steam it, then toss it with gremolata (or gremolada), a lively mixture of parsley, lemon zest, and garlic.

1 pound fresh medium asparagus spears, trimmed
1 tablespoon salt-free all-purpose seasoning

gremolata

1/4 cup finely snipped fresh parsley
1 tablespoon snipped fresh dillweed
1 teaspoon grated lemon zest
1 medium garlic clove, minced
1/8 teaspoon pepper

Put the asparagus in a steamer basket. Sprinkle with the all-purpose seasoning. Steam for 2 to 3 minutes, or until the asparagus is tender-crisp. Drain well. Place in a serving bowl and cover with aluminum foil to keep warm.

In a small bowl, stir together the gremolata ingredients. Pour over the asparagus. Toss gently to coat.

COOK'S TIP: When using fresh asparagus, discard about the bottom 1 inch of the stalk ends (breaking where the stalk bends).

asparagus and two red peppers with orzo

Serves 8; ½ cup per serving

Orzo, the rice-shaped pasta, and asparagus make an enticing side dish. Combined with colorful red bell pepper, they provide an attractive addition for any table.

6 cups water

¾ cup dried orzo

1 pound fresh medium asparagus, trimmed, cut into 1-inch pieces, or 9 ounces frozen cut asparagus, thawed forabout 2 minutes

½ medium red bell pepper, cut into thin strips

1 medium shallot, thinly sliced

¼ cup water

½ tablespoon honey or maple syrup

1 teaspoon dried oregano, crumbled

1 teaspoon white wine vinegar

¼ teaspoon crushed red pepper flakes

1 teaspoon olive oil (extra-virgin preferred)

Dash of salt

Dash of pepper

In a medium saucepan, bring the water to a boil. Stir in the orzo. Cook for 8 minutes, or until tender. Drain well.

Meanwhile, put the asparagus, bell pepper, shallot, water, honey, oregano, vinegar, and red pepper flakes in a large skillet. Bring to a simmer over medium-low heat. Simmer, uncovered, for 5 minutes, or until the asparagus is cooked but still crisp to the bite. (If cooked longer, the asparagus will lose its bright green color.)

In a medium bowl, stir together all the ingredients.

PER SERVING

calories 87
total fat 1.0 g
  saturated 0.0 g
  polyunsaturated 0.0 g
  monounsaturated 0.5 g
cholesterol 0 mg

sodium 20 mg
carbohydrates 16 g
  fiber 2 g
  sugar 3 g
protein 3 g

100 200 300 400

DIETARY EXCHANGES
1 starch

italian barley and mushrooms
Serves 4; ½ cup per serving

Using quick-cooking barley instead of traditional rice lets you add more whole grains—and a new twist—to your "pilaf."

  1 cup water
½ cup uncooked quick-cooking pearl barley
  1 teaspoon very low sodium beef bouillon granules
     Vegetable oil spray (olive oil spray preferred)
  8 ounces sliced button mushrooms
  2 medium green onions (green and white parts), minced
  1 medium garlic clove, minced
½ teaspoon dried oregano, crumbled
½ cup snipped fresh parsley (Italian, or flat-leaf, preferred)
  2 teaspoons olive oil (extra-virgin preferred)
¼ teaspoon salt
⅛ teaspoon pepper

In a small saucepan, bring the water to a boil over high heat. Stir in the barley and bouillon granules. Reduce the heat and simmer, covered, for 12 minutes, or until the barley is tender.

Meanwhile, heat a large skillet over medium-high heat. Remove from the heat and lightly spray with vegetable oil spray (being careful not to spray near a gas flame). Add the mushrooms and lightly spray with vegetable oil spray. Cook for 4 minutes, or until the mushrooms begin to lightly brown, stirring frequently.

Stir in the green onions, garlic, and oregano. Cook for 15 seconds, stirring constantly. Remove from the heat.

Stir the barley and the remaining ingredients into the mushroom mixture.

PER SERVING

calories 133

total fat 3.0 g

  saturated 0.5 g

  polyunsaturated 0.5 g

  monounsaturated 1.5 g

cholesterol 0 mg

sodium 159 mg

carbohydrates 24 g

  fiber 5 g

  sugar 2 g

protein 5 g

100 200 300 400

DIETARY EXCHANGES

1 starch; $1\frac{1}{2}$ vegetable; $\frac{1}{2}$ fat

broccoli bake with three cheeses

Serves 8; $^1/_2$ cup per serving

Fresh broccoli teams up with ricotta, Cheddar, and Parmesan cheeses to create a wonderful side dish for a group.

Vegetable oil spray

1$^1/_2$ pounds broccoli (about 3 bunches)

1$^1/_4$ cups fat-free or low-fat ricotta cheese

$^3/_4$ cup shredded fat-free or reduced-fat sharp Cheddar cheese

2 or 3 medium green onions (green and white parts), chopped

3 tablespoons egg substitute, or 1 small egg

$^1/_2$ tablespoon low-sodium Worcestershire sauce

$^3/_4$ teaspoon salt-free onion-and-herb seasoning blend

$^1/_3$ cup plain dry bread crumbs

1 tablespoon shredded or grated Parmesan cheese

$^1/_2$ teaspoon garlic powder

$^1/_2$ teaspoon dried parsley, crumbled

Preheat the oven to 350°F. Lightly spray a shallow 1$^1/_2$-quart casserole dish with vegetable oil spray.

Trim the broccoli stalks. Separate the stalks, but keep the florets attached. Steam for 6 to 8 minutes, or until tender-crisp.

Meanwhile, in a medium bowl, stir together the ricotta and Cheddar cheeses, green onions, egg substitute, Worcestershire sauce, and onion-and-herb seasoning.

In a small bowl, stir together the bread crumbs, Parmesan, garlic powder, and parsley.

To assemble, put the broccoli in the casserole dish. Spread the ricotta mixture over the broccoli. Sprinkle with the bread-crumb mixture. Lightly spray with vegetable oil spray.

Bake, uncovered, for 15 to 20 minutes, or until the broccoli is heated through and a knife inserted into the topping comes out clean.

PER SERVING

calories 101
total fat 0.5 g
  saturated 0.0 g
  polyunsaturated 0.0 g
  monounsaturated 0.0 g
cholesterol 6 mg

sodium 236 mg
carbohydrates 12 g
  fiber 3 g
  sugar 4 g
protein 12 g

100 200 300 400

DIETARY EXCHANGES
2 vegetable;
1 very lean meat

french brussels sprouts

Serves 8; $\frac{1}{2}$ cup per serving

This one-pan side dish blends brussels sprouts with the classic French flavoring combination known as mirepoix—green onions, celery, and carrots.

10 ounces small brussels sprouts (about 20)
 1 slice turkey bacon, chopped
$\frac{1}{3}$ cup sliced green onions (white part only)
$\frac{1}{3}$ cup diced celery
$\frac{1}{3}$ cup diced or shredded carrots
 1 tablespoon water (optional)

Cut the ends off the brussels sprouts and remove any outer leaves that are damaged or yellow. Put the brussels sprouts in a medium saucepan. Add cold water to cover. Bring to a boil over medium-high heat. Cook, uncovered, for 15 minutes, or until you can easily prick the brussels sprouts with the point of a sharp knife. Transfer the sprouts to a colander. Run under cold water to stop the cooking and maintain the bright color of the sprouts. Drain well.

In the same saucepan, cook the bacon over medium-low heat for about 8 minutes, or until it begins to brown. Add the green onions, celery, and carrots. Cook, covered, for 3 minutes.

Stir in the brussels sprouts. Cook, covered, for 10 minutes, or until heated through, stirring occasionally. If the vegetables begin to stick to the pan, add the 1 tablespoon water.

PER SERVING

calories 24
total fat 0.5 g
  saturated 0.0 g
  polyunsaturated 0.0 g
  monounsaturated 0.0 g
cholesterol 2 mg

sodium 39 mg
carbohydrates 4 g
  fiber 2 g
  sugar 1 g
  protein 2 g

100	200	300	400

DIETARY EXCHANGES
1 vegetable

red cabbage braised with balsamic vinegar

Serves 4; $\frac{1}{2}$ cup per serving

Eye-catching red cabbage with a touch of black-berry spread, balsamic vinegar, and lemon zest teams well with baked pork chops or poached salmon.

1 teaspoon olive oil
2 medium leeks (white part only), thinly sliced
$\frac{1}{2}$ medium red cabbage (about 1 pound), thinly sliced
$\frac{1}{4}$ cup unsweetened apple juice
2 tablespoons all-fruit seedless blackberry spread
1 tablespoon balsamic vinegar
1 teaspoon lemon zest
$\frac{1}{4}$ teaspoon pepper

Heat a medium saucepan over medium heat. Pour the oil into the pan and swirl to coat the bottom. Cook the leeks for 2 to 3 minutes, or until tender-crisp, stirring occasionally.

Stir in the cabbage. Cook for 2 to 3 minutes, or until the cabbage is tender-crisp, stirring occasionally.

Stir in the remaining ingredients. Reduce the heat and simmer, covered, for 20 to 25 minutes, or until the cabbage is tender, stirring occasionally.

PER SERVING

calories 112
total fat 1.5 g
  saturated 0.0 g
  polyunsaturated 0.5 g
  monounsaturated 1.0 g
cholesterol 0 mg

sodium 49 mg
carbohydrates 25 g
  fiber 4 g
  sugar 14 g
protein 3 g

100 200 300 400

DIETARY EXCHANGES
½ fruit; 3 vegetable; ½ fat

orange-glazed carrots

Serves 4; $\frac{1}{2}$ cup per serving

Try these sweet carrots with grilled or broiled meat or poultry.

1 medium orange
4 medium carrots, cut into $\frac{1}{8}$-inch rounds
$\frac{1}{4}$ teaspoon ground cinnamon
2 tablespoons firmly packed dark brown sugar
$\frac{1}{8}$ teaspoon salt
1 tablespoon light tub margarine

Grate 1 teaspoon zest from the orange. Set the zest aside. Squeeze the juice from the orange. Pour into a large nonstick skillet. Bring to a boil over high heat.

Add the carrots and cinnamon. Return to a boil. Reduce the heat and simmer, covered, for 8 to 9 minutes, or until tender.

Increase the heat to high. Stir in the brown sugar and salt. Bring to a boil. Cook for about 1 minute, or until richly glazed, stirring constantly. Remove from the heat.

Stir in the margarine and orange zest until completely blended.

PER SERVING

calories 76
total fat 1.5 g
  saturated 0.0 g
  polyunsaturated 0.5 g
  monounsaturated 0.5 g
cholesterol 0 mg

sodium 148 mg
carbohydrates 16 g
  fiber 2 g
  sugar 12 g
protein 1 g

100	200	300	400

DIETARY EXCHANGES
$1\frac{1}{2}$ vegetable;
$\frac{1}{2}$ other carbohydrate

cauliflower mash

Serves 4; ½ cup per serving

If you love mashed potatoes but want to cut down on carbs, this is a great solution.

- 1 pound fresh or frozen cauliflower florets (about 3 cups)
- ¼ cup fat-free evaporated milk
- ½ ounce blue cheese, crumbled
- 1 tablespoon light tub margarine
- ½ teaspoon salt
- ⅛ teaspoon pepper

Steam the cauliflower for 12 minutes, or until very tender.

In a food processor or blender, process the cauliflower and milk until smooth, scraping the side of the work bowl several times with a rubber scraper.

Transfer to a serving bowl. Stir in the remaining ingredients.

COOK'S TIP: Adding the blue cheese, margarine, salt, and pepper just before serving allows the flavors to be more pronounced.

PER SERVING

calories 64
total fat 2.5 g
  saturated 0.5 g
  polyunsaturated 0.5 g
  monounsaturated 1.0 g
cholesterol 3 mg

sodium 415 mg
carbohydrates 8 g
  fiber 3 g
  sugar 5 g
protein 4 g

100   200   300   400

DIETARY EXCHANGES
$1\frac{1}{2}$ vegetable; $\frac{1}{2}$ fat

oven-fried eggplant
Serves 6; 2 slices per serving

Try these crisp eggplant slices as an appetizer or side dish. Accompany them with low-sodium salsa and fat-free sour cream for dipping if you wish.

1 medium eggplant (at least 6 inches tall)
1/2 teaspoon salt
   Vegetable oil spray
   Pepper to taste
1/2 cup all-purpose flour
1 teaspoon dried basil, crumbled
1 teaspoon dried parsley, crumbled
1/2 teaspoon dried oregano, crumbled
1/2 teaspoon garlic powder
   Whites of 3 large eggs
3/4 cup plain dry bread crumbs

Trim the ends from the eggplant. Cut it crosswise into twelve 1/2-inch slices. Submerge in cold water with the salt for 1 hour.

Preheat the oven to 375°F. Lightly spray a baking sheet with vegetable oil spray.

Drain the eggplant. Pat dry with paper towels. Sprinkle with the pepper.

On a small plate, combine the flour, basil, parsley, oregano, and garlic powder. In a small bowl, lightly beat the egg whites. Put the bread crumbs in another small bowl. Line up the plate, bowls, and baking sheet.

Coat an eggplant slice in the flour mixture, shaking off any excess. Coat in the egg whites, then in the bread crumbs, shaking off any excess. Place on the baking sheet. Repeat with remaining eggplant.

Bake for 20 to 25 minutes, or until golden brown, turning once.

COOK'S TIP: Reheat leftovers in a 375°F oven for 5 to 8 minutes.

PER SERVING

calories 124
total fat 1.0 g
 saturated 0.0 g
 polyunsaturated 0.5 g
 monounsaturated 0.0 g
cholesterol 0 mg

sodium 323 mg
carbohydrates 23 g
 fiber 1 g
 sugar 1 g
protein 6 g

100 200 300 400

DIETARY EXCHANGES
$1\frac{1}{2}$ starch; 1 vegetable

roasted green beans and walnuts

Serves 4; $^1/_2$ cup per serving

Double roasting is the lazy way to get it done: While the beans are roasting, the nuts are toasting, bringing out the rich flavors of each.

  Vegetable oil spray
12 ounces fresh green beans, trimmed
 2 tablespoons finely chopped walnuts
 2 tablespoons finely snipped fresh parsley
$^1/_4$ teaspoon salt
$^1/_8$ teaspoon cayenne

Preheat the oven to 425°F.

  Lightly spray a large baking sheet with vegetable oil spray. Arrange the beans on the baking sheet in a single layer. Sprinkle with the walnuts. Lightly spray the bean mixture with vegetable oil spray.

Bake for 5 minutes. Stir. Bake for 5 minutes. Remove from the heat.

To serve, sprinkle with the parsley, salt, and cayenne.

braised mustard greens with pearl onions

Serves 6; ½ cup per serving

As you incorporate more leafy green vegetables into your eating plan, remember to add variety. This recipe combines peppery mustard greens, plump pearl onions, red bell pepper, and a hint of smoky flavor from imitation bacon bits.

1 teaspoon olive oil

½ medium red bell pepper, thinly sliced

1 pound fresh or frozen mustard greens, stems discarded if fresh or thawed and squeezed dry if frozen, cut into 1-inch slices

1 cup frozen pearl onions, thawed

2 tablespoons imitation bacon bits

½ cup fat-free, low-sodium chicken broth

1 tablespoon Dijon mustard

¼ teaspoon pepper

Heat a large skillet over medium heat. Pour the oil into the skillet and swirl to coat the bottom. Cook the bell pepper for 2 to 3 minutes, or until tender-crisp.

Stir in the mustard greens, pearl onions, and bacon bits. Cook for 3 to 4 minutes, or until the mustard greens are slightly wilted, stirring occasionally.

Stir in the broth, mustard, and pepper. Reduce the heat and simmer, covered, for 20 to 25 minutes, or until the mustard greens are tender.

COOK'S TIP: Look for convenient 1-pound packages of fresh greens, such as mustard and collard greens. They are prewashed and precut to save you time.

PER SERVING ···

calories 62
total fat 1.5 g
  saturated 0.0 g
  polyunsaturated 0.0 g
  monounsaturated 0.5 g
cholesterol 0 mg

sodium 105 mg
carbohydrates 10 g
  fiber 3 g
  sugar 3 g
protein 4 g

100	200	300	400

DIETARY EXCHANGES
2 vegetable; 1/2 fat

creole lentils

Serves 4; ½ cup per serving

Simmer lentils to tenderness with tomatoes, onions, peppers, celery, and okra. A touch of hot sauce adds zip.

Vegetable oil spray
1 medium green bell pepper, chopped
1 medium rib of celery, finely chopped
½ cup chopped onion
2 medium tomatoes, chopped
1 cup fresh or frozen cut okra
¾ cup water
½ cup dried lentils, sorted for stones and shriveled lentils and rinsed
½ teaspoon dried thyme, crumbled
2 medium bay leaves
¼ cup snipped fresh parsley
2 teaspoons olive oil (extra-virgin preferred)
½ teaspoon salt
¼ teaspoon red hot-pepper sauce

Heat a large saucepan over medium-high heat. Remove from the heat and lightly spray with vegetable oil spray (being careful not to spray near a gas flame). Cook the bell pepper, celery, and onion for 4 minutes, or until the onion is soft, stirring frequently.

Increase the heat to high. Stir in the tomatoes, okra, water, lentils, thyme, and bay leaves. Bring to a boil. Reduce the heat and simmer, covered, for 30 minutes, or until the lentils are tender. Remove from the heat. Discard the bay leaves.

Stir in the parsley, oil, salt, and hot-pepper sauce. Let stand, covered, for 5 minutes to allow the flavors to blend.

PER SERVING

calories 139
total fat 2.5 g
 saturated 0.5 g
 polyunsaturated 0.5 g
 monounsaturated 2.0 g
cholesterol 0 mg

sodium 317 mg
carbohydrates 22 g
 fiber 10 g
 sugar 5 g
protein 9 g

100 200 300 400 DIETARY EXCHANGES
1 starch; $1\frac{1}{2}$ vegetable; $\frac{1}{2}$ lean meat

orzo with tomato and capers

Serves 4; ½ cup per serving

This versatile Mediterranean combination is delectable both as a hot or room temperature side dish and as a cold pasta salad.

3 ounces dried orzo
1 small tomato (about 4 ounces), seeded and diced
¼ cup snipped fresh parsley
1 tablespoon capers, rinsed and drained
2 teaspoons olive oil (extra-virgin preferred)
2 teaspoons dried basil, crumbled
½ to 1 teaspoon cider vinegar
½ medium garlic clove, minced
½ teaspoon salt
⅛ teaspoon crushed red pepper flakes

Prepare the orzo using the package directions, omitting the salt and oil. Drain well.

Meanwhile, in a medium bowl, stir together the remaining ingredients.

Add the orzo. Toss gently. Serve hot, at room temperature, or cold.

stir-fried sugar snap peas with shallots and walnuts

Serves 4; $\frac{1}{2}$ cup per serving

Dress up any meal from grilled chicken to meat loaf with this super side dish of crisp, rather sweet sugar snaps enhanced with imitation bacon bits and fragrant five-spice powder.

Vegetable oil spray
2 medium shallots, chopped
8 ounces fresh or frozen sugar snap peas
2 tablespoons imitation bacon bits
1 teaspoon toasted sesame oil
$\frac{1}{4}$ teaspoon five-spice powder (optional)
1 tablespoon crushed dry-roasted walnuts

Heat a large nonstick skillet over medium heat. Remove from the heat and lightly spray with vegetable oil spray (being careful not to spray near a gas flame). Cook the shallots for 1 to 2 minutes, or until tender-crisp, stirring constantly.

Stir in the peas, bacon bits, sesame oil, and five-spice powder. Cook for 1 to 2 minutes, or until the peas are tender-crisp.

Sprinkle with the walnuts.

COOK'S TIP ON DRY-ROASTING NUTS: Place the nuts in a dry, heavy skillet and toast over medium heat until fragrant and lightly browned, 2 to 7 minutes, stirring occasionally. Remove the skillet from the heat as soon as the nuts are toasted.

PER SERVING

calories 63
total fat 3.0 g
 saturated 0.5 g
 polyunsaturated 1.5 g
 monounsaturated 1.0 g
cholesterol 0 mg

sodium 41 mg
carbohydrates 7 g
 fiber 2 g
 sugar 3 g
protein 3 g

100 200 300 400 **DIETARY EXCHANGES**
$^1/_2$ starch; $^1/_2$ fat

smashed potatoes with aromatic herbs

Serves 4; ½ cup per serving

After simmering the skin-on potatoes, add herbs and seasonings to the cooking pan, then coarsely mash the mixture for a side dish with interesting texture and taste.

1 pound red or Yukon gold potatoes (about 4 medium)

½ cup fat-free half-and-half

1 tablespoon snipped fresh parsley or 1 teaspoon dried, crumbled

1 tablespoon finely chopped or minced fresh rosemary or 1 teaspoon dried, crushed

2 teaspoons prepared white horseradish

1 medium garlic clove, minced

⅛ teaspoon pepper

½ teaspoon salt

Put the potatoes in a medium saucepan. Fill the pan with water to cover the potatoes by 1 inch. Bring to a boil over high heat. Reduce the heat and simmer, partially covered, for about 30 minutes, or until the potatoes are tender when pierced with the tip of a sharp knife. Drain, leaving the potatoes in the pan.

Add the remaining ingredients. Mash coarsely or to the desired texture with a potato masher.

COOK'S TIP: Feel free to replace the rosemary with basil, oregano, dill, thyme, savory, or sliced green onions (green part only).

PER SERVING

calories 100
total fat 0.0 g
  saturated 0.0 g
  polyunsaturated 0.0 g
  monounsaturated 0.0 g
cholesterol 0 mg

sodium 329 mg
carbohydrates 25 g
  fiber 3 g
  sugar 5 g
protein 5 g

100   200   300   400

DIETARY EXCHANGES
$1\frac{1}{2}$ starch

lemon-herb brown rice

Serves 4; $^1/_2$ cup per serving

Adding the margarine spray at the very end and not stirring it into the rice mixture lets the flavor stay on top so you can taste it with every bite.

1 cup uncooked quick-cooking brown rice
$^1/_4$ cup finely snipped fresh parsley
1 teaspoon dried basil, crumbled
$^1/_2$ to 1 teaspoon grated lemon zest
1 tablespoon fresh lemon juice
$^1/_2$ teaspoon salt
20 sprays fat-free liquid margarine spray

Prepare the rice using the package directions, omitting the salt and margarine. Transfer to a serving bowl.

Stir in the remaining ingredients except the margarine spray.

Spray the top with margarine spray. Do not stir.

PER SERVING

calories 89
total fat 1.0 g
 saturated 0.0 g
 polyunsaturated 0.5 g
 monounsaturated 0.5 g
cholesterol 0 mg

sodium 298 mg
carbohydrates 18 g
 fiber 1 g
 sugar 0 g
protein 2 g

100	200	300	400	DIETARY EXCHANGES

1 starch

pesto and pecan rice

Serves 4; ½ cup per serving

This snazzy side dish will really attract attention.

Vegetable oil spray
½ medium green bell pepper, chopped
½ cup onion, chopped
1 medium rib of celery, chopped
1 medium garlic clove, minced
½ cup uncooked brown rice
1½ cups low-sodium vegetable broth or fat-free, low-sodium chicken broth
¼ teaspoon pepper
⅛ teaspoon salt
½ tablespoon prepared pesto
½ tablespoon low-sodium vegetable broth or water
1 tablespoon chopped fresh basil leaves (optional)
2 teaspoons coarsely chopped pecans, dry-roasted

Heat a medium saucepan over medium heat. Remove from the heat and lightly spray with vegetable oil spray (being careful not to spray near a gas flame). Cook the bell pepper, onion, celery, and garlic for 3 to 4 minutes, or until the onion is soft, stirring occasionally. Transfer to a plate.

Respray the pan. Cook the rice for 1 to 2 minutes, or until lightly toasted, stirring occasionally.

Stir in the 1½ cups broth, pepper, and salt. Increase the heat to high and bring to a boil. Reduce the heat and simmer, covered, for 40 to 45 minutes, or until the rice is tender and the liquid is absorbed.

Meanwhile, in a small bowl, whisk together the pesto and 1 tablespoon broth until smooth. Stir with the bell pepper mixture into the cooked rice.

To serve, sprinkle the rice with the basil and pecans.

PER SERVING

calories 126
total fat 2.5 g
 saturated 0.5 g
 polyunsaturated 0.5 g
 monounsaturated 1.0 g
cholesterol 1 mg

sodium 123 mg
carbohydrates 23 g
 fiber 2 g
 sugar 2 g
protein 4 g

100	200	300	400

DIETARY EXCHANGES
1 starch; 1½ vegetable; ½ fat

spinach with almonds and lemon zest

Serves 4; ½ cup per serving

When you need an elegant side dish, you will love this super-speedy combination of prewashed baby spinach, dry-roasted almonds, caramelized onions, lemon zest, and Parmesan. Serve with pan-seared or grilled fish or baked pork chops.

1 teaspoon olive oil

1 medium onion, thinly sliced

1 teaspoon light brown sugar

1 medium garlic clove, minced

1 pound baby spinach (about 10 cups)

1 tablespoon low-sodium Worcestershire sauce

1 teaspoon grated lemon zest

2 tablespoons shredded or grated Parmesan cheese

1 tablespoon slivered almonds, dry-roasted

Pour the oil into a large nonstick skillet and swirl to coat the bottom. Cook the onion over medium-high heat for 7 to 8 minutes, or until golden brown, stirring occasionally. (Watch carefully so the onion does not burn.)

Stir in the brown sugar and garlic. Cook for 1 minute, or until the flavors have blended.

Stir in the spinach, Worcestershire sauce, and lemon zest. Cook for 3 to 4 minutes, or until the spinach is wilted, stirring occasionally.

To serve, spoon the spinach into a serving bowl. Sprinkle with the Parmesan and almonds.

PER SERVING ···

calories 78
total fat 3.0 g
  saturated 0.5 g
  polyunsaturated 0.5 g
  monounsaturated 1.5 g
cholesterol 2 mg

sodium 139 mg
carbohydrates 10 g
  fiber 4 g
  sugar 4 g
protein 5 g

100	200	300	400	**DIETARY EXCHANGES**

2 vegetable; $\frac{1}{2}$ fat

stewed zucchini and cherry tomatoes

Serves 4; $^1/_2$ cup per serving

Dress up meat loaf or grilled chicken breasts with this classy side dish.

2 medium zucchini (about 8 ounces)
1 teaspoon canola or corn oil
4 medium garlic cloves
2 tablespoons fat-free, low-sodium chicken broth
$^1/_2$ cup cherry tomatoes, halved
2 tablespoons chopped fresh basil leaves or
   1 teaspoon dried, crumbled
$^1/_8$ teaspoon pepper
2 tablespoons shredded or grated Romano cheese

Cut the zucchini into $^1/_2$-inch slices, preferably with a crinkle-cutter.

Heat a medium saucepan over medium heat. Pour the oil into the pan and swirl to coat the bottom. Cook the garlic for 2 to 3 minutes, or until light golden brown, stirring occasionally.

Stir in the zucchini. Cook for 1 to 2 minutes, or until the zucchini is tender-crisp, stirring occasionally.

Pour in the broth. Reduce the heat and simmer, covered, for 5 minutes, or until the zucchini is tender, stirring occasionally.

Stir in the tomatoes, basil, and pepper. Cook for 1 to 2 minutes, or until the tomatoes are warmed through.

Transfer the mixture to a serving bowl. Sprinkle with the Romano.

COOK'S TIP ON CRINKLE-CUTTERS: You can find crinkle-cutters at gourmet shops and some supermarkets. They are easy-to-use gadgets that make attractive wavy cuts on foods such as zucchini, yellow squash, cucumbers, carrots, and various melons.

PER SERVING

calories 42
total fat 2.0 g
  saturated 0.5 g
  polyunsaturated 0.5 g
  monounsaturated 0.5 g
cholesterol 1 mg

sodium 32 mg
carbohydrates 6 g
  fiber 2 g
  sugar 3 g
protein 2 g

100 200 300 400

DIETARY EXCHANGES
1 vegetable; $1/2$ fat

mixed vegetable grill

Serves 4; ¹⁄₂ cup per serving

Here is a combination of just a few of the many vegetables that are delicious when grilled—and these are very low in calories. For uniform cooking, you will need vegetables of uniform size.

Vegetable oil spray (olive oil spray preferred)
2 medium zucchini
12 medium button mushrooms
12 cherry tomatoes
10 fresh basil leaves (optional)
Fat-free liquid margarine spray
Pepper to taste
¹⁄₄ teaspoon salt
Balsamic vinegar

If using wooden skewers, soak four 8-inch skewers in cold water for at least 10 minutes to keep them from charring.

Meanwhile, spray the grill with vegetable oil spray. Preheat the grill on medium-high. Cut the zucchini lengthwise into ¹⁄₂-inch-thick slices. Trim the mushrooms so the stems are even with the bottom of the caps.

Put 6 mushrooms on one skewer; repeat. On the remaining two skewers, alternate the tomatoes and basil leaves, beginning and ending with a tomato. Lightly spray the surface of the zucchini, mushrooms, and tomatoes with the margarine spray. Sprinkle with the pepper and salt.

Grill the vegetables for 8 to 12 minutes, or until lightly charred and the desired doneness, basting occasionally and turning the zucchini occasionally, the tomatoes frequently, and the mushrooms once. Remove the vegetables from the grill as they become done. Lightly brush with the balsamic vinegar before serving.

PER SERVING

calories 35
total fat 0.5 g
  saturated 0.0 g
  polyunsaturated 0.0 g
  monounsaturated 0.0 g
cholesterol 0 mg

sodium 167 mg
carbohydrates 7 g
  fiber 2 g
  sugar 3 g
protein 4 g

100 200 300 400   **DIETARY EXCHANGES**
1½ vegetable

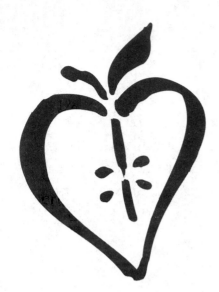

breads and breakfast dishes

Garlic Bread

Apple and Dried Cherry
  Quick Bread

Dinner Biscuits

Pan-Style Whole-Wheat Dinner Rolls

Pumpkin-Cranberry Pancakes

Peach Cornmeal Waffles

Crisp French Toast

Fruit-and-Cinnamon Oatmeal

garlic bread

Serves 4; 1 slice per serving

Don't you love the smell of garlic bread toasting in the oven? Now you can have a fantastic version that isn't drenched in calories.

 2 tablespoons light tub margarine
½ medium garlic clove, minced
¼ teaspoon dried oregano, crumbled
¼ teaspoon dried basil, crumbled
⅛ teaspoon crushed red pepper flakes (optional)
¼ 16-ounce loaf Italian bread
 2 tablespoons minced green onions (green and white parts)
 2 teaspoons shredded or grated Parmesan cheese
   Paprika

Preheat the oven to 350°F.

In a small bowl, stir together the margarine, garlic, oregano, basil, and red pepper flakes.

Cut the bread in half lengthwise. Spread the margarine mixture over the bread. Sprinkle with the green onions. Place on a baking sheet.

Bake for 15 minutes, or until the edges begin to lightly brown.

Sprinkle with the Parmesan and paprika. Cut into 4 pieces.

PER SERVING

calories 103

total fat 3.5 g
  saturated 0.5 g
  polyunsaturated 1.0 g
  monounsaturated 1.5 g
cholesterol 1 mg

sodium 225 mg
carbohydrates 15 g
  fiber 1 g
  sugar 1 g
  protein 3 g

100 200 300 400 **DIETARY EXCHANGES**
1 starch; 1/2 fat

apple and dried cherry quick bread

Serves 18; 1 slice per serving

This fruity loaf is short in stature (only about 2 inches tall) but long in taste and moistness. It's delicious as is or toasted and served with fruit spread.

Vegetable oil spray

2 cups whole-wheat pastry flour or all-purpose flour

1/3 cup firmly packed light or dark brown sugar

2 teaspoons baking powder

1 teaspoon ground cinnamon

1 teaspoon grated lemon zest

1/8 teaspoon salt

1 cup unsweetened applesauce

1/2 cup unsweetened apple juice

Egg substitute equivalent to 1 egg, or whites of 2 large eggs

1 large apple, such as Granny Smith or Braeburn, peeled and diced (about 1 cup)

1/2 cup dried cherries

Preheat the oven to 350°F. Lightly spray a 9 × 5 × 3-inch loaf pan with vegetable oil spray.

In a large bowl, stir together the flour, sugar, baking powder, cinnamon, lemon zest, and salt.

In a medium bowl, whisk together the applesauce, apple juice, and egg substitute. Add the applesauce mixture and the remaining ingredients to the flour mixture, stirring only until just combined. Do not overmix; the batter should be slightly lumpy. Spread the batter into the loaf pan.

Bake for 50 to 55 minutes, or until a cake tester or wooden toothpick inserted in the center comes out clean. Let cool in the pan for 5 minutes. Remove the loaf from the pan and let cool completely on a cooling rack.

PER SERVING

calories 77	sodium 70 mg
total fat 0.0 g	carbohydrates 18 g
saturated 0.0 g	fiber 2 g
polyunsaturated 0.0 g	sugar 9 g
monounsaturated 0.0 g	protein 2 g
cholesterol 0 mg	

100   200   300   400   **DIETARY EXCHANGES**
1 starch

dinner biscuits

Serves 8; 1 biscuit per serving

Flecked with fresh parsley and coarse pepper, these biscuits are superb.

Vegetable oil spray
1 cup all-purpose flour
1 tablespoon snipped fresh parsley or 1 teaspoon dried, crumbled
2 teaspoons baking powder
1/2 teaspoon garlic powder
1/2 teaspoon onion powder
1/4 teaspoon salt
1/8 teaspoon coarsely ground pepper
1/8 teaspoon baking soda
2 tablespoons light tub margarine (kept refrigerated until needed)
1/2 cup fat-free or low-fat buttermilk
Flour for dusting (about 2 tablespoons)

Preheat the oven to 425°F. Lightly spray an 8-inch round cake pan with vegetable oil spray.

In a medium bowl, stir together the flour, parsley, baking powder, garlic powder, onion powder, salt, pepper, and baking soda.

Using a pastry blender or fork, cut in the margarine until the margarine pieces are about pea size.

Using a fork, stir the buttermilk into the flour mixture until the mixture is just moistened. Do not overmix or the biscuits will be tough.

Lightly sprinkle a flat work surface with the flour for dusting. Put the dough on the floured surface. Turn to coat. Shape into a flat disk. With floured hands or a floured rolling pin, pat the dough to ½-inch thickness. Using a 2½-inch round cutter, cut out 8 biscuits. Place the biscuits in a single layer in the cake pan.

Bake for 10 to 12 minutes, or until the biscuits are golden brown and cooked through the center.

PER SERVING

calories 81

total fat 1.5 g

  saturated 0.0 g

  polyunsaturated 0.5 g

  monounsaturated 0.5 g

cholesterol 1 mg

sodium 232 mg

carbohydrates 14 g

  fiber 1 g

  sugar 1 g

  protein 2 g

100   200   300   400   DIETARY EXCHANGES

1 starch

pan-style whole-wheat dinner rolls

Serves 16; 1 roll per serving

Homemade yeast dinner rolls are a snap with this easy recipe. The quick-rise yeast helps speed up the rising process for fresh-baked goodness any day of the week.

1½ cups whole-wheat flour

1½ cups all-purpose flour

   ¼-ounce package fast-rising yeast

½ cup fat-free milk

½ cup water

   Egg substitute equivalent to 1 egg, or 1 large egg

2 tablespoons honey

1 tablespoon olive oil

¼ teaspoon salt

   Vegetable oil spray

2 tablespoons unsalted sunflower seeds

In a large bowl, stir together the flours. Remove 1 cup flour mixture and set aside. Stir the yeast into the flour mixture remaining in the bowl.

In a small saucepan, cook the milk and water over medium-low heat for 2 to 3 minutes, or until the mixture reaches 120°F to 130°F on an instant-read thermometer. (The yeast will not activate if the liquid gets too hot.) Alternatively, you can microwave the milk and water in a microwaveable container, uncovered, on 100 percent power (high) for 30 seconds, or until the mixture reaches the proper temperature.

Pour the milk mixture into the flour mixture. Stir in the egg substitute, honey, oil, and salt. Beat with a spoon for about 30 seconds, or until smooth.

Gradually add up to ¾ cup of the reserved flour, stirring after each addition, until the dough starts to pull away from the side of the bowl.

Sprinkle the remaining ¼ cup flour over a flat work surface. Put the dough on the floured surface. Knead for 5 to 6 minutes, or until smooth and elastic, adding more flour if needed. Leaving the dough on the flat surface, cover it with a dry dish towel. Let rest for 10 minutes.

Lightly spray a 13 × 9 × 2-inch baking pan with vegetable oil spray.

Press the dough evenly into the pan. Using a dull knife, divide the dough into 16 squares without cutting all the way through. (This will slightly separate the rolls so they will rise and bake together but break apart easily after they are baked.) Sprinkle with the sunflower seeds. Cover with a dry dish towel. Let the dough rise for 30 to 45 minutes, or until doubled in bulk.

Meanwhile, preheat the oven to 400°F.

Bake for 20 to 22 minutes, or until the rolls are golden brown and sound hollow when tapped on the top. Put the pan on a cooling rack. Let cool for 5 minutes before separating and serving the rolls.

PER SERVING

calories 109

total fat 1.5 g
 saturated 0.0 g
 polyunsaturated 0.5 g
 monounsaturated 1.0 g
cholesterol 0 mg

sodium 50 mg
carbohydrates 20 g
 fiber 2 g
 sugar 3 g
protein 4 g

100	200	300	400	**DIETARY EXCHANGES**

$1\frac{1}{2}$ starch

pumpkin-cranberry pancakes
Serves 4; 2 pancakes per serving

There's more than one way to enjoy the taste of canned pumpkin, and these pancakes will prove the point deliciously.

1 cup fat-free milk or fat-free or low-fat buttermilk
1/2 cup canned solid-pack pumpkin (not pumpkin pie mix)
1/4 cup dried sweetened cranberries
1/4 cup unsweetened applesauce
Egg substitute equivalent to 1 egg, or 1 large egg
3 tablespoons firmly packed light brown sugar
1 cup all-purpose flour
2 teaspoons baking powder
1/2 teaspoon baking soda
1/4 teaspoon ground ginger
1/4 teaspoon ground nutmeg
Vegetable oil spray

In a medium bowl, whisk together the milk, pumpkin, cranberries, applesauce, egg substitute, and brown sugar.

In a large bowl, stir together the remaining ingredients except the vegetable oil spray.

Gently stir the milk mixture into the flour mixture just until no flour is visible. Do not overmix; the batter will be slightly lumpy.

Heat a large nonstick griddle or skillet over medium heat. Remove from the heat and lightly spray with vegetable oil spray (being careful not to spray near a gas flame). Return to the heat. Pour onto the griddle about ⅓ cup batter each for 4 pancakes. Cook for 3 to 4 minutes, or until small bubbles appear all over the tops of the pancakes and the bottoms are golden brown. Flip the pancakes. Cook for 1 to 2 minutes, or until the pancakes are cooked through and golden on the bottom. Repeat with the remaining batter.

PER SERVING

calories 225
total fat 0.5 g
  saturated 0.0 g
  polyunsaturated 0.0 g
  monounsaturated 0.0 g
cholesterol 1 mg

sodium 428 mg
carbohydrates 48 g
  fiber 2 g
  sugar 22 g
protein 7 g

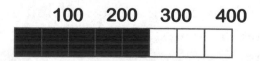

100 200 300 400

DIETARY EXCHANGES
2 starch; 1 fruit;
½ very lean meat

peach cornmeal waffles

Serves 8; 1 waffle per serving

These homey, peach-studded waffles are perfect for a weekend brunch.

Vegetable oil spray
1 1/3 cups all-purpose flour
2/3 cup yellow cornmeal
1/4 cup sugar
2 teaspoons baking powder
1/2 teaspoon baking soda
1/4 teaspoon ground nutmeg
1 1/2 cups fat-free or low-fat buttermilk
1 cup diced peaches, fresh, unsweetened frozen, or canned in fruit juice, peeled if fresh, thawed if frozen, or drained if canned
Egg substitute equivalent to 2 eggs, or 2 large eggs
1 tablespoon canola or corn oil

Lightly spray a nonstick waffle iron (Belgian or regular) with vegetable oil spray. Preheat according to the manufacturer's directions.

Meanwhile, in a large bowl, stir together the flour, cornmeal, sugar, baking powder, baking soda, and nutmeg. Make a well in the center.

In a medium bowl, whisk together the remaining ingredients. Pour into the flour mixture. Stir until just moistened. Do not overmix.

Spread a scant ½ cup batter onto the hot waffle iron. Cook for 5 to 7 minutes, or until the waffles are golden brown and cooked through. Repeat the procedure with the remaining batter, spraying the waffle iron with vegetable oil spray between batches if necessary.

COOK'S TIP: If you want to serve all the waffles at once, preheat the oven to 250°F and place each waffle in a single layer on a baking sheet as it finishes cooking. Keep the prepared waffles warm in the oven while you cook the remaining batter.

PER SERVING

calories 192	sodium 259 mg
total fat 2.5 g	carbohydrates 37 g
saturated 0.5 g	fiber 2 g
polyunsaturated 0.5 g	sugar 11 g
monounsaturated 1.0 g	protein 6 g
cholesterol 2 mg	

100 200 300 400

DIETARY EXCHANGES
2 starch; ½ fruit

crisp french toast
Serves 4; 1½ slices per serving

Coating the bread with coarsely crumbled cereal provides an interesting new way to prepare French toast. Serve it with light maple syrup if you wish.

     1 cup toasted rice flakes cereal
     1 cup egg substitute
 1½ tablespoons fat-free half-and-half
    ½ teaspoon vanilla extract
       Vegetable oil spray
     6 slices whole-wheat bread, halved lengthwise

Preheat the oven to 200°F.

Put the cereal in a large resealable plastic bag. Using a rolling pin, crush the cereal until coarse. Transfer to a large plate.

In a medium bowl, whisk together the egg substitute, half-and-half, and vanilla extract.

Heat a large nonstick skillet over medium heat. Remove from the heat and lightly spray with vegetable oil spray (being careful not to spray near a gas flame). Return the skillet to the heat.

Quickly dip one piece of bread into the egg substitute mixture. Immediately coat well with the cereal crumbs. Repeat with enough pieces of bread to make one layer in the skillet.

Cook the bread for 1 minute on each side, or until the coating is golden brown and the egg is cooked through. Transfer to an ovenproof platter and keep warm, uncovered, in the oven.

Repeat with the remaining bread slices, respraying the skillet for each batch.

PER SERVING

calories 168
total fat 2.0 g
  saturated 0.5 g
  polyunsaturated 0.5 g
  monounsaturated 0.5 g
cholesterol 0 mg

sodium 408 mg
carbohydrates 27 g
  fiber 3 g
  sugar 11 g
protein 12 g

100   200   300   400

DIETARY EXCHANGES
2 starch; 1 very lean meat

fruit-and-cinnamon oatmeal

Serves 4; 1 cup per serving

Whether it's cold and rainy outside or you just want a little comfort to start your day, this steamy bowl of oats is packed with sweet and fruity flavors, with just a hint of cinnamon to round it out.

3¾ cups water

2 cups uncooked quick-cooking oatmeal

½ cup raisins or chopped dried apricots

⅓ cup firmly packed dark brown sugar

1 teaspoon light tub margarine (optional)

1 teaspoon ground cinnamon

½ teaspoon vanilla, butter, and nut flavoring or vanilla extract

⅛ teaspoon salt

In a medium saucepan, bring the water to a boil over high heat. Stir in the oatmeal and raisins. Reduce the heat and simmer for 3 minutes, uncovered, stirring occasionally. Remove from the heat.

Stir in the remaining ingredients.

PER SERVING

calories 289

total fat 2.5 g

  saturated 0.5 g

  polyunsaturated 1.0 g

  monounsaturated 1.0 g

cholesterol 0 mg

sodium 88 mg

carbohydrates 62 g

  fiber 5 g

  sugar 31 g

protein 7 g

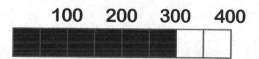

100 200 300 400

DIETARY EXCHANGES

2 starch; 1 fruit;

1 other carbohydrate

desserts

Pear and Apricot Cake

Peach and Pineapple
   Upside-Down Cake

Orange and Almond Pudding Cake

Clafouti

Raspberry Yogurt Cream Pie

Assorted Biscotti

Peach and Berry Crumble

Applesauce Oatmeal Cookies

Apple and Pear Strudel

Coconut-Lime Flan

Pumpkin Praline Mousse

Vanilla Soufflé
with Brandy-Plum Sauce

Chocolate-Hazelnut Fondue

Fruit Sauce

Blueberry Dream Dessert Squares

Citrus Freeze Bars

pear and apricot cake

Serves 8; 1 wedge per serving

This beautiful tartlike cake is simple enough to make for a weeknight snack.

Vegetable oil spray
9-ounce box single-layer white cake mix
1/2 cup water
Whites of 2 large eggs
1/4 teaspoon almond extract
1 1/2 medium pears (about 8 ounces), thinly sliced
1/4 cup all-fruit apricot spread
1/4 cup sliced almonds, dry-roasted (about 1 ounce)

Preheat the oven to 350°F. Lightly spray a 10-inch springform pan with vegetable oil spray.

In a medium mixing bowl, combine the cake mix, water, egg whites, and almond extract. Using an electric mixer, beat on high speed for 4 minutes, scraping the side with a rubber scraper frequently.

Arrange the pears in a decorative pattern in the pan. Gently pour in the batter, being careful not to disturb the pears.

Bake 30 minutes, or until the cake springs back when lightly touched in the center with your fingertips.

Immediately invert onto a serving platter. Remove the side and base of the pan. Let the cake cool completely.

Put the apricot spread in a small microwaveable bowl. Cover with plastic wrap. Microwave at 100 percent power (high) for 15 seconds, or until melted. Let stand for 15 seconds to cool slightly. Using a pastry brush, brush the spread over the pears. Sprinkle with the almonds. Cut into 8 wedges.

PER SERVING

calories 195

total fat 4.5 g

  saturated 1.0 g

  polyunsaturated 0.5 g

  monounsaturated 1.0 g

cholesterol 0 mg

sodium 217 mg

carbohydrates 36 g

  fiber 2 g

  sugar 21 g

protein 3 g

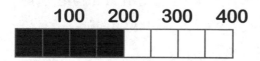

DIETARY EXCHANGES

½ fruit;

2 other carbohydrate;

1 fat

peach and pineapple upside-down cake

Serves 16; 2 x 2-inch piece per serving

Fat-free and fabulous!

Vegetable oil spray

8-ounce can sliced peaches in fruit juice

8-ounce can pineapple tidbits in their own juice

1/3 cup firmly packed light brown sugar

1 1/2 cups whole-wheat pastry flour or all-purpose flour

2 teaspoons baking powder

1/2 teaspoon ground cinnamon

1/2 cup sugar

1/2 cup unsweetened applesauce

Egg substitute equivalent to 1 egg, or 1 large egg

1 teaspoon vanilla extract

Preheat the oven to 350°F. Lightly spray an 8-inch square baking pan with vegetable oil spray.

Drain the peaches and pineapple well, reserving 3/4 cup juice. Chop the peaches.

Sprinkle the brown sugar in the pan. Arrange the peaches and pineapple on the brown sugar.

In a large bowl, stir together the flour, baking powder, and cinnamon. Make a well in the center.

In a medium bowl, whisk together the ¾ cup reserved fruit juice and the remaining ingredients. Pour into the well in the flour mixture. Stir until just combined. Spread the batter in the baking pan.

Bake for 45 minutes, or until a cake tester or wooden toothpick inserted in the center comes out clean. Let cool in the pan on a cooling rack for 5 minutes. Invert onto a plate. Let cool for 30 minutes before serving.

PER SERVING

calories 103
total fat 0.0 g
  saturated 0.0 g
  polyunsaturated 0.0 g
  monounsaturated 0.0 g
cholesterol 0 mg

sodium 62 mg
carbohydrates 24 g
  fiber 1 g
  sugar 15 g
protein 2 g

100 200 300 400 DIETARY EXCHANGES
1½ other carbohydrate

orange and almond pudding cake

Serves 16; 2 x 2-inch piece per serving

While the pudding cake bakes, the batter almost magically separates into two layers. After baking, the top part is a thin layer of spongy cake and the bottom portion is the consistency of pudding or custard.

Vegetable oil spray
1 tablespoon sugar
Whites of 2 large eggs, room temperature
1/8 teaspoon salt
1/2 cup sugar
Egg substitute equivalent to 2 eggs, or 2 large eggs
1/3 cup fat-free or low-fat buttermilk
1 to 2 tablespoons grated orange zest
1/2 cup fresh orange juice
2 tablespoons almond liqueur
1 tablespoon canola or corn oil
3/4 to 1 teaspoon almond extract
1/4 cup all-purpose flour
1 teaspoon baking soda
3 tablespoons chopped almonds

Preheat the oven to 350°F. Lightly spray an 8-inch square baking pan with vegetable oil spray. Coat the bottom and sides of the pan with 1 tablespoon of sugar, shaking out any excess.

In a medium mixing bowl, beat the egg whites and salt with an electric mixer at medium-high speed until stiff peaks form.

In a large mixing bowl, using the same beaters (no need to rinse), beat the 1/2 cup sugar, egg substitute, buttermilk, orange zest, orange juice, liqueur, oil, and almond extract at medium speed for 1 minute, or until the mixture is smooth.

Add the flour and baking soda. Beat at low speed for about 30 seconds, or until the flour is incorporated.

With a rubber or plastic scraper, fold the beaten egg whites into the batter. Pour the batter into the pan. Sprinkle with the almonds.

Place the filled baking pan in a 13 × 9 × 2-inch baking pan. Put the two pans in the oven. Fill the larger pan with hot water to halfway up the sides of the smaller baking pan. (This is known as a water bath.)

Bake for 30 to 35 minutes, or until the top of the cake is golden brown and slightly spongy to the touch. Remove the cake pan from the water bath and put on a cooling rack. Let cool for at least 15 minutes. Serve warm or at room temperature.

VARIATION: Substitute an orange liqueur for the almond liqueur; lemon or orange extract for the almond extract; or chopped walnuts with walnut extract or chopped pecans with maple extract for the almonds and almond extract.

COOK'S TIP ON WATER BATHS: Called **bain-maries** in French, water baths are used for melting ingredients such as butter or chocolate without burning them, or for baking cakes, custards, or cheesecakes where a slow and gentle process is required. To avoid spills, place the two baking pans on the oven rack before you add the water. After the water is in the pan, you can carefully slide the rack back into the oven.

PER SERVING

calories 68
total fat 1.5 g
 saturated 0.0 g
 polyunsaturated 0.5 g
 monounsaturated 1.0 g
cholesterol 0 mg

sodium 125 mg
carbohydrates 11 g
 fiber 0 g
 sugar 9 g
 protein 2 g

100   200   300   400   **DIETARY EXCHANGES**
½ other carbohydrate;
½ fat

clafouti

Serves 8; 1 wedge per serving

You'll find clafouti, usually black cherry, in many French bistros. Substituting an equal amount of other fruit makes a fine dessert, too.

    Vegetable oil spray

1 pound pitted fresh or frozen cherries

2 tablespoons firmly packed light brown sugar

1/2 teaspoon ground cinnamon

1/4 teaspoon ground nutmeg

1 cup fat-free or low-fat buttermilk

    Egg substitute equivalent to 3 eggs

2 teaspoons grated lemon zest

2 tablespoons almond liqueur or fresh lemon juice

1 tablespoon canola or corn oil

1 teaspoon almond extract

1/3 cup all-purpose flour

1/3 cup sugar

1/8 teaspoon salt

Preheat the oven to 375°F. Lightly spray an 8-inch round cake pan with vegetable oil spray.

Place the cherries in the pan. Put the pan on a rimmed baking sheet.

In a small bowl, stir together the brown sugar, cinnamon, and nutmeg.

In a food processor or blender, process the buttermilk, egg substitute, lemon zest, liqueur, oil, and almond extract on medium for 30 seconds. Add the remaining ingredients. Process on high for 30 seconds. Pour the batter over the cherries and top with the brown sugar mixture.

Bake for 55 to 60 minutes, or until puffed and golden brown and a cake tester or wooden toothpick inserted in the center comes out clean. Put the cake pan on a cooling rack. Let cool for about 10 minutes.

PER SERVING

calories 155
total fat 2.0 g
  saturated 0.5 g
  polyunsaturated 0.5 g
  monounsaturated 1.0 g
cholesterol 1 mg

sodium 117 mg
carbohydrates 29 g
  fiber 2 g
  sugar 22 g
protein 4 g

100 200 300 400

DIETARY EXCHANGES
1 fruit;
1 other carbohydrate;
1/2 lean meat

raspberry yogurt cream pie

Serves 8; 1 slice per serving

The aroma of fresh lemon and raspberries baking will make everyone in the house eager for this rich-tasting pie to come out of the oven.

   Vegetable oil spray
1 cup low-fat graham cracker crumbs
3 tablespoons stick margarine, melted

filling

2½ cups fresh or frozen unsweetened raspberries
  3 6-ounce containers fat-free or low-fat French vanilla or vanilla yogurt
¼ cup sugar
   Whites of 2 large eggs
  3 tablespoons all-purpose flour
  2 teaspoons grated lemon zest

Preheat the oven to 350°F. Lightly spray a 10-inch pie plate or springform pan with vegetable oil spray.

In a medium bowl, stir together the graham cracker crumbs and melted margarine. Press the mixture onto the bottom of the pie plate.

Sprinkle the raspberries over the crust.

In a food processor or blender, process the remaining filling ingredients for 30 seconds, or until smooth. Scrape down the side of the work bowl and process again. Pour over the raspberries.

Bake for 1 hour to 1 hour 10 minutes, or until golden brown. Serve warm or cover and refrigerate until needed.

PER SERVING ···

calories 196	sodium 152 mg
total fat 5.0 g	carbohydrates 33 g
saturated 1.0 g	fiber 3 g
polyunsaturated 1.0 g	sugar 22 g
monounsaturated 2.5 g	protein 6 g
cholesterol 1 mg	

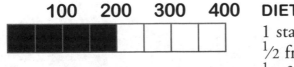

DIETARY EXCHANGES
1 starch; 1 skim milk;
1/2 fruit; 1 fat
1/2 fat

assorted biscotti

Serves 10; 2 cookies per serving

Biscotti are wonderful cookies to dunk in your favorite coffee, tea, or dessert wine. Follow the same basic instructions below for whichever of the three delectable flavors you choose.

cinnamon-walnut biscotti

dry ingredients

2 cups all-purpose flour

1/2 cup sugar

1/2 cup chopped walnuts

1/2 tablespoon baking powder

1/2 teaspoon ground cinnamon

1/4 teaspoon salt

wet ingredients

1 large egg

Whites of 2 large eggs

1/4 cup fat-free milk

....

White of 1 large egg, lightly beaten

dried fruit and marsala biscotti

dry ingredients

    2 cups all-purpose flour

    1/3 cup sugar

    1/2 cup dried cherries, chopped to the size of raisins

    1/2 cup dried apricots, chopped to the size of raisins

    1/2 tablespoon baking powder

    1/4 teaspoon salt

wet ingredients

    1 large egg

    Whites of 2 large eggs

    1/4 cup dry marsala or unsweetened apple juice

    White of 1 large egg, lightly beaten

chocolate chocolate biscotti

dry ingredients

2 cups all-purpose flour

½ cup sugar

½ cup milk chocolate morsels

¼ cup unsweetened cocoa powder

½ tablespoon baking powder

¼ teaspoon salt

wet ingredients

1 large egg

Whites of 2 large eggs

¼ cup fat-free milk (plus up to 2 tablespoons as needed)

....

White of 1 large egg, lightly beaten

Preheat the oven to 375°F. Line a rimmed baking sheet with cooking parchment.

In a large bowl, stir together the dry ingredients. For the Dried Fruit and Marsala Biscotti, be sure the pieces of dried fruit are separated.

In a small bowl, stir together the wet ingredients.

Add the wet ingredients to the dry ingredients. Stir together. If the Chocolate Chocolate Biscotti batter doesn't hold together, gradually stir in the extra milk as needed. Divide the dough in half. Form each half into a log 10 to 12 inches long. Place the logs on the baking sheet. Brush with the remaining egg white.

Bake the Cinnamon-Walnut Biscotti and the Dried Fruit and Marsala Biscotti for 15 to 20 minutes, or until the top is golden. Bake the Chocolate Chocolate Biscotti for 20 minutes. Leave the oven on.

Let cool on a cooling rack for 5 minutes. Cut each log on the diagonal into 10 slices. Place the slices with one cut side up on the baking sheet.

Bake for 10 to 15 minutes, or until the cut side of the Cinnamon-Walnut Biscotti and the Dried Fruit and Marsala Biscotti is golden and the Chocolate Chocolate Biscotti is firm to the touch.

Let cool completely on a cooling rack. Store the biscotti in an airtight container for up to two weeks at room temperature or freeze them for up to three months.

CINNAMON-WALNUT BISCOTTI

PER SERVING

calories 184
total fat 4.5 g
 saturated 0.5 g
 polyunsaturated 3.0 g
 monounsaturated 0.5 g
cholesterol 21 mg

sodium 146 mg
carbohydrates 30 g
 fiber 1 g
 sugar 11 g
 protein 5 g

100 200 300 400

DIETARY EXCHANGES
2 starch; $\frac{1}{2}$ fat

DRIED FRUIT AND MARSALA BISCOTTI

PER SERVING

calories 183
total fat 1.0 g
  saturated 0.0 g
  polyunsaturated 0.0 g
  monounsaturated 0.0 g
cholesterol 21 mg

sodium 143 mg
carbohydrates 37 g
  fiber 1 g
  sugar 14 g
protein 5 g

100   200   300   400

DIETARY EXCHANGES
$1\frac{1}{2}$ starch; 1 fruit

CHOCOLATE CHOCOLATE BISCOTTI

PER SERVING

calories 198
total fat 3.5 g
  saturated 1.5 g
  polyunsaturated 0.0 g
  monounsaturated 1.5 g
cholesterol 23 mg

sodium 152 mg
carbohydrates 36 g
  fiber 1 g
  sugar 15 g
protein 6 g

100   200   300   400

DIETARY EXCHANGES
2 starch; $\frac{1}{2}$ other
carbohydrate; $\frac{1}{2}$ fat

peach and berry crumble

Serves 4; 1/2 cup per serving

You can whip this up for a little cozy comfort, regardless of the season.

Vegetable oil spray
1 pound frozen unsweetened peach slices, thawed and halved, or 12 ounces peach slices and 4 ounces frozen unsweetened raspberries
1/3 cup dried sweetened cranberries
2 teaspoons cornstarch
2 teaspoons fresh orange juice or water
1/2 teaspoon vanilla extract
1/3 cup uncooked quick-cooking oats
1/4 cup sugar
1 tablespoon flour
1/4 teaspoon ground cinnamon
2 tablespoons light tub margarine

Preheat the oven to 350°F. Lightly spray a nonstick 8 × 4-inch loaf pan with vegetable oil spray.

In a medium bowl, stir together the peaches, cranberries, cornstarch, orange juice, and vanilla until the cornstarch is dissolved.

Pour the peach mixture into the pan.

In a small bowl, combine the remaining ingredients except the margarine. Using 2 knives, cut the margarine into the oat mixture until it has a coarse texture and the pieces are about the size of small peas. Sprinkle over the peach mixture.

Bake for 25 minutes, or until the peaches are tender. Remove from the oven.

Preheat the broiler. Broil the crumble for 3 to 4 minutes, or until the topping begins to brown. Remove from the broiler and let stand for about 30 minutes to allow the flavors to blend.

PER SERVING

calories 191
total fat 3.5 g
  saturated 0.0 g
  polysaturated 1.0 g
  monosaturated 1.5 g
cholesterol 0 mg

sodium 46 mg
carbohydrates 38 g
  fiber 4 g
  sugar 26 g
protein 2 g

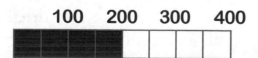

100 200 300 400

DIETARY EXCHANGES
1 fruit; $1\frac{1}{2}$ other carbohydrate; $\frac{1}{2}$ fat

applesauce oatmeal cookies
Serves 12; 2 cookies per serving

These cookies are chewy and not too sweet—the perfect after-school or anytime snack. If you need to serve a crowd, just double the ingredients.

    Vegetable oil spray
1/2 cup unsweetened applesauce
1 1/2 cups uncooked rolled oats
1 cup whole-wheat pastry flour or all-purpose flour
1 teaspoon baking soda
1/2 teaspoon ground cinnamon
1/4 teaspoon salt
1/3 cup dried apple slices, cut into small pieces
1/4 cup sugar
1/4 cup firmly packed light brown sugar
1 tablespoon plus 1 teaspoon canola or corn oil
1/4 teaspoon vanilla extract

Preheat the oven to 350°F. Lightly spray two baking sheets with vegetable oil spray.

Place a strainer over a small bowl. Pour the applesauce into the strainer and let drain for about 10 minutes. Discard the liquid.

Meanwhile, in a medium bowl, stir together the oats, flour, baking soda, cinnamon, and salt.

In another medium bowl, stir together the dried apples, sugar, brown sugar, oil, and vanilla.

Stir the drained applesauce into the apple mixture. Stir into the oat mixture.

Drop by heaping teaspoonfuls, about 2 inches apart, onto the baking sheets. Using clean hands or the back of a spoon, flatten the cookies to 1/4-inch thickness. (The dough will be sticky.)

Bake for 12 to 15 minutes, or until the cookies begin to brown. Leave the cookies on the cookie sheets for 5 to 10 minutes, or until the cookies hold their shape, before transferring to a cooling rack. Let cool completely.

COOK'S TIP ON MAKING UNIFORM COOKIES: A small ice cream scoop with a releasing handle is ideal for portioning out cookies of uniform size.

PER SERVING

calories 105
total fat 2.0 g
 saturated 0.0 g
 polyunsaturated 0.5 g
 monounsaturated 1.0 g
cholesterol 0 mg

sodium 135 mg
carbohydrates 20 g
 fiber 2 g
 sugar 10 g
protein 2 g

100 200 300 400

DIETARY EXCHANGES
1 starch;
1/2 other carbohydrate

apple and pear strudel
Serves 8; 1 slice per serving

Using frozen phyllo dough really reduces the preparation time for this mouthwatering dessert.

Vegetable oil spray

filling

4 baking apples, such as McIntosh or Rome, peeled, cored, and thinly sliced

1 Anjou or Bartlett pear, thinly sliced

1/3 cup sugar

1/4 cup raisins or diced dried apricots

1 tablespoon all-purpose flour

2 teaspoons ground cinnamon

1/4 teaspoon ground nutmeg

pastry

White of 1 large egg

2 tablespoons light olive oil

Dash of salt

6 sheets frozen phyllo dough, thawed

2 tablespoons plain dry bread crumbs

1 teaspoon sugar

Set the oven rack on the upper level of the oven. Preheat the oven to 350°F. Lightly spray a baking sheet with vegetable oil spray.

In a large bowl, stir together the filling ingredients.

In a small bowl, lightly beat together the egg white, oil, and salt.

Keeping the unused phyllo covered with a damp cloth or damp paper towels to prevent drying, lay a sheet of phyllo with one long side toward you on a flat work surface. Working quickly, use a pastry brush to lightly coat the surface of the phyllo sheet with the egg white mixture. Sprinkle evenly with $1/2$ teaspoon bread crumbs. Repeat with the remaining phyllo and bread crumbs, making a stack of the 6 phyllo sheets.

Spread the apple mixture along the long side of the dough nearest you. Starting at that side, roll up jelly-roll style into a cylinder. Place the roll with the seam side down on the baking sheet. Brush with the remaining egg white mixture. Sprinkle with 1 teaspoon sugar.

Bake for 25 to 30 minutes, or until golden brown. Remove from the oven and let cool slightly on the baking sheet. Cut into 8 slices (a bread knife works well for this). While the strudel is warm, transfer to plates.

COOK'S TIP: To serve the next day, reheat the strudel, uncovered, in a preheated 350°F oven for 10 minutes.

COOK'S TIP ON LIGHT OLIVE OIL: Light olive oil has a milder flavor than regular olive oil. The calories and the fat are the same, however.

PER SERVING

calories 191
total fat 4.0 g
 saturated 0.5 g
 polyunsaturated 0.5 g
 monounsaturated 2.5 g
cholesterol 0 mg

sodium 108 mg
carbohydrates 38 g
 fiber 2 g
 sugar 21 g
 protein 2 g

100 200 300 400 **DIETARY EXCHANGES**
1 starch; 1½ fruit;
½ fat

coconut-lime flan

Serves 12; 1 slice per serving

A sprinkling of toasted coconut enhances this melt-in-your-mouth, custard-style dessert, already bursting with lime zest, coconut extract, and gingerroot.

$\frac{1}{3}$ cup sugar

3 tablespoons water

14-ounce can fat-free sweetened condensed milk

1 cup fat-free evaporated milk

Egg substitute equivalent to 4 eggs

1 tablespoon grated lime zest

2 teaspoons grated peeled gingerroot

1 teaspoon coconut extract

$\frac{1}{3}$ cup shredded sweetened coconut

In a small, heavy saucepan, heat the sugar and water over low heat for 2 to 3 minutes, or until the sugar dissolves, stirring occasionally. Increase the heat to medium high and bring to a boil. Cook for 8 to 10 minutes, or until the mixture is a caramel color, swirling the pan occasionally to stir. (Don't use a spoon. Sugar crystals could cling to it and cause the mixture to crystallize.) Watch carefully to be sure the mixture doesn't burn. Pour into a 1-quart round flan pan or 9-inch round glass pie dish. Let cool for at least 15 minutes.

Preheat the oven to 325°F.

In a medium bowl, whisk together the remaining ingredients except the coconut. Pour over the cooled syrup. Place the flan pan on a 17 × 12 × 1-inch rimmed baking sheet. Fill the rimmed baking sheet half full with warm water. Or place the flan pan in a baking pan and add warm water to a depth of 1 inch.

Bake in the center of the oven for 1 hour, or until a knife inserted in the center comes out clean. Remove the pan from the baking sheet and set on a cooling rack. Let cool for 30 minutes. Cover with plastic wrap and refrigerate for 2 to 48 hours.

Meanwhile, in a small nonstick skillet, dry-roast the coconut over medium-low heat for 3 to 4 minutes, or until golden brown, stirring occasionally.

To unmold the flan, run a knife around the side of the pan. Invert onto a rimmed serving plate deep enough to hold the flan and the caramelized liquid.

To serve, cut into 12 slices. Sprinkle each slice with coconut.

PER SERVING

calories 156
total fat 1.0 g
 saturated 1.0 g
 polyunsaturated 0.0 g
 monounsaturated 0.0 g
cholesterol 3 mg

sodium 107 mg
carbohydrates 30 g
 fiber 0 g
 sugar 30 g
protein 6 g

100 200 300 400 **DIETARY EXCHANGES**
2 other carbohydrate;
1 very lean meat

pumpkin praline mousse
Serves 10; ½ cup per serving

An alternative to traditional pumpkin pie, this mousse is unbelievably delicious. If you're in a hurry or want to cut a few calories, leave off the praline topping.

       30-ounce can pumpkin pie mix
       (not canned pumpkin)
  8 ounces frozen fat-free or light whipped
       topping, thawed
  ½ teaspoon vanilla extract
       Vegetable oil spray

praline topping
  ¼ cup sugar
  ¼ cup chopped pecans
  ½ teaspoon ground cinnamon

  4 ounces frozen fat-free or light whipped
       topping, thawed

In a large mixing bowl, beat the pumpkin pie filling, 8 ounces whipped topping, and vanilla with an electric mixer on medium high for 2 to 4 minutes, or until light and fluffy.

   Spoon the mousse into a large serving bowl or 10 ramekins or stemmed glasses. Cover with plastic wrap and refrigerate for at least 1 hour before serving.

Meanwhile, line a small baking sheet with aluminum foil. Lightly spray with vegetable oil spray.

In a small, heavy skillet, cook the sugar over medium heat for 6 to 10 minutes, or until it dissolves and liquefies, stirring frequently with a heatproof spoon. Stir in the pecans and cinnamon. Reduce the heat to low and cook for 30 seconds to 1 minute, or until golden.

Remove from the heat and quickly spread the pecan mixture onto the foil-lined baking sheet. Let it cool completely, 10 to 15 minutes. Break the topping into small pieces.

To serve, spoon the whipped topping over the mousse. Sprinkle with the praline topping.

COOK'S TIP: You can make the praline topping several days in advance. Store it in an airtight container. Be sure to use a heatproof spoon when making the topping; a rubber spatula will melt.

PER SERVING

calories 188
total fat 2.5 g
  saturated 0.0 g
  polyunsaturated 0.5 g
  monounsaturated 1.0 g
cholesterol 0 mg

sodium 134 mg
carbohydrates 37 g
  fiber 2 g
  sugar 26 g
protein 1 g

100 200 300 400

DIETARY EXCHANGES
$2^{1}/_{2}$ other carbohydrate; $^{1}/_{2}$ fat

vanilla soufflé with brandy-plum sauce

Serves 6; 1 cup soufflé and 2 tablespoons sauce per serving

The drama of serving soufflés right from the oven is hard to beat. Adding a warm brandy-plum sauce takes this dessert to center stage.

Vegetable oil spray

1/4 cup sugar

3/4 cup fat-free milk

1/4 cup sugar

Egg substitute equivalent to 2 eggs, or 2 large eggs

1 tablespoon cornstarch

4 ounces egg whites or whites of 4 large eggs

1/8 teaspoon cream of tartar

1/4 cup sugar

brandy-plum sauce

3/4 cup fat-free or low-fat vanilla yogurt

3 tablespoons plum jam

1 tablespoon brandy

Preheat the oven to 350°F. Lightly spray six 1-cup soufflé dishes with vegetable oil spray. Sprinkle 2 teaspoons of the sugar in each dish. Turn each dish to coat thoroughly. Place the dishes on a rimmed baking sheet.

In a medium nonaluminum saucepan, stir together the milk and ¼ cup sugar. Cook over medium-low heat just to the boiling point, about 8 minutes.

In a medium bowl, whisk together the egg substitute and cornstarch until the cornstarch is completely absorbed.

In very small amounts, pour the hot milk mixture into the egg substitute mixture, whisking constantly. Transfer the mixture to the saucepan.

Cook over medium-low heat for about 12 minutes, or until the egg substitute mixture thickens into a pastry cream (custardlike thickness, like pudding before it sets), stirring constantly and vigorously to keep the eggs from scrambling and being careful to stir the entire bottom, including the edge, of the pan. Remove from the heat. Let cool for 10 minutes.

In a large glass or stainless steel mixing bowl, beat the egg whites and cream of tartar with an electric mixer at high speed for 2 minutes, or until soft peaks form. Continuing to beat at high speed, gradually add ¼ cup sugar, 1 tablespoon at a time. Beat for about 3 minutes, or until the egg whites are very stiff and resemble marshmallow creme.

Transfer the pastry cream to a large bowl. Stir in 1 cup stiff egg whites. Carefully fold in the remaining egg whites. Spoon the mixture into the prepared soufflé dishes.

Bake on the baking sheet for 19 minutes, or until the soufflés have risen about 1 inch above the rim of the dish and are lightly brown on top.

Meanwhile, in a small microwaveable bowl, stir together the yogurt and plum jam. Microwave for 1 minute at 100 percent power (high). Stir. Microwave for 30 seconds, or until warm to the touch. Stir in the brandy.

Serve the soufflés as soon as you remove them from the oven. (They will quickly begin to lose air and collapse.) After serving, spoon about 2 tablespoons sauce into the center of each.

COOK'S TIP ON PASTRY CREAM: Aluminum will discolor the pastry cream, so use a stainless steel saucepan or enamel saucepan. And stir, stir, stir while the pastry cream mixture is coming together. If bits of cooked (scrambled) eggs appear in the pastry cream, strain or push the pastry cream through a fine stainless steel sieve to remove the egg bits.

PER SERVING

calories 191
total fat 0.0 g
 saturated 0.0 g
 polyunsaturated 0.0 g
 monounsaturated 0.0 g
cholesterol 1 mg

sodium 110 mg
carbohydrates 40 g
 fiber 0 g
 sugar 38 g
protein 7 g

100 200 300 400

DIETARY EXCHANGES
3½ other carbohydrate;
1 very lean meat

chocolate-hazelnut fondue

Serves 8; $1/2$ cup fruit and marshmallows and 2 tablespoons sauce per serving

If you're a chocoholic, this recipe is for you. Strawberries, pineapple, and bananas never had it so good!

1 cup fresh strawberries, halved if large
1 cup fresh pineapple chunks
1 cup thickly sliced banana
1 cup large marshmallows

chocolate-hazelnut sauce

$3/4$ cup fat-free chocolate syrup
$1/4$ cup bottled chocolate-hazelnut spread
$1/4$ teaspoon vanilla extract

Put the strawberries, pineapple, banana, and marshmallows in separate bowls.

In a small, heavy saucepan, stir together the sauce ingredients. Heat over medium heat for 4 to 5 minutes, or until heated through, stirring frequently.

Pour the sauce into a serving dish or small fondue pot. Serve warm or at room temperature. (As it cools, the sauce will thicken slightly.)

To serve, spear the fruit and marshmallows with fondue forks or bamboo skewers and dip into the fondue.

chocolate-hazelnut sundae

Serves 8; ½ cup frozen yogurt and 2 tablespoons sauce per serving

Prepare the chocolate-hazelnut sauce as directed above. Substitute 1 quart fat-free frozen vanilla yogurt for the fruit and marshmallows. For each serving, spoon ½ cup frozen yogurt into a bowl. Top with 2 tablespoons sauce.

COOK'S TIP ON BANANAS: To keep the banana slices from turning brown, dip them in a small amount of orange, lemon, or pineapple juice.

CHOCOLATE-HAZELNUT FONDUE

PER SERVING

calories 173
total fat 2.5 g
  saturated 0.5 g
  polyunsaturated 0.5 g
  monounsaturated 1.5 g
cholesterol 0 mg

sodium 27 mg
carbohydrates 38 g
  fiber 1 g
  sugar 25 g
  protein 1 g

100	200	300	400

DIETARY EXCHANGES
$\frac{1}{2}$ fruit; 2 other
carbohydrate; $\frac{1}{2}$ fat

CHOCOLATE-HAZELNUT FONDUE

PER SERVING

calories 202
total fat 2.0 g
  saturated 0.5 g
  polyunsaturated 0.5 g
  monounsaturated 1.5 g
cholesterol 1 mg

sodium 62 mg
carbohydrates 42 g
  fiber 0 g
  sugar 34 g
  protein 4 g

100	200	300	400

DIETARY EXCHANGES
3 other carbohydrate;
$\frac{1}{2}$ fat

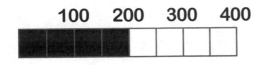

fruit sauce

Serves 8; 2 tablespoons per serving

Expand your culinary horizons by experimenting with two classic, fragrant spices—cardamom and mace. This so-easy, velvety sauce is a great place to begin.

1 medium mango, diced

1/2 cup canned apricot halves in extra-light syrup, drained

2 tablespoons fresh orange juice

1 tablespoon light brown sugar

1 teaspoon grated lemon zest

1/8 teaspoon ground cardamom or allspice

1/8 teaspoon ground mace or nutmeg

In a food processor or blender, process all the ingredients for 1 to 2 minutes, or until smooth.

Serve immediately, cover and refrigerate for up to four days, or heat in a small saucepan over medium-low heat for 2 to 3 minutes, or until warmed through, stirring occasionally.

fruit and yogurt sauce

Serves 12; 2 tablespoons per serving

For a yogurt-enhanced fruit sauce, stir $1/2$ cup fat-free or light vanilla yogurt into the finished sauce. This version is best served chilled.

COOK'S TIP ON CARDAMOM AND MACE: Cardamom pods hold several small black seeds that are very fragrant. You can grind the seeds with a mortar and pestle or purchase cardamom already ground. Visit a gourmet grocery that sells spices by the ounce so you can experiment with small amounts at a reasonable cost. Mace is the ground outer covering of nutmeg and is used to flavor both savory and sweet dishes. Its taste is similar to that of nutmeg, although a bit more intense and slightly spicy, which is why nutmeg is a handy substitute.

FRUIT SAUCE

PER SERVING

calories 33

total fat 0.0 g
  saturated 0.0 g
  polyunsaturated 0.0 g
  monounsaturated 0.0 g
cholesterol 0 mg

sodium 2 mg
carbohydrates 9 g
  fiber 1 g
  sugar 8 g
protein 0 g

100 200 300 400

DIETARY EXCHANGES
$^1/_2$ fruit

FRUIT AND YOGURT SAUCE

PER SERVING

calories 31

total fat 0.0 g
  saturated 0.0 g
  polyunsaturated 0.0 g
  monounsaturated 0.0 g
cholesterol 0 mg

sodium 8 mg
carbohydrates 7 g
  fiber 1 g
  sugar 7 g
protein 1 g

100 200 300 400

DIETARY EXCHANGES
$^1/_2$ fruit

blueberry dream dessert squares

Serves 16; 1 piece per serving

Combining the tang of blueberries and sour cream with the sweetness of sugar and dessert topping, these chilled fruit squares are a dreamy way to end a meal.

    Vegetable oil spray
1 cup low-fat graham cracker crumbs
3 tablespoons stick margarine, melted

filling

2/3 cup sugar
2 envelopes unflavored gelatin (1/4 ounce each)
1 cup hot water
2 cups fat-free or low-fat blueberry yogurt
1 cup fat-free or light sour cream
1/2 cup fat-free milk
1 envelope dessert topping mix
1 teaspoon vanilla extract
2 cups fresh or frozen blueberries, thawed and patted dry with paper towels if frozen

Preheat the oven to 350°F. Lightly spray a 13 × 9 × 2-inch baking pan with vegetable oil spray.

In a medium bowl, stir together the graham cracker crumbs and margarine. Press the mixture onto the bottom of the pan.

Bake for 10 minutes. Let cool for about 20 minutes.

Meanwhile, in a medium saucepan, stir together the sugar and gelatin. Pour in the water. Cook over medium heat for about 5 minutes, or until the mixture is syrupy and the gelatin is dissolved, stirring constantly. Pour into a large bowl and refrigerate for about 15 minutes, or until completely cooled.

Fold the yogurt and sour cream into the sugar mixture.

Put the milk, topping mix, and vanilla in a medium mixing bowl. Using an electric mixer, beat on high for about 3 minutes, or until stiff. Fold into the yogurt mixture. Fold in the blueberries. Pour into the prepared crust.

Refrigerate, uncovered, for about 4 hours, or until firm. Cut into 16 pieces.

PER SERVING

calories 143
total fat 3.0 g
  saturated 1.0 g
  polyunsaturated 0.5 g
  monounsaturated 1.5 g
cholesterol 4 mg

sodium 90 mg
carbohydrates 26 g
  fiber 1 g
  sugar 19 g
protein 4 g

100 200 300 400

DIETARY EXCHANGES
$\frac{1}{2}$ skim milk; 1 other carbohydrate; $\frac{1}{2}$ fat

citrus freeze bars

Serves 15; 3 x 1¾-inch bar per serving

A nice balance of sweet and tart makes this a dessert you'll want to keep on hand in your freezer. Best of all, it takes only minutes to prepare.

Vegetable oil spray
25 reduced-fat vanilla wafers
14-ounce can fat-free sweetened condensed milk
Egg substitute equivalent to 1 egg (do not use unpasteurized egg)
1 to 2 teaspoons grated lime or lemon zest
⅔ cup fresh lime or lemon juice
8 ounces frozen fat-free or light whipped topping, thawed
5 reduced-fat vanilla wafers

Lightly spray a 9-inch square baking pan with vegetable oil spray. Arrange the 25 cookies in a single layer in the pan. (There will be spaces between the cookies.)

Pour the milk and egg substitute into a medium bowl. Add the lime zest and lime juice. Stir for 3 to 4 minutes, or until the mixture begins to thicken. Fold in the whipped topping. Pour over the cookies in the baking pan.

Crumble the remaining 5 cookies over the filling. Cover with plastic wrap and put in the freezer for about 4 hours, or until frozen.

To serve, let thaw for 4 to 5 minutes, or just until the bars are cuttable. Cut into 15 bars.

PER SERVING

calories 135

total fat 0.5 g

  saturated 0.0 g

  polyunsaturated 0.0 g

  monounsaturated 0.0 g

cholesterol 1 mg

sodium 70 mg

carbohydrates 28 g

  fiber 0 g

  sugar 21 g

protein 3 g

100   200   300   400

DIETARY EXCHANGES
2 other carbohydrate

Part III

APPENDIXES

APPENDIX A:
shopping

When you want to lose weight and eat healthfully, a trip to the grocery store can feel like walking into the lion's den. It doesn't have to be that way. Never before have so many healthful options been so widely available. Concentrate on the multitude of foods you can enjoy. The variety they provide is key to spicing up your daily eating plan and making sure you get all the nutrients your body needs. Since food appeals to almost all our senses—sight, smell, touch, and taste—let grocery shopping be part of the sensory experience.

make the "thyme" to grocery shop

Consider doing your major grocery shopping once a week if you don't already. It will take a bit of time, but so does making those daily stops. The fewer shopping trips, the less opportunity for temptation. Also, planning ahead can help you fit in the proper daily and weekly amounts of various food groups (see the American Heart Association guidelines on pages 66–71 and "Part II: Menu Planning and

Recipes," pages 150–155). It will be worth the effort in executing healthful meal planning. As you incorporate grocery shopping into your weekly schedule, it will become part of your routine. Try it; let shopping become an important stop on your path to success!

general tips for the trip

- Avoid shopping when you feel hungry. Grab a healthful snack beforehand to suppress your appetite. That way, unhealthful foods won't be so tempting.

- Don't buy what advertisers are selling if it's not what you need. Remember that they spend a lot of money and brainpower to make you want to buy their products.

- Don't be enticed by sales or specials. Recognize that saving a few cents on a "good deal" will cost you much more than money if it adds useless calories to your diet.

- Bring a grocery list—even if you need only a few items—and stick to it unless you see some fresh products you want to include.

- Organize your list by category to save time going back and forth between departments.

- Identify foods that you buy out of habit but could eliminate or cut back on, such as ice cream or sugary drinks. If you don't buy them, they won't be in your kitchen to tempt you.

- Read the Nutrition Facts label on food products for serving size and servings per container, plus number of calories and amount of total fat, saturated fat, cholesterol, sodium, and more for each serving. These numbers make it easier for you to monitor your calorie consumption.

- Be careful of those marketing labels on the front of the package. Just because a product proudly proclaims it is low fat, low carb, or low sodium doesn't necessarily mean it's your best choice. The food may be loaded with sugar, fat, sodium, or calories. Keep in mind that ingredients are listed in order from greatest to least amounts.

mapping out a shopping plan

Think about the layout of your favorite grocery store. Processed foods usually are in the middle aisles, so plan to do most of your shopping along the perimeter, where the produce, dairy items, and seafood and meats are likely to be. Now, with your list in hand, it's time for your shopping trip!

vital veggies and flavorful fruit

Make the produce department your first stop. Think color when shopping for fruits and vegetables. Be sure to include dark green vegetables, such as broccoli, spinach, and dark green lettuces. Carrots, sweet potatoes, oranges, grapefruit, cantaloupe, and winter squash healthfully fulfill the need for foods in the yellow and orange palettes. For red, enjoy tomatoes, red bell peppers, and strawberries. Be adventurous and try new fruits and vegetables often. Aim for at least five servings each day from the vegetables and fruits category.

the main grain

For some of your four or more daily servings of grains and other starches, you might want to start with bread or rolls to complement your dinner. The most nutrient-rich breads are made of 100 percent whole grains. Look for whole wheat as the first ingredient on the label. Multi- and whole-grain and pumpernickel breads and rolls are other good choices. Limit your consumption of white breads since they have far less nutritional value than those made from whole grains. The same is true for pasta. When possible, choose the whole-wheat varieties instead of those that are more processed. When buying rice, choose wild or brown varieties. They are much more nutritious and flavorful than white rice, which loses many of its nutrients during processing.

gone fishin'!

Next, stop by the seafood department. Ask what's the freshest catch and, if you won't be preparing it right away, how to store it. Try to have at least two servings of fish, preferably fatty fish, per week. Salmon and tuna, both rich in omega-3 fatty acids, are excellent choices.

chicken little

When buying poultry, remember that white meat is leaner than dark meat, and one portion of boneless, skinless chicken or turkey should be about 4 ounces raw. Even the chicken breast halves that you buy in the grocery store are likely to be more than one serving.

the meating place

Choose lean cuts of meat and keep serving sizes to about 4 ounces raw, after trimming all the visible fat and removing any bones. That 1-pound sirloin should feed four people, not one or two! Choose cuts of beef marked Select; they are leaner than Prime or Choice. Round steak, sirloin steak, flank steak, and tenderloin are all good choices. As an alternative to red meat, try pork. For the leanest cuts, choose tenderloin, center-cut roasts, and loin chops.

hi-ho, the dairy-o

Be sure to plan on three or more daily servings of dairy products (see page 68 for details), preferably fat free or low fat. The difference in calories between those and whole-milk dairy products is huge. Products such as fat-free half-and-half or fat-free evaporated milk can be a great help in satisfying your craving for that rich dairy taste without the calories.

fit fats

Fats and oils are essential, even while you are dieting. Knowing what to use and in what amount is key. The less solid the fat, the better it is for you. That's because the softer the margarine, the less hydrogenated it is and the less trans fat it contains. When using margarine, fat-free spray is best. Squeeze and tub margarines are better choices than stick margarine, and light stick margarine is better than regular. Choose a margarine with unsaturated vegetable oil listed as the first ingredient. Check the label to be sure the margarine has fewer than 2 grams of saturated fat per tablespoon and 0 grams of trans fat. When using oil, choose polyunsaturated and monounsaturated oils to replace saturated fats. Select oil with a maximum of 2 grams of saturated fat per tablespoon. Olive oil and canola oil are good choices; other acceptable choices include almond, corn, safflower, sesame, soybean, sunflower, and walnut oils. Be sure to pick up at least one variety of nonstick vegetable oil spray for cooking. Limit yourself to 5 teaspoons of fat (most of them monounsaturated and polyunsaturated) each day. Remember to count what is in prepared foods, such as salad dressing and baked goods, as well as in margarine and oil. Avoid saturated fats, such as butter, shortening, coconut or palm oil, and lard.

hydration station

When buying beverages, be especially watchful for the hidden calories. Instead of high-calorie sodas and fruit drinks, buy club soda, flavored waters, and sugar-free drinks. Use fresh lemons, limes, or oranges to add a punch of flavor. Drink fruit juice or vegetable juice sparingly to fulfill your servings of healthful fruits, and look for 100 percent unsweetened varieties. These juices are more nutritious by far than many other beverages, but they don't provide the fiber you'll get by eating the fruit or vegetable the juices come from.

the other fast food

Feel fishy tonight but don't have any seafood at home? Be open to supplementing your weekly shopping trip with spur-of-the-moment choices that fit into your eating plan.

- Stop at the grocery store for healthful dinner ingredients instead of picking up fast food. Just concentrate on what you need for one meal so you're not tempted to fill your cart with junk food. Before you get to the store, jot down a quick list to keep yourself focused.

- Keep frozen or pantry-ready meals on hand so you have some fallback choices.

- Have the makings of a few low-calorie appetizers (see pages 244–269 for examples) on hand for last-minute guests.

- Make extras of your favorite recipes and freeze individual portions. It's an easy way to keep track of portion size, and you'll increase your "bank" of available options for last-minute meals and snacks.

  As you transition to more healthful eating habits, your shopping patterns—and what you put in your shopping cart—will change. Even small differences in those habits can yield big results. Congratulate yourself as you see how much progress you make.

foods to have on hand for preparing a quick meal

It's a good idea to stock your kitchen with products you can easily use to prepare a speedy and healthful meal. Think about the food groups and serving sizes mentioned on page 68. Look again at the menus we created (pages 158–229) and the ones you came up with on your own. Then combine your choices from the categories below for a quick answer to the "what's for dinner" question.

VEGETABLES

Fresh vegetables
Frozen vegetables (without sauce)
Canned vegetables (no-salt-added)
Packaged salad greens

FRUITS

Fresh fruit
Frozen fruit (unsweetened)
Canned fruit (in water, its own juice, or extra-light or light syrup)

BREADS, GRAINS, AND STARCHES

Frozen waffles (fat-free or low-fat)
Cereals (whole grain, hot and cold)
Sweet, white, or red potatoes
Beans, such as navy, pinto, red, black, or kidney (no-salt-added if canned)
Whole-wheat pasta
Whole-wheat couscous

Brown rice

Whole-wheat flour tortillas (fat-free or low-fat)

SEAFOOD

Fresh tuna or canned tuna (in distilled or spring water or in pouch)

Fresh salmon, canned salmon, or salmon in pouch

Fresh or frozen halibut, swordfish, or trout

MEATS AND POULTRY

Chicken breasts

Lean ground beef

Ground chicken or turkey (ground without skin)

Sirloin or flank steak

Lean pork chops

Pork tenderloin

MEAT SUBSTITUTES

Meatless (soy protein) sausage

Frozen vegetarian burgers (reduced-fat)

DAIRY

Cheese (fat-free or low-fat)

Plain yogurt (fat-free or low-fat)

Sour cream (fat-free or low-fat)

Canned evaporated milk (fat-free)

Fat-free milk

MISCELLANEOUS

Liquid egg substitute

Tomato paste (no-salt-added)

Meatless spaghetti sauce (fat-free, reduced-sodium)

Tomato sauce (no-salt-added)

Dry red or white wine (regular or nonalcoholic)

Salad dressing (fat-free or light)

Plain dry bread crumbs

Salsa (low-sodium)

Olive, canola, or corn oil

Fat-free spray margarine

Light tub margarine

Whole-wheat flour

Vinegar, such as balsamic, red wine, or plain rice

All-purpose seasoning (salt-free)

Cream of mushroom soup, condensed (low-fat, reduced-sodium)

Cream of chicken soup, condensed (low-fat, reduced-sodium)

Canned chicken broth (fat-free, low-sodium)

Canned beef broth (fat-free, no-salt-added)

Canned vegetable broth (low-sodium)

Soy sauce (low-sodium)

Tomato or mixed-vegetable juice (low-sodium)

american heart association food certification program

Look to the American Heart Association Food Certification Program for additional help in food selection. The program's heart-check mark is an easy, reliable tool you can use to quickly identify products that are heart-healthy. The heart-check mark on food packages indicates that the product meets the American Heart Association food criteria for saturated fat and cholesterol for healthy people over age two.

For a list of certified products, visit heartcheckmark.org. Use the online "Grocery List Builder" to create and print a heart-healthy shopping list you can take to the store.

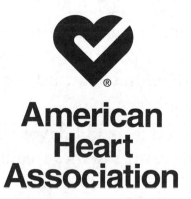

American Heart Association

Meets American Heart Association
food criteria for saturated fat and cholesterol
for healthy people over age 2.

APPENDIX B: cooking

How do you cook healthfully without sacrificing flavor? Our recipe developers are charged with creating delicious dishes that meet the American Heart Association standards for heart health. They have learned lots of ways to add flavor but not calories, and they are passing some of their expertise along to you.

tricks of the trade

Use the following tricks of the trade for a more healthful approach to cooking.

THE MEAT OF THE MATTER

- Remove and discard all visible fat before cooking meats and poultry. Either cook poultry without the skin or discard the skin before serving the poultry.

- Marinate foods to add flavor and tenderize meat and poultry. Wines (regular or nonalcoholic, but not sodium-laden cooking wines), fruit or vegetable juices, and low-calorie, low-sodium broths, flavored with different vinegars, herbs, and spices, are all good choices for the marinade.

- After you roast or broil meats, use a fat separator to remove fat from the drippings. If you don't own that handy utensil, pour the drippings into a cup. Cover and refrigerate overnight. The hardened fat will rise to the top and will be easy to remove. Use the remaining rich essence to make natural gravy or to flavor other meat-based dishes.

- Use the same trick for stews and some soups. Cover and refrigerate them overnight, then remove the hardened fat. Such foods usually taste better the next day anyway, and you'll be doing your body a favor.

- Try shredding or finely chopping vegetables to stretch ground poultry or ground meat. You'll cut calories and your grocery bill!

EAT YOUR VEGGIES

- Wrap cooked veggies in edible pouches of lettuce or steamed cabbage leaves. Add herbs, spices, or low-calorie sauces for extra flavor.

- Steam or microwave vegetables with only a small amount of liquid so they retain their flavor and nutrients.

- Bake vegetables in a little low-fat or fat-free stock, or in wine or water. Experiment with herbs to vary the flavor.

- Add chopped fresh herbs or ground spices rather than margarine to season cooked vegetables.

DRESS UP THE SAUCES IN LOW-CAL STYLE

- Thicken soups, stews, sauces, and gravies with pureed cooked (even leftover) vegetables. Add gingerroot, lemon or lime zest, chile peppers, or garlic to flavor basic sauces.
- Mix fat-free or low-fat buttermilk, plain yogurt, fat-free sour cream, flavored vinegars, or fruit juices into regular salad dressings and sauces to cut back on the calories and fat.
- To capture flavor without adding unnecessary calories, reduce sauces by boiling the liquid until it is about half the original volume. For a creamier sauce, remove the sauce from the heat and add a small amount of fat-free half-and-half or fat-free evaporated milk.

tools of the trade

Having the right equipment to work with can make low-calorie cooking easier to do. Here is a list of some of the tools we find helpful.

- Nonstick pots and pans, including a large skillet with a tight-fitting lid.

- Good-quality, sharp knives. You're more likely to cut yourself with a dull knife, and you'll waste a lot of time with all that extra sawing back and forth.

- A roasting pan with a rack.

- A ridged stovetop grill pan, especially if you don't have an outdoor grill.

- A collapsible metal steamer or a set of Chinese bamboo steamers. A spaghetti cooker can double as a steamer.

- A fat separator.

- A kitchen scale.

- A citrus zester or kitchen rasp.

- A pump bottle. If you spray oil onto foods, you'll need less than if you drizzle the oil.

- Measuring cups and spoons. It's easy to overestimate amounts when you don't measure. You can accumulate a lot of calories and a lot of fat very quickly by eyeballing ingredients.

How many of these do you have in your kitchen? If you have none or only a few, consider gradually adding them to your arsenal of weapons for fighting the battle of the bulge. They are a fairly small price to pay for helping you attain—and maintain—your ideal weight.

APPENDIX C: eating out

For most of us, it's easier to eat healthfully when we prepare our own food than when we eat out. Given today's busy schedules, however, it isn't realistic to expect to cook all your meals at home. But don't let eating out stress you out. You **can** enjoy the experience of eating out without totally derailing your healthful eating plan. The strength of your commitment to that plan is the key. If you regularly apply the same techniques of substitution or portion control in a restaurant as you should at home, you can continue your journey to successful weight loss.

ask and you shall receive

Many restaurants are happy to provide you with what you want—you just need to ask! The worst that will happen is that the kitchen staff won't be able to make the changes.

- **Can you broil, grill, or poach my order? Would you please use as little fat as possible?**
- **Would you explain how this is prepared?** Food preparation terminology may be unfamiliar to you. (See the list on pages 691.)

- **May I have a lunch-size portion?** Even at dinnertime this option may still be available.

- **May I substitute salad for french fries? Fat-free milk for cream?**

- **May I have soft corn tortillas?** Eat these instead of the fried tortilla chips served in Mexican restaurants.

- **May I have a to-go box with my meal?** Restaurant portions are so large these days that it's easy to eat almost twice what you need without thinking.

- **Would you take the bread basket away?** Have your server remove the temptation after your companions have helped themselves and given their okay.

- **May I have the sauce/salad dressing/gravy on the side?** These food toppers often drown the food they are meant to complement, and they contribute lots of expendable calories. Dip the tines of your fork into the sauce, dressing, or gravy before spearing each bite. You'll be surprised at how much less you can use.

the filling station

Here are a few suggestions for filling up without filling out.

- Drink a glass or two of water while you wait for your food to be served. It will help take the edge off your hunger.

- Eat slowly! Did you know that it takes about 20 minutes for your brain to register the signal from your stomach that it is full? Putting your utensils down between bites will help you slow down.

- Consider eating something low in calories—and preferably high in fiber (it's filling)—before leaving for the restaurant if you are very hungry. A small apple is one of many great choices.

- Consider having two low-fat appetizers instead of an entrée. It may help you watch portion size but still be satisfied and full.

mulling over the menu

It's important when eating out to take some time to study the menu and find the best options. Be the first at your table to order. Then stick to your decision regardless of what your companions select.

By becoming familiar with the following terms, you can make better meal selections when eating out.

LOW-CALORIE MENU TERMS

au jus	broiled	poached
baked	grilled	roasted
braised	lean	steamed

HIGH-CALORIE MENU TERMS

au gratin	bisque	fried
basted	breaded	hollandaise
battered	buttered/buttery	Parmesan
béarnaise	creamed/creamy	scalloped
béchamel	crisp	tempura

fitting in fast foods

We know that eating fast food is a reality for many Americans. Fast-food restaurants are quick, inexpensive, and conveniently located. As our society moves into a more health-conscious age, many of these restaurants are offering healthful options to consumers. If you eat at fast-food restaurants, try the following.

- Eat only part of what you order.
- Split an entrée with a companion.
- Be extra calorie-conscious for the next few meals.
- Ask for special preparation, such as no sauce or cheese.

- Order the kid's meal; the portion is smaller than the adult's meal.
- Order à la carte rather than the "meal" option.
- Opt for a salad; use the dressing sparingly, and watch for hidden calories in items such as croutons and cheese.
- Choose the fruit option, if available, for the side item.
- Ask for the nutrition guide at the restaurant to compare food options.
- Review the nutrition guides on restaurants' websites.

nutritional averages of comparable foods from fast-food restaurants

Although many fast-food restaurants are offering better choices than before, some of the other menu items, such as the ones shown below, can derail your diet plan.

ITEM	CALORIES	TOTAL FAT	SODIUM
Biscuit with bacon	336	20 g	587 mg
Cheeseburger, extra-large (9.8 ounces)	1,030	79	1,200
Chicken Caesar salad (about 12 ounces)	555	34	1,406
Chicken fingers (5.5 ounces)	495	30	1,265
Chocolate croissant	420	24	235
Chocolate milkshake (13.9 to 14.5 ounces)	460	13	315
French fries (about 4 ounces)	373	19	845
Fried fish (1 piece)	230	13	700

ITEM	CALORIES	TOTAL FAT	SODIUM
Hamburger, junior-size (3 to 3.6 ounces)	247	12	392
Hamburger (quarter-pound)	400	20	855
Meatball sub (6-inch)	500	24	1,260
Onion rings, regular order (3.3 to 4 ounces)	350	18	365
Pizza, 1 slice, medium			
Cheese	290	14	590
Ham	260	12	610
Pepperoni	257	12	548
Vegetable	270	12	510

APPENDIX D: common foods by calorie count

Use this handy list when you are looking for ways to round out your meal or find a healthful snack. For a more complete list, you may want to consult a book or website dedicated to calorie counts.

0–49 CALORIES	
1 medium apricot	17
½ cup cooked artichoke hearts	40
½ cup cooked asparagus	25
½ cup canned sliced bamboo shoots	13
¼ cup barbecue sauce	47
½ cup canned beets	27
1 large bell pepper	44
½ cup blackberries	31
½ cup blueberries	41
1 medium breadstick (hard)	41
½ cup cooked broccoli	22
½ cup shredded raw green cabbage	9
½ cup cubed cantaloupe	27

1 raw baby carrot	6
½ cup raw cauliflower	13
1 celery rib	10
1 ounce low-fat Cheddar cheese	49
10 sweet cherries	43
1 medium cucumber	46
¼ cup liquid egg substitute	30
1 fortune cookie	28
1 medium dill pickle (3¾ inch)	12
½ cup fat-free, sugar-free flavored gelatin	10
½ medium grapefruit	38
10 grapes	35
½ cup cooked green beans	22
10 small jelly beans	40
1 medium kiwifruit	46
1 cup torn lettuce (average of various types)	6
1 tablespoon reduced-calorie mayonnaise dressing	37
1 piece melba toast, any flavor	20
1 cup sliced raw button mushrooms	15
½ cup cooked oat bran	44
3 large black olives	15
3 extra-large green olives	15

1 medium peach	37
2 tablespoons picante sauce or tomato-based salsa	9
1 plum	36
1 cup light microwave popcorn	21
10 pretzel sticks	10
1½ cups mixed salad greens	14
½ cup cooked spinach	21
½ cup strawberries	27
½ cup cooked yellow summer squash	18
1 medium tomato	27
½ cup cubed watermelon	23
½ cup sliced raw zucchini	9

50–99 CALORIES

1 medium apple	72
6 ounces apple juice	87
½ cup unsweetened applesauce	53
10 dried apricot halves	84
½ cup cooked barley	97
7 ounces alcohol-free beer	50
½ cup canned pickled beets	75
½ cup cooked black-eyed peas	99
¾ cup bran flakes (without milk)	90

2 tablespoons light chocolate syrup	50
1 medium ear yellow corn, cooked	77
6-inch corn tortilla	56
½ cup 1% cottage cheese	82
1 ounce feta cheese	75
3 ounces cooked flounder	99
½ cup cooked lima beans	97
½ cup mango slices	54
8 ounces fat-free milk	90
1 ounce part-skim mozzarella cheese	72
1 medium orange	70
6 ounces orange juice	84
3 ounces cooked orange roughy	75
1 medium pear	97
½ cup cooked green peas	67
½-ounce chocolate-covered peppermint patty	50
½ cup pineapple tidbits canned in juice	75
6 ounces pineapple juice	98
1 small (1-ounce) whole-wheat pita	76
3.5-ounce refrigerated fat-free, sugar-free pudding cup	90
1-ounce slice pumpernickel bread	80
1-ounce slice raisin bread	71
3 ounces cooked sole	99

1 cup plain soy milk	81
4-inch-square frozen buttermilk or plain waffle	88
1-ounce slice whole-wheat bread	70
1/2 cup cooked whole-wheat spaghetti	87
3 1/2 ounces red wine	74

100–149 CALORIES

1/12 angel food cake (from mix)	140
11 animal crackers (1 ounce)	126
2 ounces whole-wheat baguette	140
1 medium banana	105
1/2 cup cooked dried beans	114
12 ounces light beer	100
1 1/2 ounces bourbon	105
1/2 cup cooked brown rice	108
3 ounces roasted chicken breast, without skin	142
8 ounces hot cocoa, made with fat-free milk and 1 tablespoon light chocolate syrup	115
1 1/4 cups corn flakes (without milk)	110
1 whole-wheat English muffin	134
10 frozen french fries, baked	111
10 small gumdrops	135
1 medium multigrain hamburger bun (1 1/2 ounces)	113

2 tablespoons butterscotch or caramel ice cream topping	103
8 ounces frozen lemonade, prepared with water	100
¾ cup regular or quick oatmeal, prepared with water	111
1 ounce grated Parmesan cheese	129
3 ounces roasted lean pork tenderloin	139
1 medium baked potato with skin (5 ounces)	145
1 ounce baked potato chips	110
3 ounces drained canned Sockeye salmon with bones	130
3 ounces cooked sea bass	105
½ cup fruit sorbet	130
½ cup cooked green soybeans (edamame)	127
1 medium baked sweet potato	130
3 ounces white tuna canned n distilled or spring water	109
1 turkey hot dog without bun (1.5 ounces)	109
6 ounces fat-free or light yogurt, no sugar added	111

150–200 CALORIES

1 ounce dry-roasted almonds	169
3½-inch plain bagel	195

1 ounce dry-roasted cashews	163
3 ounces broiled flank steak without fat	192
3 ounces broiled 90% lean hamburger patty	173
2½-ounce martini	156
1 ounce dry-roasted peanuts	170
1 ounce dry-roasted pecan halves	196
1 ounce dry-roasted pistachios	172
3 ounces cooked Atlantic or coho salmon	156
3 ounces roasted dark meat turkey without skin	170
1 ounce dry-roasted walnut halves	185

APPENDIX E:
food diary page

Date: _____ ☐ Mon. ☐ Tues. ☐ Wed. ☐ Thurs. ☐ Fri. ☐ Sat. ☐ Sun.

TIME & PLACE	FOOD OR BEVERAGE (type and amount)	CALORIES	WHAT PROMPTED YOU TO EAT?
breakfast			
snack			

lunch

snack

dinner

snack

TOTAL Daily Calories: _____

APPENDIX F:
activity diary page

Date: _____ ❏ Mon. ❏ Tues. ❏ Wed. ❏ Thurs. ❏ Fri. ❏ Sat. ❏ Sun.

TIME OF DAY	ACTIVITY	DURATION	LEVEL OF EXERTION	LEVEL OF ENJOYMENT

TOTAL Daily Activity Minutes: _____

Notes:

If You Did Not Exercise Today, Why?

❏ **Not enough time**

❏ **Didn't want to**

❏ **Other**

Level of Perceived Exertion

0 = Nothing at all

1 = Very, very light

2 = Very light

3 = Light

4 = Moderate/brisk

5 = Somewhat hard

6 = Hard

7 = Very hard

8 = Very, very hard

9 = Extremely hard

10 = Absolute maximal effort

Level of Enjoyment

1 = Did not enjoy

2 = Neutral

3 = Did enjoy

APPENDIX G: equivalents

INGREDIENT	MEASUREMENT
Almonds	1 ounce = $1/4$ cup slivers
Apple	1 medium = $3/4$ cup chopped, 1 cup sliced
Basil leaves, fresh	$2/3$ ounce = $1/2$ cup chopped, stems removed
Bell pepper, any color	1 medium = 1 cup chopped or sliced
Carrot	1 medium = $1/3$ to $1/2$ cup chopped or sliced, $1/2$ cup shredded
Celery	1 medium rib – $1/2$ cup chopped or sliced
Cheese, hard, such as Parmesan	4 ounces = 1 cup grated $3 1/2$ ounces = 1 cup shredded
Cheese, semihard, such as Cheddar, mozzarella, or Swiss	4 ounces = 1 cup grated
Cheese, soft, such as blue, feta, or goat	1 ounce, crumbled = $1/4$ cup
Cucumber	1 medium = 1 cup sliced

Lemon juice	1 medium = 3 tablespoons
Lemon zest	1 medium = 2 to 3 teaspoons
Lime juice	1 medium = 1½ to 2 tablespoons
Lime zest	1 medium = 1 teaspoon
Mushrooms (button)	1 pound = 5 cups sliced or 6 cups chopped
Onions, green	8 to 9 medium = 1 cup sliced (green and white parts)
Onions, white or yellow	1 large = 1 cup chopped 1 medium = ⅔ cup chopped 1 small = ⅓ cup chopped
Orange juice	1 medium = ⅓ to ½ cup
Orange zest	1 medium = 1½ to 2 tablespoons
Strawberries	1 pint = 2 cups sliced or chopped
Tomatoes	2 large, 3 medium, or 3 small = 1½ to 2 cups chopped
Walnuts	1 ounce = ½ cup chopped

APPENDIX H: health implications of overweight and obesity

National attention is focusing more and more on the increasing rate of weight gain in the United States. We are experiencing an epidemic of obesity. About 135 million American adults age 20 years and older are overweight or obese. According to the National Institutes of Health, more than half of American adults are at a weight that is considered unhealthy. Each year, an estimated 300,000 Americans die of causes related to obesity. Cardiovascular disease accounts for a large number of these deaths, making obesity an important concern for the American Heart Association.

heart health and weight: how they relate

Obesity occupies an unusual position as a health issue. It is considered a disease itself, yet it also is a risk factor for illnesses such as heart disease—including heart attack, congestive heart failure, sudden cardiac death, and angina or chest pain. In addition to contributing to the risk of heart attack, obesity puts added strain on the heart, which can lead to other potentially fatal conditions, such as cardiomyopathy (weakness of the heart muscle), an enlarged heart, or irregular heart rhythms.

Being overweight or obese also makes you more prone to the conditions that are independent risk factors for heart disease. Obesity can lead to increased blood levels of harmful LDL cholesterol and triglycerides (the chemical form of most fats) and decreased levels of HDL cholesterol, or the "good" cholesterol.

High levels of HDL cholesterol are linked with lower risk for heart disease and stroke, so a low HDL level can indicate increased risk. Adults who are obese are twice as likely to have high blood pressure as those who are at a healthful weight. High blood pressure increases the heart's workload, causing the heart to enlarge and weaken over time. The risk of developing diabetes is greater in people who are overweight or obese. When diabetes is present with other risk factors, such as high blood pressure and high blood cholesterol and triglycerides, the risk of heart disease and stroke is especially great. Other conditions associated with excess weight include gallbladder disease, arthritis, some types of cancer, sleep apnea, and breathing problems.

Obesity is now recognized as a major risk factor for coronary heart disease, which can lead to heart attack.

risk factors for heart disease and stroke

In addition to overweight and obesity, other factors influence your risk of heart disease or stroke. Some risk factors result from circumstances that can't be controlled. However, you can make changes, such as losing weight, to modify the factors that **can** be controlled to lessen your risk.

risk factors you can't control

- **Age**—With increased age comes increased risk.

- **Sex**—Men are more prone to heart disease earlier in life. After menopause, however, women's incidence of heart disease increases.

- **Heredity**—Genetic influences predispose some people to particular health risks. If a parent, sibling, or grandparent has had heart disease, especially at an early age, you're at higher risk. Race also plays a role. For example, African-Americans have a greater risk of heart disease and stroke than whites.

risk factors you can control or treat

Fortunately, there are ways you can manage controllable risk factors. Hereditary risk often shows itself in clinical conditions that you can treat. If high blood pressure, high blood cholesterol, or diabetes runs in your family, work with your healthcare professional to help prevent or control these conditions. Losing weight and being physically active, as we recommend in this book, will help lessen your risk: A loss of just 10 or 20 pounds can make a significant difference in your blood pressure and cholesterol levels, and regular exercise will help you control or prevent high blood pressure, high blood cholesterol, and diabetes. Quitting smoking is another important step in reducing your risk of heart attack and stroke.

HIGH BLOOD PRESSURE

High blood pressure is often called the "silent killer" because it usually has no symptoms. In fact, many people have hypertension for years without knowing it. When high blood pressure exists with obesity, smoking, high blood cholesterol levels, or diabetes, the risk of heart attack or stroke increases significantly.

Have your blood pressure checked at least every two years. Normal blood pressure levels are below 140/90 mm Hg (millimeters of mercury). If your blood pressure is 140/90 mm Hg or higher on two or more separate visits, you should be treated for high blood pressure. A new classification, "prehypertension," has been created to describe blood pressures between 120 and 139 mm Hg systolic (the top number in a blood pressure reading) or 80 and 89 mm Hg diastolic (bottom number). If your blood pressure falls into this range, it is a signal that you should adopt health-promoting habits, such as eating well to lose weight and increasing the amount of physical activity in your life. If lifestyle changes don't bring your blood pressure levels down to normal, your physician may prescribe medication.

Most Americans consume more sodium each day than needed to maintain the body's balance of fluids and electrolytes. For many people, reducing the amount of dietary sodium may lower high blood pressure and the risks of heart disease and stroke that come with it. If you have high blood pressure or there is a history of it in your family, your doctor may recommend a limit lower than the 2,300 mg recommended for healthy adults.

HIGH BLOOD CHOLESTEROL

Be sure to have your blood cholesterol levels checked regularly by a healthcare professional. Your total blood cholesterol measurement is broken down to determine the levels of harmful LDL and helpful HDL cholesterol present in your blood. Excess LDL cholesterol and other substances can build up on the inner walls of your arteries as plaque. This condition can lead to heart disease, including heart attack and stroke. Low levels of HDL cholesterol are linked to a higher risk of heart disease.

To reduce your risk, you should aim for an LDL level of less than 130 milligrams per deciliter (mg/dL), with less than 100 mg/dL being the optimum. Women should aim for an HDL level greater than 50 mg/dL; men should aim for 40 mg/dL or more. Although a total blood cholesterol of 200 mg/dL or more is considered high, the ideal level is 175 mg/dL or less.

If your blood levels of LDL cholesterol are elevated, try to limit your intake of saturated fat to no more than 10 percent of daily calories and of dietary cholesterol to less than 300 mg each day. If you have heart disease or are at high risk for developing it, limit saturated fat to no more than 7 percent of calories and cholesterol intake to less than 200 mg a day. To lower your blood cholesterol, it is important to limit your intake of saturated and trans fats, but it is also prudent to watch your intake of foods rich in dietary cholesterol, such as egg yolks, animal fats, organ meats, and shellfish.

Changing to a healthful diet alone is often enough to lower LDL cholesterol. You may need medication as well, however, especially if you are one of the people whose bodies are programmed to make too much cholesterol. If so, take the cholesterol lowering medications recommended by your doctor and follow a low-saturated fat, low-cholesterol diet.

the skinny on dietary fats and cholesterol

Including fats in your diet is essential to good nutrition, but eating too much of certain fats—saturated fat, trans fat, and cholesterol—raises the level of LDL cholesterol in your blood. As you make food choices, cut back on the harmful saturated and trans fats and replace them with more helpful polyunsaturated or monounsaturated fats, which help lower blood cholesterol levels when the saturated fat content of the diet is low.

- Saturated fats are found in meats, poultry, whole-milk dairy products (such as cream, butter, and cheese), lard, and tropical vegetable oils, such as coconut, palm, and palm kernel oils.

- Trans fats are created when vegetable oils are hydrogenated to make them more solid. Commercial products containing hydrogenated or partially hydrogenated vegetable oils include vegetable shortenings, stick margarines, and baked goods such as cookies and crackers.

- Polyunsaturated fats are found primarily in corn oil, safflower oil, walnuts, and fish. Monounsaturated fats are found in olive oil, canola oil, peanut oil, olives, and avocados. Most unsaturated oils and fats contain varying percentages of both polyunsaturated and monounsaturated fats.

DIABETES

The hormone insulin converts the sugars and starches from food into energy. Diabetes results when too much glucose builds up in the blood. This happens when your body doesn't make enough insulin, can't use its own insulin as well as it should, or both. Diabetes is a serious disease in itself, as well as a risk factor for heart disease. Type 2 diabetes, the most common, develops when the body doesn't make enough insulin, and doesn't efficiently use the insulin it makes. This scenario of inefficient use is called **insulin resistance.** Obesity and physical inactivity can lead to the problem of insulin resistance.

Type 2 diabetes can often be prevented or controlled by careful weight management and physical activity. Your healthcare professional can determine your blood glucose level with a simple blood test. If you have diabetes, work with your doctor or dietitian to develop an individualized diet. It's also important to keep your blood pressure below 130/80 mm Hg to help prevent damage to your blood vessels.

CIGARETTE SMOKING

Compared with nonsmokers, if you smoke you are two to four times more likely to develop coronary heart disease and more likely to experience sudden cardiac death. Exposure to second-hand smoke can also significantly increase your risk of death due to heart disease. If you are a smoker who wants to lose weight, you may be afraid you will gain even more pounds if you quit. You may feel that it will be too much to stop smoking and change your eating habits at the same time. Consider, however, the high price you pay in terms of your health if you smoke. Try to find a way to integrate quitting into your weight-loss plan. As soon as you stop smoking or reduce the smoke in your environment, your risk of heart disease will drop dramatically.

recent advances in obesity research

With the increased attention to the problem of obesity and its effect on public health, more research is focusing on the physiological basis for weight gain. Several studies have shown promising results that may lead to a better understanding of why some people seem destined to battle the bulge while others can apparently eat at will.

For example, researchers are investigating the recent finding that chronic lack of sleep may be linked to the escalating prevalence of overweight and obesity (see the following box). One possible explanation is that those who are up late are also likely to be eating and drinking into the night, therefore consuming more calories than they are burning in the extra time spent awake. In addition, however, several studies have shown that levels of two appetite-regulating hormones, leptin and grehlin, are altered in sleep-deprived individuals. These changes are likely to increase appetite and may account for the correlation.

a connection between sleep and weight?

In a study presented at the Annual Scientific Meeting of the North American Association for the Study of Obesity in November 2004, researchers found that subjects who slept four hours or less each night were 73 percent more likely to be obese than those who slept for seven to nine hours a night. The subjects who averaged five hours of sleep per night had a 50 percent greater risk to be substantially overweight, and those who slept six hours per night reduced their risk to 23 percent.

Studies like these continue to expand our knowledge of the delicate balance between biology and behavior. To keep informed on the latest developments in research on obesity and health, visit the American Heart Association website at americanheart.org.

APPENDIX I:
american heart association national center and affiliates

For more information about our programs and services, call 1-800-AHA-USA1 (1-800-242-8721) or contact us online at www.americanheart.org. For information about the American Stroke Association, a division of the American Heart Association, call 1-888-4STROKE (1-888-478-7653).

NATIONAL CENTER
American Heart Association
7272 Greenville Avenue
Dallas, TX 75231-4596
214-373-6300

AFFILIATES
FLORIDA/PUERTO RICO AFFILIATE
St. Petersburg, FL

GREATER MIDWEST AFFILIATE
Illinois, Indiana, Michigan, Minnesota, North Dakota, South Dakota, Wisconsin
Chicago, IL

HEARTLAND AFFILIATE
Arkansas, Iowa, Kansas, Missouri, Nebraska, Oklahoma
Topeka, KS

HERITAGE AFFILIATE
Connecticut; Long Island, New York; New Jersey; New York City
New York, NY

MID-ATLANTIC AFFILIATE
District of Columbia, Maryland, North Carolina, South Carolina, Virginia
Glen Allen, VA

NORTHEAST AFFILIATE
Maine, Massachusetts, New Hampshire, New York State (except New York City and Long Island), Rhode Island, Vermont
Framingham, MA

OHIO VALLEY AFFILIATE
Kentucky, Ohio, West Virginia
Columbus, OH

PACIFIC/MOUNTAIN AFFILIATE
Alaska, Arizona, Colorado, Hawaii, Idaho, Montana, New Mexico, Oregon, Washington, Wyoming
Seattle, WA

PENNSYLVANIA/DELAWARE AFFILIATE
Delaware, Pennsylvania
Wormleysburg, PA

SOUTHEAST AFFILIATE
Alabama, Georgia, Louisiana, Mississippi, Tennessee
Marietta, GA

TEXAS AFFILIATE
Austin, TX

WESTERN STATES AFFILIATE
California, Nevada, Utah
Los Angeles, CA

INDEX